THE CARELESS ATOM

THE

CARELESS

ATOM

by

SHELDON NOVICK

HOUGHTON MIFFLIN COMPANY
BOSTON

Library of Congress Catalog Card Number:
68–9768

Printed in the United States of America

This book is for Sherwood

There is an understandable drive
on the part of men of good will
to build up the positive aspects of nuclear energy
simply because the negative aspects
are so distressing.

Dr. Alvin Weinberg
Director, Oak Ridge National
Laboratory (1956)

ACKNOWLEDGMENTS

IT WOULD BE DIFFICULT to acknowledge my full indebtedness to Dr. Barry Commoner without saddling him with responsibility for any errors or failings in what follows. For the past four years I have been his student as well as his assistant, and what little I know about the tangled relationship between science and society I learned from him. Those of my readers who are acquainted with his work will easily see the great debt which this book owes him.

Another debt is owed to the Committee for Environmental Information, which in a direct way made this book, and many other more important enterprises like it, possible.

It was an article by Lin Mattison and Richard Daly which first drew my interest to reactors, and many of the ideas presented here were first suggested in long discussions with Lin, to whom I am also grateful for access to his extensive files.

Special thanks are due to David Pesonen, who started it all. I am indebted to his writings, more of which I hope will soon be published, as well as to our conversations, particularly for much of the material in Chapter III.

Linda Mattison's comments, corrections, and suggestions came at a time when they were much needed, and appreciated.

Professor Harold Green was kind enough to read the manuscript and to make a number of useful corrections and suggestions. For these, and his kind encouragement on other occasions, I am deeply grateful.

I particularly want to thank Dr. Bernard Spinrad for his kindness and courtesy in commenting on the manuscript before publication.

Miss Eva Schneider was of very great assistance in the preparation of early drafts of the manuscript, often under trying circumstances. My thanks are also very much due to Miss Lenore Harris, whose help through all stages of this project was invaluable. Miss Joy Wolfe and Mrs. Elayne Drey were also of assistance in typing.

None of the kind people mentioned here are to be held responsible for any of the statements which follow, nor for any errors which they may have been unable to keep me from making.

SHELDON NOVICK

CONTENTS

THE CARELESS ATOM

I

ACCIDENTS HAPPEN

ON DECEMBER 12, 1952, an experiment was being conducted at the NRX reactor, at Chalk River, Ontario. The atomic plant had been turned on at low power. One of the reactor operating crew was working in the basement of the building at an unrelated task. By mistake, he opened three or four valves he should not have; three or four (no one now recalls) of the shutoff rods lifted out of the reactor, diminishing the margin of safety.

Like atomic plants intended for electric power production, Chalk River reactor was controlled by a number of long rods inserted among the fuel tubes containing uranium, which when inserted or withdrawn, changed the rate of the nuclear chain reaction. Twelve of the rods were equipped to move very quickly; any seven of these "shutoff" rods, when inserted into the reactor, would shut it down.

When the rods withdrew, red lights began appearing on the control desk upstairs. The supervisor at the control desk telephoned to the basement to tell the operator there to stop whatever he was doing; then, leaving his assistant in charge at the control desk, the supervisor went downstairs to see what was going on.

According to the official report of the accident by W. B.

Lewis for Atomic Energy of Canada, Ltd.,[1] when the supervisor reached the basement, "He recognized the operator's mistake and was horrified at the possible consequences if the operator had continued to open these wrong valves. . . ." The supervisor then closed the valves which his subordinate had opened, assuming that the shutoff rods would then drop back into place. And, in fact, the red warning lights at the control desk went out; but the rods had only dropped a little way, enough to turn off the warning lights but not enough to reestablish the needed condition of safety. The cause of this mechanical failure has never been established—the ensuing accident obliterated its traces.

Having, as he thought, corrected the error, the supervisor telephoned upstairs to his assistant. He meant to tell the assistant to push buttons 4 and 3 on the control desk; this would have returned the whole system to normal. Instead, he said, "Push buttons 4 and 1," and immediately realizing his mistake, tried to correct it. But the assistant had already set down the phone to carry out the order. Although the reason for the order could not have been clear to him, there seemed nothing dangerous about executing it: the red warning lights had gone out.

Pushing button 1 resulted in raising four more of the shutoff rods out of the reactor; with three or four rods still withdrawn (although no one knew this yet) a total of seven or eight of the shutoff rods were out of action. The result was complete loss of the safety margin which should have been there; the level of atomic reaction occurring deep in the reactor fuel, instead of remaining steady from moment to moment, began to increase slowly.

It took a few seconds for the staff in the control room to realize that this was happening, and it was a complete surprise, but there was still no alarm. About twenty seconds after he pushed button 1, the assistant, realizing something was wrong, pushed another emergency button which should have resulted in all the shutoff rods dropping back into the reactor, shutting it down. But two of the red lights stayed on, and in fact, of the seven or eight rods which were already withdrawn, only one dropped back, and that one moved very slowly; it took about a minute and a half to fall the ten feet required.

The control room staff was now seriously concerned. The assistant hurriedly called his supervisor in the basement urging him to do something to get the rods down; meanwhile the instruments recording reactor power still showed a steady increase. As the power went on rising, it became clear that emergency measures would be needed. The precious heavy water contained in the reactor vessel would have to be dumped. The heavy water was necessary for the maintenance of the chain reaction; dumping it would stop the reactor, whatever else happened. One of the physicists in the control room was already reaching for the dump switch when the assistant supervisor gave the word.

It took some time for the heavy water to run out of the reactor; in about thirty seconds, however, instruments showed that power had dropped down to zero, and everyone breathed a sigh of relief. But the consequences of the accident had hardly begun to be felt. Down in the basement, through an open door, the supervisor could see water gushing into the room below the reactor; this was highly radioactive cooling water. Another staff member rushed to the control room to report a rumble and a spurt of water up through the top of the reactor.

At this point automatic alarms began sounding in the reactor building; radioactivity in the air had been detected by the instruments. A frantic telephone call from another building (the chemical extractions plant) revealed that high levels of radio-activity were being experienced there. Sirens were sounded, warning personnel to remain indoors. Within a few minutes the project head gave the order for the evacuation of the entire plant. Only those present in the control room donned gas masks and remained.

The whole accident inside the reactor took place in about seventy seconds, and resulted in the release, from nuclear re-action alone, of as much energy as is contained in the explosion of a half ton of TNT — although this release occurred over a period of several seconds rather than within the fraction of a second required for a violent explosion. The main immediate effect was quickly to raise the temperature of some of the ura-nium fuel past its melting point, and to cause some mild explo-sions of steam. These expelled some water from the fuel area, which in turn caused a further increase in the energy release; the water normally interfered somewhat with the atomic reac-tion, and its removal speeded up an already dangerous proc-ess.

In the rapidly increasing temperature, molten uranium and molten aluminum from the tubes which contained the fuel both mixed with the surrounding water and steam. The result was a series of chemical reactions, releasing more energy. More seri-ously, the reaction of uranium with water released free hydro-gen; air flowing into the reactor met with the hydrogen and at the high temperature caused an explosion. This explosion lifted the 4-ton gasholder dome four feet into the air and jammed it among surrounding structures.

Due to the effective functioning of emergency procedures, no one at the plant was injured during the accident, and although many were exposed to radiation, the exposures were relatively mild. The reactor core was destroyed.

The Chalk River reactor is very different in design and operation from the atomic power plants being built today. It shows clearly, however, two of the forces involved in a serious accident: the sudden release of energy by an uncontrolled atomic chain reaction, and the additional potential for explosion created by the chemical reaction of reactor materials with air and water under the suddenly high temperatures and pressures. Many of the materials used in modern reactor cores, in addition to uranium itself, react chemically with water at high temperatures.

To some extent, the Chalk River accident was caused simply by human error, and although reactor designs may change, people will always run them, and the chance of human error is always there. When it combines with mechanical failure, as at Chalk River, totally unforeseen situations may arise, and improbable results follow. In order to diminish the risk of human error, modern nuclear power plants have highly elaborate and highly complex automatic safety equipment. But these have their problems too. For complex mechanical systems sometimes behave in unforeseen and unwanted ways — as seems to have happened in the power blackout of the whole Northeast in October 1965.

All of which simply goes to say that "accidents do happen," a lesson which should not be difficult to learn in the reactor business, which has suffered a number of bad ones. Five years after Chalk River, there was another near-catastrophe, this time in England, at Windscale Pile No. 1, a reactor used for military purposes. This accident was far more serious than the one at Chalk River, and resulted not only in the total loss of the reactor, but in the release of large amounts of radioactivity into the air. Fortunately the plant was in a sparsely populated area.

Pile No. 1 is fueled with natural uranium, and is cooled, not by water as are the Chalk River and most American plants, but by air drawn through it by huge blowers and expelled, after being delayed and filtered, through high smokestacks. The heart of the reactor is a 50-foot cube of graphite, in which are inserted the long tubes of uranium fuel.

The intense radiation in a reactor induces sometimes surprising changes in the materials exposed to it. Graphite (the same material used for pencil leads) swells, and many of its physical characteristics change. The graphite is storing some of the energy of the radiation which falls on it; this energy may be released again at some unexpected time, heating the graphite and surrounding materials. The stored energy which may sometimes be released spontaneously from the graphite is named for Eugene P. Wigner, the physicist.

Since unexpected releases of heat within the complex mechanism of a reactor may cause serious damage, some means of dealing with this difficulty is needed. Quite by accident, the British discovered that heating the graphite slightly might trigger the release of the stored energy; the addition of some heat tends to trigger the release of even more heat.

In 1952, a spontaneous release of Wigner energy occurred in Windscale Pile No. 1, while the pile was shut down. Since that time regular procedures for controlling the release of Wigner energy have been carried out. On October 7, 1957 such a procedure was begun.[2]

At 1:03 A.M. the pile was shut down and the main blowers were turned off. Throughout the day a series of routine checks of the instrumentation were made, to make sure that the pile was shut down, and to test the monitoring devices within the pile.

So that the reactor operators will know what is happening within the tons of uranium which make up the core, a number of sensing devices are distributed through the fuel and the moderator. Some of these are thermocouples, which measure the temperature at different points in the uranium and graphite. The thermocouples of Pile No. 1 were carefully checked during the day of October 7 and defective ones replaced. At 7:25 P.M., all air flow through the reactor core was cut off, and the pile was started up at a low level to heat the graphite moderator. Early the next morning, the pile was again shut down.

During the morning of October 8, it seemed to the operators of the pile that the heating had not been sufficient to trigger a Wigner release, and that in fact the graphite was cooling instead of heating itself further. Examination of the records afterward showed that some of the thermocouples in the graphite did indeed show cooling, but that others registered a rising temperature.

The physicist in charge decided that a second nuclear heating was called for, and this was begun at 11:05. "The operator slipped a little bit," according to one report, "and ran the rate of reaction faster than the rules called for; however, this was not considered a very serious violation of the procedures. The rate of heating was not considered dangerous. It was merely a little bit faster than that normally carried out."[3] During the first few minutes of the heating, it was seen that the temperatures in the uranium were rising much more rapidly than was allowed under normal conditions, and therefore control rods were inserted to dampen the chain reaction and allow the uranium to cool somewhat.

Unknown to the operators of the pile, however, serious damage had already been done. Deep within the pile one or more fuel elements had seriously overheated, and their steel jackets had melted or cracked.

The second heating triggered an overall release of Wigner energy, and the temperature of the pile went on rising during Wednesday, October 9. But in the front lower portion of the pile, uranium had been exposed to the air by the failure of the fuel-element cladding, and under the high temperatures it began to burn.

The burning of these fuel elements gradually led to the failure of other nearby cartridges; the fire slowly spread, and by the following day was affecting about 150 channels.

During Wednesday, the pile instruments showed nothing wrong, except that at one point the graphite moderator was heating somewhat too rapidly. By ten o'clock the temperature recordings had risen to the point at which certain routine measures were prescribed for cooling the pile, including drawing small amounts of air through the core. Still no serious problem was detected by the reactor staff.

Before dawn on Thursday morning, instruments within the pile's smokestack indicated a rise in radioactivity, but the physicist in charge assumed that this was a normal result of the cooling air being discharged, and took no action. At noon radioactivity was detected on the roof of the weather station. The temperature of the pile continued to rise, and still more cooling air was drawn through. The smokestack meters showed a much sharper rise in radioactivity, and the pile operators realized that some of the fuel elements must have failed. There was still no hint of the fire raging within the reactor's core.

At 1:45 P.M., an attempt was made to discover where in the pile the fuel failure had occurred, but the scanning gear was jammed and could not be moved. The radioactivity of air coming from the pile continued to increase, as did the temperature. By this time the general manager of the pile was informed, and he instructed the works general manager that a bad burst had occurred. The works general manager directed that the affected fuel elements be identified and removed as soon as possible.

That afternoon, radiation workers in protective clothing entered the reactor enclosure. The radiation level of the air was checked, and then the workers stepped onto a hoist which lifted them to a point at the face of the pile where instruments indicated the highest temperatures. A plug in the wall of the pile was removed, showing four uranium channels. The uranium cartridges were seen to be at red heat.

The heat had distorted the fuel cartridges so badly that they could not be removed. Push rods came out with molten uranium dripping from them. Surrounding cartridges were removed in an attempt to contain the fire, but the temperature of the burning region remained very high. Although the fire was contained in about 150 channels, the possibility existed that further Wigner releases would occur in other regions of the pile, adding to the total heat.

At midnight, the decision was made to use water to cool the pile. This was a difficult decision to make, for water striking the glowing uranium might cause an explosion. An AEC official reported later, "They will not guarantee that they could do it a second time without an explosion."[4] The chief constable of Cumberland was warned of the possibility of an emergency; men in the factory were warned to stay indoors and wear face masks. By 7:00 A.M. of October 11 it was decided that all factory personnel should be under cover. It took until nine o'clock to institute safety precautions, and then the water was turned on. There was no explosion.

Pouring of water from hoses continued for twenty-four hours until, by Saturday afternoon, the pile was quite cold.

As a result of the accident, Windscale Pile No. 1 was a total loss. But more importantly, large amounts of radioactivity had been released from the smokestacks between October 10 and 12.

The immediate serious hazard was from iodine 131 released from the fuel of the reactor, where it was formed as a product of the breakdown of the uranium. Radioactive iodine was deposited over 200 square miles of neighboring farmland, fortunately a very sparsely inhabited area. Cows grazing in this area were removed from pasture, and the milk produced after the accident destroyed.

Drifting south and east, however, the radioactive cloud from the stacks of Windscale spread over a large area indeed. The total radioactivity released was probably about a tenth of that released during the explosion of the atomic bomb at Hiroshima, and affected a large portion of England and Northern Europe. The Danish, Netherlands, Belgian, and French governments were concerned with the increases in radioactivity in their countries as a result of this accident in northwest England.

Although Windscale Pile No. 1 was even more different from modern power reactors than the Chalk River plant, the history of its accident teaches the same lesson: there will always be an element of human failure no matter how carefully a reactor is designed; and a reactor is such a complex mechanism that very often it will behave in unexpected ways. In this case, for instance, temperature-measuring devices were distributed in the regions of highest temperature during normal operation; but during the accident, heating occurred in other areas and went undetected for more than a day.

A number of other serious reactor accidents have occurred. In 1961, another and more tragic accident occurred at a small research and training reactor in an isolated spot in Idaho. The reactor exploded, killing the three men who were tending it, and discharging some radioactivity to the surrounding area.

In 1964, T. J. Thompson of the Massachusetts Institute of Technology wrote that there had been nine serious reactivity accidents since 1949 in nonmilitary installations alone. "To date, nine [reactor fuel] cores have been destroyed or seriously damaged. . . . Three reactors have been put out of action by accidents and never revived." [5] Late in 1966 there was still another serious accident, at the Enrico Fermi plant at Lagoona Beach, Michigan; as we shall see, this accident was potentially the most serious of all.

II

TURNING SWORDS
INTO PLOWSHARES

ENRICO FERMI SPLIT THE ATOM IN 1934, but didn't know it. In the following four years the uranium atom was split again and again by scientists in Rome, Paris, and Berlin, but still no one recognized what was happening. Fermi wrongly believed he had created a new element, but the results were puzzling. He had bombarded uranium with the newly discovered neutron. The uranium became radioactive and seemed to take on new chemical properties, as if it had been transmuted to a new element — but the new properties were not what would have been expected.

The results were so puzzling, in fact, that the experiment was performed repeatedly by Fermi in Rome, and by other leading physicists. There was excited activity throughout the world, and no one paid any attention to an article which appeared in the German *Journal of Applied Chemistry*. The article was by a young husband-and-wife team of chemists, Ida and Walter Noddack, and they thought that Fermi was wrong. In the article they suggested: "It is conceivable that when heavy nuclei [uranium] are bombarded with neutrons those nuclei might break up into several large fragments. . . ."[1] This accurate suggestion was dismissed by Fermi and by everyone else. For it seemed obvious that the atom could not be split by the homely apparatus that Fermi had used. All the principles of physics made it clear that the nucleus of the atom could only be broken apart by vast forces, far greater than anything which scientists had been able to muster at that time.

Most physicists believed that uranium was absorbing neutrons from Fermi's device. The neutron is one of the two main components of the weight of the atom, and has no electrical charge. If the uranium in Fermi's crucible had simply absorbed neutrons, it would have been converted to a new element, and it was this that Fermi was expecting. When he did find new radioactivity and new chemical properties in the uranium exposed to his neutron gun, he assumed these were the properties of the new element. This explanation was so broadly accepted that physicists all over the world set eagerly to work to isolate the new material and explain its puzzling properties.

The properties were puzzling because there was no new element. The neutrons from Fermi's gun had not simply been absorbed by the uranium atoms; the uranium atoms had absorbed them and then split into two parts; it was these fragments that Fermi had observed. Yet physicists and chemists were repeating Fermi's experiment in an attempt to isolate and explain the surprising characteristics of the new element supposedly being created.

There was, in fact, a race to identify the new element, a race in which the winner would almost certainly receive a Nobel Prize. The leading contenders in the race were two women, Lise Meitner and Irène Joliot-Curie, who for many years had been bitter rivals. There had been sharp exchanges between them at normally sedate professional gatherings, and Fräulein Meitner had on several occasions cast doubt on the accuracy of results proceeding from Mme. Joliot-Curie's laboratory.

Women prominent in the field of physics were then as rare as they are today. Otto Hahn, a chemist who maintained a thirty-year collaboration with Lise Meitner, describes her arrival at his laboratory in the Emil Fischer Institute in Berlin, in 1907:

> In those days women were not allowed to work at the Fischer Institute. When I put the matter to Emil Fischer, he granted permission to Miss Meitner to work with me in the carpenter's shop on the ground floor of the Institute, where the radio-active measurements were carried out; he requested her, however, not to enter the study rooms on the upper floor as that would be setting a precedent.[2]

The close association between Hahn and Meitner continued until 1938 when Lise Meitner, who was Jewish, was forced to leave Berlin. The two were so much thought of as a team that when, at a professional congress, someone approached Miss Meitner with the words, "We have already met," she absentmindedly replied, "I think you must be taking me for Professor Hahn."

Irène Joliot-Curie also had a collaborator, her husband, Pierre Joliot, who assumed his wife's distinguished name when they married. Her mother, the famous Mme. Curie, was the only person at that time to have received two Nobel Prizes, one in chemistry and one in physics, and it was believed the daughter wished to equal this achievement. She came very close indeed, having already received one Nobel Prize for the discovery of artificial radioactivity. The discovery of the first man-made element would certainly result in a second prize.

Fermi's experiment was repeated many times in both laboratories, where extensive and refined chemical techniques were used to separate the radioactive materials that resulted from

neutron bombardment. Each time these separations were carried out, the result was a substance which simply could not be
an element further up the atomic chain from uranium; yet despite these clear indications, no physicist could accept what
was obviously happening — nuclear fission. As late as 1938,
Ernest Lawrence, the inventor of the cyclotron, announced
that it was as unrealistic to expect useful energy from the atom
as to try to cool the ocean and use the heat extracted for practical purposes. Einstein, Planck, Bohr — all the leading physicists
of the day — believed fission under ordinary circumstances to
be impossible.

In the autumn of 1938, Lise Meitner slipped across the German border into the Netherlands, never to return. But Hahn
remained in Berlin, carrying on his separation experiments with
a colleague, Strassman. Work went on in Paris under the direction of the Joliot-Curies, and shortly after Lise Meitner's departure from Berlin, they published a paper explaining some of
their previous results as errors. The results were not errors,
however — they only seemed so because of the supposed im-
possibility of lighter elements being created from uranium. It
could only have been a matter of time before the Joliot-Curies
would realize the correctness of their observations, but almost
immediately the paper came to the attention of Strassman, who
hurried with it to Otto Hahn.

"I'm not interested in our lady friend's latest writings," Hahn
replied when shown the paper. But he was finally persuaded
to read it, and becoming excited, immediately set to work with
Strassman. Within weeks he had confirmed the fact of nuclear
fission, for which he, and not Meitner or Joliot-Curie, was to
receive the Nobel Prize in 1944. He and Strassman definitely
established that, mixed with their irradiated uranium, were mi-

nute quantities of barium, an element which weighs a little more than half as much as uranium, and could only have been formed by the splitting of the uranium atom. Just before Christmas of 1938, Hahn and Strassman prepared a report of their work which was published the following month. So reluctant were they to oppose the prevailing doctrines of physics, that despite the incontrovertible evidence they refused to draw a conclusion from their work.

"As chemists," they wrote, they could only conclude that barium was present in the uranium extract, "[but] as nuclear chemists, closely associated with physics, we cannot decide to take this step in contradiction to all previous experience in nuclear physics." [3]

Hahn immediately wrote to Lise Meitner, describing the results which had been made possible by the hint provided by her rival, Mme. Joliot-Curie. The implications of these experiments were immediately apparent to Meitner, spending Christmas in exile in the tiny Dutch township of Kungelv with her young nephew, O. R. Frisch. Frisch was also a physicist and a refugee, who had fled Germany to work with one of the patriarchs of physics, Niels Bohr, at his institute in Copenhagen. Avidly discussing the report from Hahn in long walks through the snow, aunt and nephew worked out the explanation of the splitting of the uranium nucleus; they quickly submitted a letter to the British journal *Nature,* which was published days after the Hahn and Strassman report. In this letter the word "fission" was first used; it was borrowed from biology where the term describes the process by which cells divide.

Events moved quickly after that. Frisch returned to Denmark, and immediately recounted the new discoveries to Niels Bohr, who was to depart the same day for the United States.

When Bohr heard Frisch's story, he slapped his forehead and cried, "How could we have overlooked that so long?" So excited did the discussion between the two physicists become that Bohr nearly missed the ship for New York, where he was to meet with Albert Einstein, another refugee of Fascism, who had settled at the Institute for Advanced Studies in Princeton.

On Monday, January 16, Bohr arrived in New York. In Princeton he told a friend, twenty-seven-year-old physicist John Wheeler, of the Hahn-Strassman experiments. Wheeler immediately arranged for a meeting to be held in Princeton the following Wednesday, at which Bohr was to tell about the splitting of the atom. Enrico Fermi, who had started it all, was not present at that meeting. He had arrived in New York just three weeks before Bohr, to take up his work at Columbia University; having just accepted a Nobel Prize in Stockholm, Fermi had decided not to return to Fascist Italy, and had brought his family to America. A young colleague, Willis Lamb, then a twenty-five-year-old physics instructor at Columbia, brought him the news of the revelations Bohr was making in Princeton, the explanation of the five-year-long mystery of Fermi's own experiments.

Fermi immediately designed an experiment to confirm the new results, but he did not wait for the confirmation. He had a date to meet with Bohr the next morning in Washington, at a conference on theoretical physics. Fermi apparently had no doubt that fission had indeed taken place; his meeting with Bohr in Washington on the morning of Thursday, January 26, 1939, was the first step on the road which would lead him to Alamogordo and the nation to Hiroshima, and a nuclear arms race.

That Thursday morning Fermi and Bohr sat at the back of a

classroom in George Washington University, talking excitedly, oblivious to the meeting going on around them. They knew that discoveries of vast importance to physics had been made, but they had not yet realized the importance of nuclear fission to a world at war. For the practical importance of atomic energy depended on two factors, one of which would be resolved in weeks; the other would not be settled for years.

The first factor was the possibility of a chain reaction. A uranium nucleus, struck with a neutron, splits. The neutron has less than one electron volt of energy; fragments of the split atom carry 200 million electron volts. This is clearly an unprecedented multiplication of force. But an atom is, after all, very small. The energy released by the fission of a single uranium atom can only be detected by sensitive instruments.

But what if, when the uranium nucleus splits, it produces two new neutrons? Each of these would then split two more atoms, which would produce four neutrons to split four atoms, which would produce eight neutrons, and so on. If, as Fermi and Bohr had already realized, fission produced neutrons, a chain reaction would be possible, and a single neutron would act like a match to touch off an atomic fire of unprecedented power. On March 3, 1939, the Hungarian physicist Leo Szilard performed an experiment at Columbia University which confirmed Fermi's prediction that neutrons would be produced by fission: the practical release of atomic energy was possible.

But there was still another difficulty to overcome, and in the early days of 1939 it seemed to the physicists nearly insurmountable. It became clear in those early discussions that only a tiny fraction of natural uranium could be fissioned. More than 99 percent of uranium as it is found in nature is in the form of U-238, the isotope which has 238 protons and neutrons in its nucleus. About seven-tenths of one percent of the mineral is U-235, an isotope with three fewer neutrons. Only this seven-tenths of one percent could be split by neutrons. U-238 would not fission — and, furthermore, it would absorb neutrons without being split, and would thus interfere with a chain reaction occurring in the U-235.

There would be no difficulty if there were an easy way of separating the two isotopes of uranium, but this was, and is, an enormously difficult job. The two isotopes of uranium do not differ in any way except for the tiny difference — three parts in 238 — in their atomic weights. The chemical properties of the two forms are identical, and they cannot be separated by ordinary chemical means. Methods of separating isotopes in minute quantities for laboratory work were known, but doing so on a commercial scale seemed to the physicists very difficult. But should it be possible, the implications were clear.

A chain reaction, if it were possible at all, would occur very quickly, releasing a great deal of energy in a very short period of time. And this is simply a definition of an explosion. An atomic bomb was possible — and this would be as obvious to German physicists as to the newly arrived Americans. It was obvious also to a *New York Times* science reporter named William Laurence. On February 24, Fermi and Bohr were again at a meeting together, this time the annual meeting of the American Physical Society at Columbia University. Laurence was covering the meeting for the *Times,* and when he heard Fermi suggest that a chain reaction was possible, he immediately saw the implications.

"Could not a small quantity of uranium 235, say just one kilogram, be used as a bomb equal to thousands of tons of TNT?" Laurence asked Fermi and Bohr after the meeting.

In his book, *Men and Atoms*,[4] Laurence says that Fermi replied, "We must not jump to hasty conclusions," in an attempt to discourage curiosity, for plans were already being discussed to alert the United States Government to possibilities in nuclear fission. Unaware of the scientists' efforts along these lines, and believing that the Germans might be stealing a march, Laurence began accumulating material for a newspaper article which he hoped would focus American attention on the atom. The painstaking accumulation of the evidence that German scientists were indeed working on fission took a full year. On May 5, 1940, the story appeared on the front page of the *Times*:

VAST POWER SOURCE
IN ATOMIC ENERGY
OPENED BY SCIENCE

Relative of Uranium Found to
Yield Force 5 Million Times
as Potent as Coal

Germany Is Seeking It

The article described accurately the enormous power latent in uranium for commercial application and for destruction. To Laurence's surprise, there was no reaction from the U.S. Government at all. Persuaded of the importance of his message, Laurence tried again, this time by submitting a similar article to the *Saturday Evening Post*, which was accepted only when it had been certified as accurate by an imposing array of the country's most prominent physicists. The article finally appeared in September of 1940 — and again, there was no reaction from Washington. The accuracy of Laurence's statements was attested to somewhat later by the Government, however. As Laurence writes,

> Early in the Spring of 1945, after I had been invited to join the inner circle of the atomic-bomb project, I learned, to my amazement, that the [*Saturday Evening Post*] article had been classified as secret and that I would not be permitted to carry it around with me. A copy in my briefcase was stamped "Secret" and solemnly locked in a large safe.[5]

Although Laurence did not know it, similar efforts to bring the atom to official attention were being made by scientists, and meeting with as little success. Fermi approached the Navy Department and was rebuffed. Finally, in 1941, on the eve of the Japanese attack on Pearl Harbor, atomic energy was brought to President Roosevelt's attention through a letter signed by Albert Einstein. By the following year the Manhattan Engineer District, the code name for the all-out effort to produce an atomic bomb, had come into being.

Far more attention was given in those early days of atomic energy to its commercial applications than is now realized, when nuclear weapons have come to overshadow so much of our thought. The French government, for instance, seemed to have been primarily interested in postwar commercial applications of atomic energy. In 1939, Joliot-Curie approached the French Minister of Munitions, who showed great interest in atomic energy. Patents were quickly filed in Swiss patent offices. German scientists apparently also devoted much effort, during the war, to industrial applications of fission. In this country too the difficulties of producing a nuclear weapon seemed very great, if not insurmountable; without the threat of a German atom bomb, we would not have tried to build ours before the end of the war. Industrial applications seemed to hold more promise. As late as 1941, there was still no major effort devoted to weapons development in this country, but in that year Arthur Holly Compton, famous for his work on X-rays, approached General Electric regarding potential industrial atomic development. He reports that GE was quite interested.[6] But by December of that year, the Federal Government preempted the nuclear field, and we entered the war ourselves.

In March of 1939, when Szilard and others confirmed the fact that neutrons were produced each time a uranium nucleus fissioned, it was clear that an atomic bomb was possible in theory. Yet the construction of such a bomb seemed terribly difficult because of the necessity for separating fissionable uranium 235 from the overwhelming amounts of uranium 238, which seemed a near impossible task. And in fact, if this were the only way of making an atom bomb, the attempt might never have been made.

To use atomic energy for industrial purposes, such as the production of electricity, it would not be necessary to separate the two isotopes of uranium, and might not even be desirable to do so. When the nucleus of the U-235 atom splits, two or three neutrons on the average are expelled at enormous speeds. In a block of natural uranium, there are 139 atoms of U-238 for each atom of U-235. It is therefore most likely that these speeding neutrons, if they do not escape entirely, will strike not another U-235 atom, but an unfissionable U-238. They will be absorbed, and the chain reaction will end before it has begun.

But U-235 has a peculiar characteristic which will be best understood by golfers: they know that when putting, if they hit the ball too hard, it will go right over the hole without dropping in. Only a slowly moving ball will be "captured." So with

U-235 — a neutron moving slowly has a greater chance of being captured by a U-235 atom and splitting it than a fast neutron like those produced by fission. U-238, on the other hand, usually absorbs only fast neutrons. Slow neutrons therefore usually bounce harmlessly off U-238 until they hit a U-235 atom.

It is possible to sustain a chain reaction in natural uranium without separating the U-235 and U-238, by slowing the neutrons produced by fission. Slowing down neutrons is not as difficult as it sounds. Fermi had done it in those historic experiments of 1934, simply by passing the neutrons through water or graphite before they hit his uranium "target." The water slowed the neutrons because each neutron collided with many water molecules before it could escape.

Fermi applied this principle in the first major construction of the Manhattan Project, in 1942. He and his colleagues worked in an abandoned squash court under Stagg Field at the University of Chicago. A brass plaque for years hung modestly on a wire fence at the site, commemorating the achievement of the group:

ON DECEMBER 2, 1942
MAN ACHIEVED HERE
THE FIRST SELF-SUSTAINING CHAIN REACTION
AND THEREBY INITIATED THE
CONTROLLED RELEASE OF NUCLEAR ENERGY

What Fermi and his group had done was to build the world's first nuclear reactor, the distant ancestor of the huge nuclear power plants now rising outside the country's major cities. It was a surprisingly simple device: a pile of graphite blocks in which blocks of uranium metal and uranium oxide were placed in alternate layers of the graphite. When an atom of U-235 in one of the blocks of uranium fissioned, usually two or three neutrons would streak away at enormous speed and go crashing into the surrounding graphite where, after repeated collisions, they would be slowed but not absorbed. Eventually the neutrons would pass through another of the blocks of uranium; already moving too slowly to be easily absorbed by U-238, the neutrons would bounce off these atoms until finally they would encounter an atom of U-235, split it and start the process all over again.

Some of the neutrons, of course, would escape from the pile without ever encountering a U-235 atom. Others would be absorbed by impurities in the uranium and graphite. But if one neutron found its way back to a U-235 atom for each atom which split, the chain reaction would be "self-sustaining": it would go on at a steady, constant rate. If two of the neutrons produced in each fission went on to split other U-235 atoms, the reaction would grow very quickly to the point of an explosion.

In order to keep the reaction under control, long rods of cadmium were inserted into the pile; these were its only moving parts. Cadmium is a material which absorbs neutrons; as long as the "control rods" were fully inserted, they would absorb too many of the neutrons for a chain reaction to occur. On December 2, 1942, these rods were slowly withdrawn. The number of neutrons free in the pile slowly increased until there were slightly more neutrons colliding with U-235 atoms and splitting them than there were the moment before. The number of fissions began to increase geometrically, and a recording pen that Fermi and his fellow scientists watched began tracing a slow curve that turned upward at an ever increasing rate. The pile was "critical." Fermi signaled to the young physicist George Weil to reinsert the cadmium control rod; Eugene Wigner produced a bottle of Chianti and toasts were drunk from paper cups. The atomic age had begun.

The first reactor, or "pile" as it was then called, was not built with industrial applications in mind. It was a test of a method of producing plutonium for atomic weapons, but it was also the forerunner of modern nuclear electric power stations.

Ordinary power plants make electricity from the heat of burning coal, oil or gas, or from the power of falling water. Atomic power plants make electricity from the heat of splitting atoms.

Nuclear power plants are now usually called reactors, simply because they are little more, at bottom, than containers in which atomic reactions go on. The typical nuclear power reactor holds many tons of uranium in a cylindrical steel container. When enough uranium sufficiently rich in U-235 is assembled in one place and is interspersed with water or similar material to slow or "moderate" neutrons, it undergoes atomic reaction and becomes very hot. The problem in an ordinary power plant is to keep the fire going; in an atomic power plant the problem is to keep it from getting out of hand. The steel vessel filled with uranium would simply go on getting hotter and hotter until it exploded, unless control devices were inserted.

The reactor at its simplest is therefore a steel vessel containing uranium: the uranium fuel is ordinarily packed into long narrow tubes which are collected in bundles called "fuel assemblies." Long control rods among the fuel tubes regulate the rate of reaction — and hence the heat produced. Water is pumped into the vessel and comes in contact with the hot fuel tubes. Steam is produced and drawn off, and from there an atomic power plant is just like any other. The steam turns the blades of turbines, which drive generators which make electricity.

This seems a simple and cheap way to make electric power, for uranium releases huge amounts of energy when its atoms split. One pound of uranium 235 contains the energy of millions of pounds of coal. In the late 1940's, when atomic power plants were first being discussed publicly, highly respected individuals predicted that the atom would make electricity too cheap to meter. And although this has not turned out to be quite the case, atomic power plants are becoming cheaper and are appearing on the outskirts of our largest cities — New York, Boston, Chicago, Los Angeles, Detroit, and San Francisco. By the early 1970's there will be more than a hundred of these plants operating, most of them enormous, capable of producing a million kilowatts of power, more than enough power for a city of a million inhabitants. By the end of the century, half of all America's electricity is expected to come from the atom.

And yet, despite the optimistic prophecies of the 1940's, the present economic success of nuclear power plants has been a surprise to nearly everyone. During its first eight years of operation, the Atomic Energy Commission, civilian successor to the wartime Manhattan Project, was preoccupied with the problems of developing and building nuclear weapons. It was not until the mid-1950's that pressure from Congress and industry forced an expanded program of civilian atomic power plant development. As late as 1961, fully two-thirds of the AEC's reactor budget was devoted to military applications.

The principal military applications of reactors were for use in nuclear submarines and for the production of plutonium.

The second application prompted construction of the world's first reactor at the University of Chicago during the Second World War. In the early days of the Manhattan Project, two approaches were taken toward atomic weapons construction. The first was the attempt to isolate essentially pure uranium 235 from the nonfissionable and hence nonexplosive, but far more abundant, uranium 238 with which it is mixed in nature. This was considered an extremely difficult and uncertain task, and a second back-up method was also tried.

Fermi and his co-workers had shown that when natural uranium, a mixture of U-235 and U-238, was combined with graphite, the U-235 could sustain a chain reaction despite the presence of large quantities of U-238, which acted like an impurity, absorbing neutrons and thus poisoning the chain reaction. It had long been known, however, that when U-238 absorbed neutrons it was converted to a new element. This new element, plutonium, had first been produced in literally microscopic quantities by a group headed by Dr. Glenn Seaborg, at Berkeley, California, by bombarding uranium 238 with neutrons produced in a cyclotron. Seaborg therefore reached the goal (and eventually the Nobel Prize) which had been sought so long, but by the wrong paths, by Lise Meitner and Irène Joliot-Curie. But his results were far more important than those two distinguished ladies could have guessed. As had been predicted by L. A. Turner of Princeton, plutonium was like uranium 235 — it could sustain a chain reaction and therefore could be used to construct an atom bomb.

Only infinitesimal quantities of plutonium could be produced by Seaborg's method; but Fermi's atomic pile represented a means of making far more. A pile, or reactor, could be built as large as one liked, which meant that enormous numbers of neutrons could be produced in a controlled chain reaction, and these could transform the uranium 238 which was a constituent of the reactor into plutonium. The plutonium could then be extracted by conventional chemical processes.

This method was proved a success during the war. Enormous plutonium production reactors were built near Richland, Washington, on the Columbia River. At the peak of wartime construction, 45,000 workers were engaged at the reactor site. By 1945, enough plutonium had been produced to build the bomb (called "fat man" by its builders) which destroyed the city of Nagasaki. The devastation of Hiroshima, however, was accomplished with a bomb made of uranium 235 which had been separated from the more common but less explosive form of the element by a process called gaseous diffusion.

Although U-235 has proved to be the cheaper of the two bomb materials, this country has constructed fourteen plutonium production reactors. Nine of these were built at the wartime site of Hanford, near Richland, Washington; five were built on the Savannah River in South Carolina. These supplement the gaseous diffusion plants for separation of U-235 which produce most of our atomic weapons.

Although the size and characteristics of the plutonium production reactors are classified information, they are clearly very big. Published estimates indicate that on the average each plant produces well over one million kilowatts of heat energy. This is the heat produced in the chain reaction, and for most of the reactors it is simply a dangerous nuisance. If this waste heat were to be harnessed, however, it could be used to produce large blocks of electric power.

The possibility of using plutonium production reactors for a second purpose, electric power generation, and thus making them far more economical, was obvious from the outset, but in fact it was not realized except in one case, the New Production Reactor completed in 1965. Electric power from this plutonium production reactor is generated and distributed by the Washington Public Power Supply System.

The pressures of stockpiling Cold War weapons prevented the AEC from paying much attention to electric power production until fairly recently, but it was always clear that this aspect of reactors would not be indefinitely ignored. During the 1950's there was considerable uneasiness among the private, or investor-owned, utilities over the Federal Government's growing investment in reactors which could be used for power production. It was probably the concern among the private utilities over this potential new source of public power that accounted for their eagerness, in the 1950's, to participate in the atomic energy program.

Reactors for plutonium production therefore provided the basic principles and the initial economic impetus toward nuclear power plants. With major reactor development efforts in other military applications, it is not surprising that the form civilian plants eventually took was also heavily influenced by military projects.

The most obvious application for atomic power plants is in military submarines. Unlike conventional oil-burning engines which need air for combustion, reactors require no air for their operation. Reactors are compact. They do not need to be refueled except at long intervals. In short, they are ideal for a submarine which must stay under water for long periods of time.

Several reactor designs were experimented with for submarine propulsion, but the final choice was a type called the "pressurized water" reactor, built by the Westinghouse Electric Corporation. In this type, cooling water is circulated through the reactor under pressure, so that it does not boil. After leaving the reactor core, this water passes through pipes in a boiler, where steam is produced, before being returned to cool the reactor again.

Westinghouse has now become one of the two manufacturers which supply the majority of reactors for civilian power production. All Westinghouse plants, including the country's first reactor to produce power for commercial use, have been developed from the power plants which drive nuclear submarines and surface ships. This is not to imply that Westinghouse has taken undue advantage of its position as a defense contractor. The basic design of the pressurized water reactor, like the designs of other types, is in the public domain and freely available from the AEC.

Westinghouse is also one of the principal suppliers of conventional electric generating equipment; its main rival is the General Electric Company. With a potential market for reactors provided by private utilities trying to forestall federal atomic power generation, and with its chief competitor engaged in reactor development, General Electric quickly came up with a rival model, the boiling water reactor. This was a type first developed for research purposes at the Atomic Energy Commission's Argonne Laboratory. It differed from the pressurized water reactor in that there was no separate boiler — the steam was generated right in the reactor core and drawn off to the turbines.

GE and Westinghouse dominated the reactor field from the outset, and continue to do so. Of the reactors ordered through

1967, the two firms divided 80 percent about equally between them. The remainder were supplied by Combustion Engineering and Babcock and Wilcox, two major suppliers of conventional boilers.

While atomic energy was under military control, and then for eight years more under the Atomic Energy Act of 1946, only the Government could build or own reactors. A new Atomic Energy Act passed in 1954 opened the door to private ownership. In 1955, the Atomic Energy Commission announced the Cooperative Power Reactor Demonstration Program, through which utilities could obtain heavy federal assistance in building nuclear plants. Shortly thereafter, two utilities announced plans to build reactors with their own funds, although receiving substantial indirect subsidies from the Government in the form of reduced fuel costs, design assistance, waste disposal services, and others. The Consolidated Edison Company, which supplies New York City, announced plans to build a Westinghouse reactor on the Hudson River; Commonwealth Edison announced that it would build a General Electric reactor near Chicago. Ten other utilities, both investor-owned and publicly owned, announced plans for small plants under the cooperative demonstration program, and received substantial direct and indirect assistance.

The dozen atomic power plants which were to be built by utilities alone or in cooperation with the AEC ran into trouble from the outset. The Fermi plant at Lagoona Beach, Michigan, near Detroit, never succeeded in producing substantial amounts of electric power. The plant at Hallam, Nebraska, after a long history of difficulties, was finally shut down, and at this writing is being dismantled, while a coal-burning plant rises to replace it. All of the other plants experienced technical difficulties,

soaring costs, and long delays. A mood of gloom settled over
the nuclear industry.

By 1963, the prospects for civilian atomic power looked
bleak. Manufacturing firms which had entered the nuclear
field during its first flowering, five years before, were announcing plans to withdraw. Utilities seemed to have lost interest
in reactors, and violent legal battles were being fought with
citizens' groups contesting the safety of those reactors which
were being built. A highly respected study by the economist
Philip Mullenbach, for the Twentieth Century Fund, summed
up the prevailing attitude:

> . . . the fact is that private utilities, eight years after the passage
> of the 1954 [atomic energy] act, had constructed only two full-
> scale plants without heavy government assistance, and these two
> were among the very first announced. The evidence raises the
> question whether the private utilities are prepared even at this
> late date to make the large investments called for by full-scale
> nuclear power.[7]

Yet at almost the same time these words were published,
the New Jersey Central Power and Light Company announced
that it had reached an agreement with General Electric to purchase a reactor capable of generating more than 500,000 kilowatts, twice the size of any previously built. The utility
planned to ask for no federal assistance — but what was more
surprising, its calculations showed that the nuclear plant would
produce power more cheaply than a coal plant at the same site.
This was the first plant to be chosen on strictly economic
grounds: for the first time, nuclear power could compete with
coal.

It may be that General Electric had stolen a march by pro-

viding guaranteed prices and performance for the New Jersey
plant to be built at Oyster Creek that meant no profit, and
perhaps a loss, to the manufacturer. Although the plant is
not yet in operation, it has already suffered a number of technical setbacks which have put it far behind schedule, and
which will put its cost to both manufacturer and utility beyond
that which had been announced.

Nevertheless, the Oyster Creek announcement was heralded
as the long-awaited breakthrough in reactor economics. By
1965, when it seemed clear that both General Electric and
Westinghouse were willing to sell reactors on similar terms for
other locations, a flood of orders began pouring in which has
not yet abated. By April of 1968, about 100 reactors were
operating, under construction, or being ordered. During 1966
and 1967, more than half the generating capacity of new
plants ordered in the United States was nuclear, and this pace
has continued into 1968.

The plants being ordered now are twice the size of Oyster
Creek, and it is hoped by the manufacturers and the utilities
that the economies of size will, in fact, make those new plants
cheaper than coal plants in almost all parts of the country.
Whether or not the economic realities will confirm these predictions is yet to be seen. The sudden and largely unexpected
rush to reactors has created some far more serious problems.

Because of military, political, and economic pressures, it has
never been possible to question seriously the present need for
atomic power, nor to choose among the various routes to that
goal which are available. With few exceptions, there has been
no public discussion whatever of the benefits and risks of our
present nuclear power program. One of those exceptions, and
the most notable is, as might be expected, in California.

III

EARTHQUAKES AND ACCIDENTS

CALIFORNIA ROUTE 1 IS A TWO-LANE HIGHWAY; going north from San Francisco it edges the Pacific Coast, in a series of roller-coaster curves on the hills which rise from the sea there. For a while it flattens out as it skirts inland of Tomales Bay. Then the open sea is in view again for a while and the hills return. About fifty miles north of San Francisco, the highway passes the tiny town of Bodega Bay. The Bay is formed by a rocky peninsula, Bodega Head, which arches in a curve west and south and ends in a granite hammerhead. This isolated and beautiful spot was to be the site of one of the country's most controversial peacetime atomic ventures.

A left turn from Route 1 will take you into the small fishing village of Bodega Bay. The Bay is the first harbor of refuge north of San Francisco, and it is crowded with fishing boats. There is a new four-lane road around the shore of the harbor. It runs past a cluster of piers and houses on the east shore and sweeps on to the west shore, the inner side of the peninsula. Here the houses quickly disappear; the road runs on over what was once a series of rocky tidal pools rich in marine life. A stranger wonders what optimistic town plan produced this four-lane road running down deserted Bodega Head.

The road runs past a long galvanized-wire fence and finally

ends in a parking area. But there is nothing here, and seemingly nothing within the fence. Very near the end of the peninsula, in an indentation in the granite hill on the harbor side, is a large circular hole, now filled with water, and a heap of gravel long abandoned. There are no placards or other signs to mark this as the location of what was to have been the Pacific Gas and Electric Company's Bodega Bay Atomic Park. After more than six years of planning and battle the Pacific Gas and Electric Company on October 30, 1964, announced that it had abandoned plans for a nuclear-powered electric generating plant at Bodega Bay. On the following day the San Francisco *Chronicle* reported:

> The site, only 1000 feet west of the San Andreas fault, was dropped as the location for a 325,000-kilowatt nuclear plant because of fears that dangerous radiation would be released in case of a severe earthquake.

In making his brief announcement, Robert H. Gerdes, then president of P. G. & E., stated, according to the *Chronicle*, "We would be the last to desire to build a plant with any substantial doubt existing as to public safety." [1]

The statement must have been a difficult one for Gerdes to make, for the investment in the Bodega Bay Atomic Park had already reached $4 million in planning and construction costs alone. The additional investment of the private utility's talent, time, and money in the six-year battle against public opposition to the nuclear reactor at Bodega will probably never be known.

Early in 1958, Pacific Gas and Electric began bargaining for land on Bodega Head. To the country's largest privately owned utility, with assets in the billions, this must have seemed a minor element of routine. Several months before, P. G. & E. officers had met privately and in secret with the Board of Supervisors of Sonoma County. Supervisor E. J. ("Nin") Guidotti later recalled, "We were all aware of the possibility that [the plant] would be nuclear." [2] But no public announcement was made.

P. G. & E. had announced that it planned to add some nuclear plants to its generating capacity, but it did not say whether the Bodega site would house one of the new plants. At this time there was only one nuclear plant in the country producing commercial electric power, the Shippingport atomic plant in Pennsylvania. P. G. & E. was therefore perhaps a little hesitant about public reaction to a neighboring atomic power plant; whatever its reasons, the announcement that the Bodega plant was to be nuclear did not come until nearly three years after the utility began acquiring land. The secrecy with which these early steps were taken did not avoid local opposition to the plant, however. Opposition began almost at the outset, and stemmed at first from Rose Gaffney, who owned a little more than four hundred acres of Bodega Head.

Bodega was then a very beautiful and largely undisturbed place, with a long if quiet history. A Russian sealing station had been there. The Mexicans and the Americans followed in slow succession; there is no drama in Bodega's history. It was a beautiful peaceful spot, and Rose Gaffney's title to her land was originally granted in Mexico City, not Washington, D.C. It is dry, rocky ground. In recent years Mrs. Gaffney had derived a small income from it by renting it for pasturage; a small dairy herd grazed the hills which were brown in summer, green in winter.

nouncement the already organized opposition focused on a new issue: safety. For the site of the plant was only 1000 feet from the San Andreas fault, the most active source of earthquakes in the country, and the cause of the 1906 earthquake which devastated San Francisco.

In 1965, Dr. Edward Teller, often called the "father of the H-Bomb," and not otherwise noted for his caution in advocating the military development of atomic energy, wrote in 1965: "In principle, nuclear reactors are dangerous. . . . By being careful, and also by good luck, we have so far avoided all serious nuclear accidents. . . . In my mind, nuclear reactors do not belong on the surface of the earth. Nuclear reactors belong underground." [3] It is easy to see the cause of Dr. Teller's trepidation. As we shall see, the results of a serious accident involving a reactor could be disastrous; if anything could cause such an accident, an earthquake might.

A reactor like the one planned for Bodega is a complex and temperamental device, under the best of circumstances. It would seem unreasonable to expect such a device to go on functioning safely during an earthquake; yet this is precisely what the designers of the P. G. & E. plant intended. For it was clear that sometime during the lifetime of the reactor there might be another severe earthquake at the San Andreas fault. Light warning tremors are a commonplace in the area; severe earthquakes have occurred several times, the worst having been in 1906. The earthquake which more recently devastated the Alaskan coast was due to the same system of faults.

The world's worst earthquake zones lie in a circle around the Pacific Ocean. The earthquakes which periodically rack the western coast of the United States, and the devastating earthquake which struck Alaska on Good Friday of 1964, all lie within this circum-Pacific ring of earthquakes and volcanoes.

Earthquakes are not very well understood, nor are their causes certain. They are reminders that the crust of the earth which seems so solid and immutable is in slow but constant change, and that the seemingly fixed continents are slowly rearing upward or sinking back into the sea. The slow massive movements of the earth's crust sometimes become visible to us, when growing stresses in the crust cause earthquakes.

Past geological stresses have left long cracks or faults in many parts of the world. The earthquake ring around the Pacific is a network of such faults, some of which may run for hundreds of miles. When the slow shifting in the earth's crust builds up stress in the rock, it may give suddenly, often along the line of such a fault. This sudden readjustment is an earthquake; close to the fault the earth on both sides snaps away with great force in a whiplash motion. This sudden snapping release is accompanied by the enormous vibration of readjustment, as one side of the fault grinds against the other. During the 1906 earthquake in San Francisco, the earth shifted along the fault 20 feet in some places; the west side of the fault was two or three feet higher than the east side after the earthquake.

The San Francisco earthquake was due to shifting on the San Andreas fault, the most active earthquake zone in the country, along the shoreline of California. At Bodega it actually runs through the Bay. The proposed site of the atomic power plant which Pacific Gas and Electric planned to build at Bodega was about 1000 feet from the edge of the San Andreas fault zone, despite a clear regulation of the Atomic Energy Commission that "no facility should be located closer than one fourth mile from the surface location of a known active earthquake fault." This means that the Bodega plant was to have been 320 feet closer than it should have been.

Pacific Gas and Electric maintained that the reactor could be built to ride out any major earthquake which might occur during the plant's lifetime. The Atomic Energy Commission's prestigious Advisory Committee on Reactor Safeguards gave preliminary agreement to the plan, but, late in 1964, the AEC's own staff expressed some doubts, and P. G. & E. withdrew their application. Yet for three years they had maintained the safety of the atomic plant in the face of growing opposition and technical disagreement.

Bodega Head is an ancient granite formation, and at first sight would seem to provide the solid rock anchorage which is ideal for structures which hope to ride out the shock of a nearby earthquake. Even though the proposed site was close to the San Andreas fault, it was thought to be outside the "zone of fling" — the area bordering the fault where the earth snaps away during an earthquake. The Bodega site would only suffer the shocks, transmitted through the ground, of the earthquake readjustment, but there would be no shifting on Bodega Head itself. In principle it seemed possible to build a building which would ride out the shock waves, although what effect such drastic shocks would have on the delicate mechanism of a reactor was hard to foretell. P. G. & E. maintained in its original application that no matter what damage was suffered by the reactor core itself during an earthquake, the containment structure to be provided would assure that there would be no release of radioactivity to the outside air to pose a hazard to nearby residents.

This approach is typical of all builders of modern power reactors. It is generally recognized that our understanding of reactors is not good enough for us to rule out absolutely the possibility of a drastic mishap in the reactor itself, and correspondingly each reactor is equipped with a number of devices designed to reduce the consequences of such an accident, should it happen. In many reactors the ultimate line of defense is the containment sphere, a steel or concrete dome designed hopefully to contain all or most of the radiation which would be released in a major reactor accident.

The Bodega reactor was to have a different sort of containment, a "pressure suppression" system, which had only been tried once before at the far-smaller installation at Humboldt Bay, California. This would provide a huge doughnut-ring suppression pool, half filled with water, around the reactor. Any build-up of pressure in the reactor, as in an accident, would vent harmlessly into the pool; radioactive wastes would be contained in the pool and in a steel drywell which surrounded the reactor core.

Opposition to the reactor had originally been in terms of conserving the unique natural qualities of Bodega Head. When serious safety problems about the Bodega site began to appear, the Northern California Association to Preserve Bodega Head and Harbor, led by David Pesonen, was able to marshal an impressive body of expert testimony and independent information. An early problem to appear was that the site of the reactor, supposed to be solid rock, was in fact the sloping side of an ancient canyon which had long ago filled with sediment. Preliminary borings on the site showed almost 60 feet of silt, clay, and sand. Dr. Pierre Saint-Amand, a professional seismologist from the Naval Ordnance Testing Station, China Lake, California, a man very well known in this field, and later a member of the team sent by the governor of California to

survey the effects of the Alaskan earthquake and to make recommendations to prevent similar damage to structures in
California, was retained by Pesonen's group to give an independent evaluation of the reactor site. Saint-Amand's report
read in part:

> It is generally thought that it is better to build upon solid rock
> than upon alluvium. This is certainly true at a distance from the
> causative fault. However, at near fault distances, where fling is
> important, rock may be as bad or worse. Clearly the worst pos-
> sible situation is to build upon a combination of the two. At the
> Bodega Head site the rock is severely crushed, broken and
> mylonitized. It could scarcely be classed as good foundation
> material. It will transmit well high-frequency vibrations, and
> then plastically deform in response to regional readjustment of
> strain; it will probably also undergo mass movement due to its
> own weight during the long-period oscillations. In addition,
> the alluvium, a loosely aggregated clay-rich soil, will certainly
> yield at a different rate than the rock, subjecting the installation
> to widely varying dynamic loads and permitting the several parts
> of the installation to settle different amounts, probably resulting
> in serious damage from changes in level and position to intercon-
> necting structures, to the cooling system, and to the reactor itself.
> A worse foundation situation would be difficult to envision.[4]

This report was made during 1963; shortly after it was issued,
a team from the United States Geological Survey visited the
site. By this time preliminary construction had begun, including the first excavation of the shaft in which the reactor itself would be housed. USGS investigators Schlocker and Bonilla
first visited the site in the summer of 1963, and then were called
back to it in October. A fault running through the reactor
shaft itself had been discovered.

The two geologists remained at the site while construction progressed. When the shaft was 142 feet in diameter and 73 feet below sea level, Schlocker and Bonilla examined the shaft and reported, in January 1964, that running through the reactor site was,

> an important zone of weakness that could undergo differential movement if stressed to a degree comparable to the stress applied to granitic rocks on [nearby] Point Reyes peninsula during the 1906 earthquake.[5]

As David Pesonen noted later in a pamphlet, "One of the most important findings of this report . . . was that during the 1906 earthquake there had been significant faulting of the rock on Point Reyes, *outside* the commonly accepted San Andreas Zone."[6] What had happened at nearby and geologically similar Point Reyes could easily happen at the reactor site on Bodega Head.

This discovery put a very different light on the problem of the safety of the site. P. G. & E.'s own former consultant, geologist Dr. William Quaide, stated to a San Francisco *Chronicle* reporter: "There is a chance that the fault could break beneath the plant's site in case of an earthquake. I think the probability is low. . . . But it is necessary to face the moral issue: 'If there is even a slight chance of danger, should we go ahead and build the plant?' "[7]

P. G. & E. insisted on the low probability of movement along the fault through the reactor site, and in its own report on the situation noted that there was no evidence of movement along the fault "during the last 40,000 years."[8]

The otherwise unsuitable characteristics of the site became

submerged in the debate over whether there would actually be slippage along the fault running through the reactor site. Dr. George Housner, P. G. & E.'s consultant on design and a widely respected professor of structural engineering at the California Institute of Technology, reported to the Company in 1961:

> Since it is quite impossible to desi~ a power plant to survive without damage the large permanent ground surface displacements that might occur if earthquake fault slippage occurred on the site, this possibility must be given special consideration.[9]

The Atomic Energy Commission eventually insisted that this serious possibility must be taken into account, and asked P. G. & E. to amend its application for a construction permit. The company responded by submitting Amendment 7 to its Hazards Analysis, offering a novel design to "accommodate movement along [the fault on the site], even though the possibility of such movement occurring is not considered to be credible." The novel design, never before used in a civilian structure, was apparently based on the design of underground siloes which protect this country's intercontinental ballistic missiles against nuclear attack.

The tenacity with which Pacific Gas and Electric clung to the Bodega site despite the mounting evidence of its unsuitability is quite puzzling. Some support, it was true, was given by the AEC's Advisory Committee on Reactor Safeguards which approved the site. It was only in the face of almost certain disapproval by the Atomic Energy Commission itself that the application for the reactor was withdrawn. Although $4 million had been invested in the Bodega site, the multibillion dol-

lar utility would certainly have weathered the loss easily.
What may have been more important was the utility's much
greater commitment to nuclear power in general. Plans called
for an increasing reliance of the company on nuclear plants
in California, where air pollution problems and looming natural
gas shortages seemed to leave no other alternative (Los Angeles has already ruled that no more conventional power
plants may be built in its area).

Most suitable sites for nuclear plants in arid California are
along the seacoast, for power plants require enormous quantities of cooling water. Yet the San Andreas fault zone runs up
and down nearly the whole length of the California coast. A
defeat for the company at Bodega Head might mean far greater
difficulty in obtaining licenses for other sites. And public opposition could be expected to redouble.

Public opposition to reactors in California has, indeed, been
reinforced. Reactors proposed for other California sites have
run into strong opposition. The reactor proposed for Malibu
found knowledgeable and well-organized public resistance. A
similar pattern is being repeated at the Diablo Canyon reactor
site. At Malibu, a geologic situation similar to that at Bodega
has been discovered — old faults traverse the site — and the
AEC has again asked for consideration of ground displacement
at the site. The Los Angeles Department of Water and Power,
at this writing, is still considering whether to try again with a
"novel design concept" or to abandon the site.

Despite continual difficulties, however, the reactor program
in California is struggling forward. The most spectacular event
has been the announcement of plans by the Los Angeles Department of Water and Power, and other groups, to construct
two huge reactors on a man-made island just off the Orange

County shore, in one of the most populous areas of the state, just 24 miles from Los Angeles' Civic Center. The two plants jointly will produce six times as much power as the Bodega reactor would have, and will also produce 150 million gallons of fresh water from sea water each day for Los Angeles. The project is being conducted jointly with, and partly financed by, the Atomic Energy Commission and the Department of Interior's Office of Saline Water. Congress has recently made available $72 million in federal funds for the project. The remainder of the project's $4.5 million cost will be borne by the local community. Soaring costs have dampened the original enthusiasm for this project, however, and some of the participants have apparently withdrawn.

In view of the continuing California reactor program, it may be worthwhile to take a closer look at the possibilities for accident in the now defunct Bodega plant. The best analysis of accident potential in a nuclear reactor is contained in a study of the Bodega plant in the April 1964 issue of *Nuclear Information*, by Lindsay Mattison and Richard Daly.[10] The following account is drawn largely from that report.

The Bodega reactor was to have been of the boiling-water variety being marketed by General Electric. Cooling water would be drawn in from Bodega Bay and passed into the reactor; steam at high temperature and pressure would be drawn directly from the reactor core and carried through some 200 feet of pipe to the turbines and generator in an adjoining building, where the electrical power would actually be produced. The 529 uranium fuel tubes in the reactor core would be protected from the water by metal jackets, and contained in a steel reactor vessel through which the water would flow. A pear-shaped steel drywell would provide a protective container for the reactor vessel, and the drywell in turn would be hooped with the circular pressure suppression system. In case of an accident, steam from the reactor vessel would pass through eight pipes into the pressure suppression pool, preventing undue strain on the drywell.

During a violent earthquake, the reactor building might be damaged, and one or several of the numerous pipes leading from the reactor core out of the drywell could be smashed. One possible spot for such a break would be the steam pipe leading to the turbines. If the accident also ruptured the pipes carrying coolant to the core and simultaneously rendered emergency cooling mechanisms inoperative, the result would be the rapid melting of the reactor's fuel.

This melting would occur whether the reactor were operating at the time or not. If the reactor were operating, the temperature of the fuel at full power would quickly rise past the melting point through the energy being liberated by nuclear fissioning. If the reactor were to be shut down in time, a meltdown would still result although more slowly, because of the heat derived from breakdown of the radioactive waste products accumulated in the fuel.

"The maximum accident seen by P. G. & E. as possible at its Bodega Reactor," according to Mattison and Daly, "would release 80 million curies of fission products, but contain them in the drywell." A curie is the radioactive equivalent of a gram of radium. Eighty million curies is a staggering quantity — a Hiroshima-size atomic bomb would release only a few hundred thousand curies. "The findings of various geologists point to the possibility that the reactor drywell container would be breached by on-site earth movement in the event of an earthquake, releasing fission products to the atmosphere. What would be the effect on people in the area if all 80 million curies did disperse?"

Neither Mattison and Daly, nor anyone else, consider the dispersal of such catastrophic quantities of radioactive material to be likely. Even under the conditions of a violent earthquake beneath the plant, it is hard to see how all of this material could be dispersed over a large area. Most of it is in solid or liquid form, even at the temperatures of a reactor meltdown. Only a very violent explosion could disperse this material in small enough particles for it to be borne by the wind. Since the reactor vessel would have been surrounded not only by a drywell, but also by a reactor building, the explosion would have had literally to demolish both drywell and building. Even a building cracked and distorted by an earthquake, even one that had collapsed over the reactor, would act to trap a large portion of the radioactivity.

A more likely, if still improbable, circumstance, would be the slow release of the gaseous portion of the reactor's accumulated radioactivity. A slow leakage of radiation from an earthquake-damaged reactor would result in smaller exposures to radiation over longer periods of time than the accident which is described below. An accident which resulted in even one percent of the releases assumed in what follows, although still unlikely, is not to be dismissed lightly.

> In the event that winds on Bodega Head blew to the East and Northeast, an unlikely but possible situation, the following exposures could occur. In the town of Bodega Bay, some two miles from the reactor, nearly everyone would die the first day.
>
> For those without shelter the external gamma radiation exposure could rise to 3,120 rads the first day and 14,000 rads could be accumulated in the following 90 days. The AEC suggests

half of any population exposed to 350 to 500 rads will die within a week. . . . Some twenty miles from the site, the city of Santa Rosa has 31,000 residents. There, exposures could be 72 rads the first day and some 4,600 rads in 90 days. From inhalation while the cloud passes, the beta radiation to the lungs could be 320 rads the first day and 960 the first week. Thyroid doses from inhalation in Santa Rosa could be 4,700 rads. The Federal Radiation Council recommends that for the general population a thyroid dose of .5 rads *yearly* should not be exceeded. . . .

For the San Francisco metropolitan area — fifty miles from the reactor — the external doses could be 15 rads on the first day and 104 in 90 days. The lung dose could be 84 and 250 rads, for the first day and week respectively. The thyroid dose could be 1240 rads. . . .

One may conclude that people within five miles downwind of the reactor would probably be killed and within twenty miles many of the people exposed would be very sick. Beyond that distance a few would be sick within the first week and such long term effects as increased leukemia, thyroid cancer, and congenital malformations would eventually make their appearance. For distances of hundreds of miles from such a release of radioactivity the AEC . . . suggests, "Probable destruction of standing crops, restrictions on agriculture for the first year." [11]

These predictions are based on calculation techniques developed in an AEC study of the consequences of reactor accidents, and assume a number of pessimistic weather conditions, such as thermal inversions (where a layer of cold air is trapped under a warmer one) and steady winds. The AEC has recently published more elaborate methods for calculating the effects of such an accident, but the Mattison and Daly study remains substantially accurate.

The accident which is assumed for these calculations is quite unlikely under normal conditions. Certainly the populations at risk would be evacuated within hours. For such an accident to occur, the normal water cooling of the reactor must be shut off, and the emergency cooling systems must all fail to function. In addition, the various devices for containing radioactivity from the reactor core must fail to function effectively — the reactor vessel, drywell, and pressure suppression pool, as well as the reactor building itself. Whether all these things would happen during an earthquake at the reactor site itself is a matter for speculation, but it seems at least conceivable. As we pointed out earlier, even if an accident were to occur, the actual releases of radioactivity are not likely to be as great as those assumed for the study. As Dr. Quaide pointed out, the decision in such circumstances is a moral one: If there is even a slight chance of danger, should we go ahead and build the plant?

This is a decision which will have to be faced more and more frequently in California. Because of the state's air pollution and fuel problems, most future power plants are expected to be nuclear, and because of cooling-water requirements will be sited on the earthquake-prone coast. A virtual rerun of the Bodega dispute is already going on at Malibu in Los Angeles County, where a complex of four reactors has been proposed by the Los Angeles Department of Water and Power. The first reactor, half again as large as the Bodega plant was to be, was scheduled for operation in 1968, but public opposition and difficulties in licensing have already pushed that date farther into the future.

As at Bodega, opposition to the plant at first centered on conservation issues, providing a context of debate in which safety problems appeared and then predominated. A group called Malibu Citizens for Conservation was formed and

achieved a membership of more than 1000 (the 1964 population of Malibu was only 9000). On January 29, 1963, the
Department of Water and Power submitted their proposal for
the first Malibu plant to the AEC. By the end of 1964, the
failure of the Bodega project, the Alaskan earthquake, and a
dam disaster in nearby Baldwin Hills all lent impetus to the
citizens' group opposing the reactor, and an impressive array
of scientific and technical advice and evidence was mar-
shaled.

The reactor was to be built in a beautiful coast location, Corral Canyon; a brochure from the Department of Water and
Power describes it this way: "The site is sheltered on three
sides by the canyon's surrounding terrain rising 650 feet above
the canyon floor. The fourth side faces the ocean, which is
across U.S. Highway 101. . . . The nuclear power station
will be attractively designed with good architecture and landscape to provide a pleasing appearance." [12]

The protective sound of those high canyon walls is misleading, however. Consulting geologist Thomas L. Bailey reported
to the citizens' group: ". . . the proposed site for a Nuclear
Reactor Plant in lower Corral Canyon is a geologically unstable
area subject to severe landsliding. . . ." [13] Closer examination revealed even more disturbing aspects of the site. Dr.
Thomas Clements, for thirty years head of the Department of
Geology at the University of Southern California, reported:

It is the opinion of the undersigned that the lower part of Corral
Canyon is crossed by a large overthrust fault. As a result, the
rocks of this area are highly fractured, crushed and squeezed
and, therefore, are weak and unstable. . . . the writer recommends that the site be abandoned.[14]

Dr. Barclay Kamb, Professor of Geology and Geophysics, California Institute of Technology, after making a comprehensive survey of the site, concluded:

> The disturbed zone at Corral Canyon passes directly beneath the proposed reactor installation. . . . In relation to the possible range of exposure to fault hazards in Southern California, the Corral Canyon site ranks as among the more hazardous possible.[15]

These geologists and others submitted their opinions to the Los Angeles Department of Water and Power (LADWP), but with little effect. In July of 1964 they were submitted to the Los Angeles County Board of Supervisors, which was being asked to reverse the granting of a zoning exception for the plant. The Board was also presented with a report from the LADWP's own consultant, Dr. Richard Jahns, then Dean of the School of Earth Sciences, Stanford University. Dr. Jahns stated:

> In this writer's opinion, the possibility of fault movement within the site area during the planned life of the power station is remote. With the understanding that the reactors and other critical structures would be engineered for appropriate earthquake resistance and that *none of them would be placed across a recognizable fault*, it is also this writer's opinion that the site is a satisfactory one . . . [emphasis added].[16]

The Board of Supervisors unanimously denied the zone exception for the power plant, stating that

> In the face of these conflicting reports . . . it appears that no one can predict with any certainty what degree of safety could or would be built into the Atomic plant. . . . We cannot, in good

The California State Department of Recreation had long wanted Bodega Head as a park; the University of California was considering setting up a marine biology laboratory. But for the time being, control of the area was vested in the County Board of Supervisors, and they had probably already agreed, in private, to P. G. & E.'s plans for the area. When in 1958 Rose Gaffney refused to sell her land to the utility, P. G. & E. quietly went to court and, still with no public announcement, initiated condemnation proceedings. A utility has the right of eminent domain — Mrs. Gaffney could be forced to sell her land.

The long battle which Mrs. Gaffney fought to keep from meeting P. G. & E.'s demands disrupted what might have been a smooth and orderly progress to a nuclear plant. Coupled with opposition in the town of Bodega Head and Sonoma County over a variety of issues, ranging from different plans for the development of the harbor area to a general concern over preserving the natural beauty of Bodega Head, Mrs. Gaffney's vociferous reluctance delayed and publicized P. G. & E.'s plans to the point that organized public opposition on a large scale became possible. A remarkably effective organization, the Northern California Association to Preserve Bodega Head and Harbor, whose membership eventually numbered in the thousands, came into existence, and was headed by a young Sierra Club staff member named David Pesonen.

Opposition to the Bodega plant quickly centered on conservation issues; Bodega Head had unique scientific and recreational values which would be destroyed by the plant. It was not until the summer of 1961 that P. G. & E. finally announced what had already been widely assumed in the press — the power plant at Bodega was to use atomic fuel. With this an-conscience, approve such an action which may result in dire consequences, including the possibility of loss of many lives.[17]

There is some question as to whether the LADWP requires a zone exception in order to build its plants, and the utility has announced its intention to proceed in the face of the County Supervisors' opposition. The Supervisors countered by passing a resolution to intervene in the Atomic Energy Commission proceedings regarding licensing of the plant.

Dr. Jahns's report has recently reappeared in the controversy, however. In pronouncing the site satisfactory so long as there were no faults underlying the reactor itself, he foreshadowed the most serious difficulty which the utility would encounter. During excavation, a fault running through the reactor site itself was discovered. The situation was then precisely comparable to that at Bodega. The utility maintained that the fault was inactive and had suffered no movement for at least 10,000 years; the citizens' group maintained that slippage on the fault could very well occur during the lifetime of the reactor.

Again, the Atomic Energy Commission expressed its doubts about the design of the plant in the presence of a fault. After a long series of hearings and reviews, in March 1967 the AEC insisted that the LADWP resubmit its application, showing a design which would protect the reactor against ground displacement. Despite their own consultant's report which insisted that no reactor would be placed across a fault, the LADWP has indicated it has no plans to move the plant. "We can design for ground displacement," a utility official told a trade publication. "There's nothing hard about that." Pacific Gas and Electric had ducked the issue by withdrawing their application. The Los Angeles utility has apparently decided to

face it at Malibu. "Anywhere you go in California," the
LADWP official told the reporter, "you usually have a fault.
Moving [the reactor] won't buy you anything." [18]

This gloomy estimate has been confirmed by a Department
of Interior study of another LADWP reactor site, Bolsa Island,
where LADWP and private utilities plan to build the two
huge power and fresh-water plants for the Los Angeles area.
The Bolsa Island project also has a long history.

In July of 1964, President Johnson directed the Secretary of
the Interior, in cooperation with the Atomic Energy Commission, to develop a program for the large-scale desalting of sea
water. On September 22, the Secretary's report was delivered
to the President and on April 5, 1965, he submitted legislation
to Congress accompanied by a message which expressed what
seemed to be his strong and continuing interest in accelerated
efforts to increase the country's supply of fresh water. Johnson
asked for a five-year extension of the current water-desalting
program and an increase in funding of $200 million over that
period; the program covered a wide range of research and
development problems, but gave heavy emphasis to the possibility of using very large nuclear reactors in dual-purpose
plants for desalination and the production of electric power.
The program was passed by Congress with little change, and
on September 2, 1965, President Johnson announced, while ·
dedicating a dam at Summersville, West Virginia, "The Administration has just asked Congress' approval to share in construct-
ing the world's largest nuclear-fueled desalting and electric
power plant in the Los Angeles area."

Sea water can be turned into fresh water simply by distilling
it. More than 800 plants are in operation throughout the world,
turning sea or brackish water into fresh water, most of them

operating on this simple principle in one form or another. The problem is cost — it takes a great deal of heat energy to boil water, and energy from coal or atoms is expensive. One way around the cost difficulty is to build very large nuclear plants, which also produce electricity and in which the unit cost of power drops as the plants get larger.

In April of 1964 an Office of Science and Technology task force headed by Dr. Roger Revelle reported to the President that if nuclear plants were sufficiently large, and were used for both power production and desalination, the combined savings would allow fresh water costs low enough to compete with natural supplies in some areas.[19]

The eventual result of that report was the Bolsa Island proposal: two reactors which would between them produce as much power as the Hoover Dam, 1,800,000 kilowatts, and 150,000,000 gallons of water per day — enough for a city the size of San Francisco. Clearly, there are very few places in the country which could absorb such an installation, and where water scarcity and cost could make it useful. The Los Angeles area was seemingly ideal, but unfortunately had already committed itself to a multibillion dollar system to bring water through aqueducts from Northern California. According to Frank Di Luzio, then Director of the Office of Saline Water, testifying before a House subcommittee, the Los Angeles complex would not have considered the desalting plant for another decade without considerable federal encouragement.[20] This has taken the form of a more than $72 million subsidy for the $400 million installation, the remainder of the cost to be borne by the Los Angeles Department of Water and Power, the Metropolitan Water District, the San Diego Gas and Electric Company, and the Southern California Edison Company. Actual costs of the project are now estimated at $750 million, far greater than original guesses, and the fate of the plant is again in question.

If the Los Angeles area was ideal for the project in one way, it was a problem in others. The sprawling nature of the city would force a reactor installation quite far away if it were not to be built in a heavily populated district, and the costs of transporting water and power would be great.

For economic purposes therefore, an ideal location for the plant is a man-made island to be built 3500 feet from the shore of Orange County and 24 miles from the heart of Los Angeles. This puts the plant close to its market; whether it takes it far enough away from the people is another question. The serious problem of whether a man-made island will be a reasonable foundation for a nuclear plant in the earthquake-ridden area also remains open to question. A recent Interior Department survey of the site recommends taking into account the possibility of ground displacement on the site during an earthquake. The moral question which the utilities faced at Bodega and Malibu will be faced again to a greater or lesser extent at Bolsa Island. Can even the small risk of catastrophic accident which is unavoidable in the present state of technology be accepted?

This question is growing more critical, as the number and size of nuclear plants planned for California grow. Sites for nuclear plants have been purchased in Mendocino County, Point Arena, Montezuma Slough, South Moss Landing, sites just north of San Diego and south of Sacramento, Nipomo Dunes, Diablo Canyon, Cayucos Beach, as well as Malibu and Bolsa Island; Southern California Edison has recently announced plans for a $200 million nuclear generating facility in Santa Barbara, California, north of Los Angeles; the plant will generate 1,000,000 kilowatts. Reactors are already operating at Vallecitos, San Onofre, and Humboldt Bay; other projects will probably have been announced by the time these words are printed. Unfortunately, California utilities, both public and private, seem to have decided the question to their own satisfaction. There has been little public discussion of the various alternative solutions to California's growing air pollution and fuel and water problems.

If citizens' groups opposed to reactors learned many lessons in the battle of Bodega Bay, so did the utilities. Pacific Gas and Electric, still smarting after its loss at Bodega, led the way in establishing procedures for heading off controversy, and has so far been succeeding quite well. Recognizing that organized public opposition generally centers around conservation groups, P. G. & E., when it proposed to build a reactor at its site on Nipomo Dunes, a beautiful area on the coast just south of San Luis Obispo, met first with the most influential of California's conservation organizations, the Sierra Club.

Some members of the Sierra Club's Board of Directors felt strongly about preserving the natural beauty of Nipomo Dunes, and the Board assured P. G. & E. there would be opposition to a nuclear power plant there. A compromise was eventually reached, in which the Board voted not to oppose a reactor at another P. G. & E. site, Diablo Canyon, a few miles to the north, if the utility would scrap the Nopomo Dunes plan. P. G. & E. then went on to gain the acquiescence of a number of other conservation groups to the Diablo Canyon site, and simultaneously worked through a special task force to gain state acceptance through the State Resources Agency. According to P. G. & E. President Sibley, "Advance cooperation with governmental agencies, responsible conservation interests and other segments of society brings out points of difference at an early date. . . . We feel strongly that . . . this is very much a part of advance planning." [21] Sibley was quoted as referring to the granting of State and AEC approvals for the San Onofre plant without "headline problems" as attesting to the success of this approach.

The greatest success has been in gaining state and local government acquiescence. In fact P. G. & E. and the State Resources Agency, a government coordinating agency, after a joint meeting in the summer of 1964, established a joint task force to secure prior state approval of the utility's plans. This approach was soon copied by other California utilities interested in reactor development. "I'm not aware of any utility not being enthusiastic about the role of this sitting committee," stated the chairman of the task force, Harold D. Bissell.[22]

Government cooperation is only half the story, however. The government-utility task force early came to an agreement on the Malibu reactor site which is nevertheless now being hotly contested. "The public doesn't always see it our way," said Bissell.[23]

The public apparently doesn't see it their way at Diablo Canyon, either. Despite the efforts of Pacific Gas and Electric to line up conservation groups in advance, a storm is brewing over this site. Opposition is being led by the Scenic Shoreline Preservation Conference, Inc., which formed around a minority of the Sierra Club's Board of Directors who disagreed with the decision to trade Diablo Canyon for Nipomo Dunes. The group is headquartered in Santa Barbara, which is itself shortly to be the site of another large nuclear installation: California utilities may apparently expect continuing opposition.

Nor is California the only area in the country where reactors have been greeted with public opposition. On December 10, 1962, the Consolidated Edison Company of New York applied to the Atomic Energy Commission for a license to construct a 700,000 kilowatt reactor (twice the size of the proposed Bodega plant) in the heart of New York City. The reactor was to be in the Ravenswood district of Queens on the shore of the East River, just opposite Manhattan at 72nd Street. The proposal for the "Ravenswood Reactor" drew a fire of criticism, led by the Scientists' Committee for Radiation Information. In one of its reports the group stated, "Although the probability of a serious nuclear accident may be very low, it should be emphasized that major accidents in nuclear facilities differ qualitatively from those in conventional industrial facilities. A major accident in a conventional industrial facility would not contaminate a large area with long-lived, highly potent toxicants. By contrast, a nuclear reactor produces the most toxic contaminants . . . [an accident] would be a catastrophe of staggering proportions. . . .

"The foregoing considerations could be overlooked if the reactor were to be located in a remote region. They are issues of paramount importance, however, when a public utility plans to construct a reactor in a huge metropolitan district." [24]

David Lilienthal, past Chairman of the Atomic Energy Commission, commented more succinctly on this proposal to put a reactor into one of the most densely populated areas on earth. According to the *New York Times*, he called it "a very risky business." [25] An ordinance barring reactors from the city was introduced before the City Council. In the face of the growing and articulate opposition, and with the likelihood of difficulty in obtaining the requisite AEC approval, Con Ed withdrew its proposal; the reason publicly given was that power could be obtained more cheaply via long-distance transmission lines from hydroelectric stations in Labrador.

The same utility has suffered difficulties over another nuclear plant 24 miles north of New York City on the bank of the Hudson River, the Indian Point No. 2 plant, at the same site where Con Edison has been operating the far smaller Indian Point No. 1 reactor since 1962. (Although now operating reliably, this first plant was plagued by operating difficulties and unanticipated costs during its first years of operation; the Public Utilities Commission has recently been asked to consider whether Con Ed showed faulty judgment in building it.) The second plant has been opposed by local conservation groups, and suit has been filed against the Con Ed Board of Directors for allegedly gambling the utility's resources on an untried and uncertain technology.

A number of other controversies have arisen across the country. The most spectacular of all battles was the struggle over the Enrico Fermi Atomic Power Plant in Lagoona Beach, Michigan, near Detroit. The governor of Michigan, a leading senator, labor unions and citizens groups were united in opposition to the reactor; litigation eventually reached the Supreme Court, which in a divided decision sided with the reactor proponents. The plant was constructed, but never operated properly, and finally, in October 1966, suffered a near-disastrous accident which may have put it permanently out of commission.

Despite such scattered opposition, the nuclear power program has recently undergone enormous expansion. Beginning in 1965, a trickle of orders from utilities turned quickly into a flood which by the end of 1967 showed no sign of abating. In 1966, twenty-one new, large nuclear power stations were ordered; in 1967, the number of new orders had jumped to 32. Most of these plants would be in the range of 800,000 to 1,100,000 kilowatts, five times the size of the largest reactors then in operation. By the middle of 1968, more than 100 nuclear power plants were being planned, but only 12 privately owned plants were in commercial operation, all but two of them smaller than 200,000 kilowatts.

As we have seen, this flood of orders has taken even the nuclear industry by surprise, for only fairly recently it seemed that the difficulty of assuring safety and reliability in nuclear plants might make them commercial impossibilities.

IV

THE PROBLEM OF INSURANCE

ASSURING SAFETY has been an obstacle to commercial nuclear power since the early days of the program. On March 22, 1957, Harold Vance, Acting Chairman of the Atomic Energy Commission, sent a letter to Carl Durham, Chairman of the Joint Congressional Committee on Atomic Energy. Enclosed with the letter was an advance copy of a study done by the AEC which would soon be famous. The report was titled, "Theoretical Possibilities and Consequences of Major Accidents in Large Nuclear Power Plants," and was based on research done at the AEC's Brookhaven National Laboratory under the direction of Kenneth W. Downes. It was an attempt to predict the damage which would be done to the public should a major reactor accident occur. "Since the beginning of the reactor program," Vance said in his letter, "the experts and the Congress and the public and the [Atomic Energy] Commission have all been concerned with the causes and the possible magnitude of damage from reactor accidents and with means of prevention." [1]

The study, which is now generally known simply by its AEC document number, "WASH-740," focuses on what was in 1957 considered to be a "typical" reactor of the near future — one about half the size of the proposed Bodega reactor, and a sixth of the size of most plants now being planned. "The reactor is assumed to be located near a large body of water, most likely a river, about 30 miles from a major city." The Acting Chairman of the AEC summarized the report in the following way:

> For the three types of assumed accidents, the theoretical estimates indicated that personal damage might range from a lower limit of none injured or killed to an upper limit, in the worst case, of 3400 killed and about 43,000 injured.
>
> Theoretical property damages ranged from a lower limit of about one half million dollars to an upper limit in the worst case of about seven billion dollars. This latter figure is largely due to assumed contamination of land with fission products.
>
> Under adverse combinations of the conditions considered, it was estimated that people could be killed at distances up to 15 miles, and injured at distances of about 45 miles. Land contamination could extend for greater distances.
>
> In the large majority of theoretical accidents considered, the total assumed losses would not exceed a few hundred million dollars.[2]

Although this report is now more than ten years old, its conclusions are still important. In 1965 the AEC reexamined the study, in the light of the somewhat different and far larger reactors then being planned. A letter from the Chairman of the Atomic Energy Commission to the Joint Committee on Atomic Energy, dated June 18, 1965, refers to the new research, and although insisting that the likelihood of a serious accident was even lower than it had been in 1957, concludes that "the theoretically calculated damages [of such an accident] would not be less and under some circumstances would be substantially more than the consequences reported in the earlier study."[3]

The nature and details of the AEC's new study are not known, for despite persistent rumors that a whole new report updating WASH-740 had been prepared (the forthcoming report had even been publicly referred to by one of the Commissioners[4]), nothing has been released, nor did Chairman Seaborg give the basis for the remarks in his letter. The "circumstances" under which still more serious accidents might happen are therefore unknown.

The original WASH-740 attempted to define the likelihood, as well as the severity, of a disastrous accident. The following surprising statement is made: "Nuclear reactors have been operated since December 2, 1942, with a remarkable safety record." [5] a footnote amplifies this remark: "All the half-dozen 'runaway' incidents (Chalk River, Borax, EBR-1, etc.) experienced thus far, either inadvertent or planned, have occurred in research or experimental test reactors — in contrast to the steadily operating power reactors considered here."

This footnote provides the only mention in the entire 105-page report of accidents which had already occurred. It is even misleading. *All* the reactors built in this country at the time the report appeared, and which were for the purpose of generating electricity, were experimental. They are listed by the AEC in its annual summary of the reactor program under the heading "Experimental Reactor Systems." None of these, nor any other civilian reactors in the U.S. at the time, could be characterized as "steadily operating": at the time the report was published, three of the six reactors in civilian use had already been shut down.[6]

The report goes on to say: "This record of safety, although highly reassuring, does not afford a dependable statistical basis for estimating the probability of occurrence of serious reactor accidents in the future." WASH-740's authors therefore proceeded to solicit the guesses of an unnamed group of "outstanding leaders in reactor technology and associated fields" as to the likelihood of a major accident. These anonymous experts' estimates ranged "from one chance in 100,000 to one in a billion per year for each reactor." Despite this reassuring opinion, the report goes on to list some of the factors which might lead to a serious accident:

1. Many power reactor systems will operate under high pressures. High pressure systems are subject to failure.

2. The cumulative effect of radiation on physical and chemical properties of materials, after long periods of time, is largely unknown.

3. Various metals used in reactors such as uranium, aluminum, zirconium, sodium and beryllium, under certain conditions not at present clearly understood, may react explosively with water, also present in many reactors . . . Chemical reactions of enough violence to rupture the containment vessels, with release of fission products, could occur.

4. After initial operation, many of the vital components become inaccessible for inspections. In non-nuclear plants, serious accidents are often averted through detection of incipient failure.

5. Much remains to be learned about the characteristics of nuclear systems.[7]

Nothing at all is said about human error, the principal or contributing cause of all the accidents which had already occurred, and something which could be expected with certainty to continue as a permanent and major hazard. Another serious omission is a class of hazards which were, and remain, the most grave in the reactor program. These are the special hazards associated with a particular design, the liquid-metal-cooled fast reactor. This latter omission is surprising, in view of the fact that the first commercial prototype of this kind of reactor was, at the time of the report's appearance, receiving enormous amounts of publicity. This was the Enrico Fermi Atomic Power Plant near Detroit, Michigan, of which we will have more to say in a later chapter.

The report is therefore weakened by the omission of the worst classes of reactor hazards, the absence of any discussion of past accidents, and the inclusion of anonymous but optimistic guesses as to the unlikeliness of a reactor accident occurring. In this light, the drastic damage estimates produced appear still more disturbing.

WASH-740 appeared at a critical point in the reactor program. The Atomic Energy Act of 1954 had stated as one of its purposes "a program to encourage widespread participation in the development and utilization of atomic energy for peaceful purposes. . . ." The participation that was to be encouraged was that of private industry, and in fact the little-debated 1954 Atomic Energy law was prepared largely in response to widespread feeling that the Government should relax its total monopoly of the industry. Under the Eisenhower Administration, in 1953, the Joint Congressional Committee on Atomic Energy held extensive hearings on "Atomic Power Development and Private Enterprise." The Atomic Energy Commission came in for severe criticism at this time for not having pursued the peaceful applications of atomic energy more vigorously, and a general feeling emerged that the cost-cutting abilities of private industry would soon produce economic nuclear electric power. Both Republican and Democratic spokesmen testified that it was time to turn over to free enterprise at least part of the "nationalized" atomic energy industry.

Legislation permitting private enterprise in the nuclear field had been drafted during the Truman Administration, but had not got off the ground. Encouraging private industry to enter the nuclear field was entirely in accord with the objectives of the Eisenhower Administration, however, which had committed itself to keeping the government out of the power business wherever possible, and to an Atoms for Peace program. In 1953, Eisenhower appointed investment banker Lewis L. Strauss Chairman of the Atomic Energy Commission; Strauss had been a member of the first Commission and Eisenhower's personal advisor on atomic energy affairs. In his autobiography,[8] Strauss describes his own opposition to federal involvement in electric power production (a principle which was later to make him a major figure in the Dixon-Yates dispute).

Chemical and manufacturing firms were understandably eager to capitalize on the enormous investments in atomic energy they had made through military programs; in some cases these investments of manpower and resources were made quite involuntarily. General Leslie R. Groves, head of the Manhattan Engineer District, describes the persuasion that was necessary to induce the Du Pont Corporation to manage construction of the plutonium production reactors built during the Second World War, and afterwards, a massive and enormously risky project for which Du Pont received no compensation beyond expenses.[9]

Other industrial companies, on the other hand, which were not participating in the government's secret research programs in atomic power production, were afraid of being excluded from what everyone was sure would eventually be a huge and

lucrative industry. The manufacturers and prospective manufacturers of reactors were therefore eager for the freeing of
atomic energy from federal domination. The only difficulty
was in finding customers for privately manufactured reactors.
Normally conservative utility companies were very reluctant
to embark on this still uncharted sea of nuclear energy.

Admiral Strauss describes in his autobiography the early attempts he made to persuade privately owned power companies
to participate in the reactor program. His efforts met their
first success when he persuaded the Duquesne Power and
Light Company to join with the AEC in construction of the
first nuclear plant to produce commercial power. Most of the
risk was borne by the AEC, which paid for, owned, and operated the nuclear portion of the plant, at Shippingport, Pennsylvania. It went into operation in December of 1957.

This first AEC venture was followed by a dozen projects involving varying degrees of federal assistance. Privately owned
utilities received design assistance, and indirect subsidies in
fuel costs and waste disposal services. Publicly owned utilities
received direct assistance in construction funds. The most
spectacular and controversial of the attempts to build reactors
with private funds, the Enrico Fermi plant near Detroit, seemed
to be foundering in 1957 in a wave of protests and legal difficulties involving the safety of such plants.

The question of safety was, in fact, closely tied to that of
private utility participation. By 1957, Windscale, Chalk River,
and other incidents had brought home the fact that reactor
accidents could happen.

A serious reactor accident would cause extensive damage
to persons and property far from the reactor itself — damage
for which the owner of the reactor would almost certainly be

liable. The WASH-740 report gives some idea of what such damage could amount to. No public or private utility could face the prospects of such catastrophic loss. In a report accompanying the Price-Anderson Act, which will be discussed shortly, the Joint Committee on Atomic Energy stated: "It was brought to the attention of the Joint Committee in the 1956 hearings, which the Joint Committee is required to hold under section 202 of the Atomic Energy Act of 1954, that the problem of possible liability in connection with the operation of reactors is a major deterrent to further industrial participation in the program . . . the problem of liability has become a major roadblock." [10]

The Joint Committee immediately set about trying to remove the roadblock. The problem was to find insurance adequate to cover the risks of reactor operation; the first step was obviously to establish the nature of the risks. On July 6, 1956, the Joint Committee asked the AEC to establish the outside limits of such risks; the eventual response to this request was WASH-740, published almost a year later. But the Joint Committee did not wait to see the study they had requested. Hearings were begun in May of 1956, to which representatives of the atomic energy industry and insurance industry were invited; a unique piece of legislation, the Price-Anderson Act, was introduced by the Committee later in the year. Congress failed to act that year on the bill, however, and hearings continued in 1957.

The problem was simply that insurance companies politely but firmly declined to insure reactors for anything like the full amount of risk. Testifying before the Joint Committee, several insurance company executives made the point that there was simply not enough experience with reactors to make normal insurance possible; since no estimate of the likelihood of an accident could be made, the insurance companies could have no basis on which to issue a policy. The potential risk was far greater than any ever assumed before. One insurance executive put it quite strongly:

> The catastrophe hazard is apparently many times as great as anything previously known in industry and therefore poses a major challenge to insurance companies. . . . We have heard estimates of catastrophe potential under the worst possible circumstances running not merely into millions or tens of millions but into hundreds of millions and billions of dollars.

> It is a reasonable question of public policy as to whether a hazard of this magnitude should be permitted, if it actually exists. Obviously there is no principle of insurance which can be applied to a single location where the potential loss approaches such astronomical proportions. Even if insurance could be found, there is a serious question whether the amount of damage to persons and property would be worth the possible benefit accruing from atomic development.[11]

The Joint Committee had reached an impasse; in order to have private industry participate in the reactor program, utilities would have to own and operate their own reactors. This they declined to do unless adequate insurance were available. But insurance companies refused to assume the risk.

Instead of accepting the very reasonable judgment that if reactors were uninsurable they were not ready for commercial application, the Joint Committee proposed a unique solution to their problem. In order to open the atomic energy field to "private enterprise," the Federal Government would itself provide the insurance which private companies would not. This may sound like an odd sort of free enterprise — the taxpayer assuming the risk and private industry accepting the profits. Nevertheless, in 1957, Senator Clinton Anderson and Congressman Melvin Price of the Joint Committee introduced into the Senate and House what shortly became Public Law 88–703, the "Price-Anderson Act."

This curious bill has received surprisingly little attention in the press. It provides a straightforward federal subsidy to a multibillion dollar industry. It represents an intrusion of the Federal Government into the power industry and into the insurance industry which establishes a radical precedent, and it effectively passes the risks of the reactor industry on to the taxpayer. Section 170 e. of the Atomic Energy Act is amended to read:

> The aggregate liability for a single nuclear incident (reactor accident) . . . shall not exceed the sum of $500,000,000 together with the amount of financial protection required. . . .

This means that the operator of a reactor must obtain as much private insurance as he can (the "financial protection required"). The Atomic Energy Commission will then provide $500 million of protection on top of that. (Technically, the AEC "holds harmless" the reactor operator for "public liability" up to this amount.) But by law, the reactor operator and the Federal Government *are not liable* for any damages in excess of that $500 million plus private insurance. In other words, if the WASH-740's maximum of $7 billion in property damage in a single accident were realized, only one-fourteenth of the damage would be covered. This "limitation of liability" clause assures private utilities that no matter how bad an accident is, they will not suffer any financial loss.

The law does provide, however, that utilities owning reactors must buy as much insurance privately as they can. We have already seen that insurance companies were rather reluctant to provide any insurance at all. Under considerable prodding from the Joint Committee, two combines of insurance companies were formed, one including the country's mutual insurance companies, the other including stock companies. Between them they included every major insurance company in the nation, and a third organization, the Mutual Atomic Energy Reinsurance Pool, was formed to draw on the insurance capacities of Europe. These combines, which effectively drew on all the insurance resources of the Western world, together agreed to provide up to $60 million insurance for each commercial reactor.

It is clear that this is merely a token of private insurance when measured against the government-provided $500 million. Even ten years later, despite constant urging from the Joint Committee, the insurance companies have only been willing to increase their participation to $74 million.

This faint private insurance participation is therefore overshadowed by a massive federal intrusion into the reactor industry. This subsidy not only exposes the taxpayer to risks he has heard very little about, but it allows the rapid expansion and commercial use of a technology that is simply not yet ready for commercial application. The consequence is an enormous safety hazard which would have been avoided if the atomic energy industry were forced to assume responsibility for its own risks.

The Federal Government may also be providing an indirect subsidy to private utilities; this can be judged from a comparison of the insurance premiums being paid private companies and the fees being paid the AEC. According to agreements in force in 1964, the Commonwealth Edison Company of Chicago was to pay $233,000 a year to private insurance companies for $60 million of insurance. For the $500 million protection provided by the AEC, they were to pay only one-tenth of that, $21,000, in "annual indemnity fees." The Consolidated Edison Company of New York was to pay $266,500 for their $60 million private insurance, and only $17,550 for the AEC's $500 million. The Yankee Atomic Electric Company of Boston was to pay $125,000 to private companies and $18,000 to the AEC.[12] Even accepting the greater likelihood of small accidents (which would be paid for by private insurers), the imbalance is striking.

An interesting sidelight to this is provided by the widely varying premiums charged by insurance companies for different reactors. The insurance combines maintain their own staff for evaluating individual reactor hazards, and these studies are presumably the basis of the premiums. Thus Yankee Atomic's reactor is slightly larger than Consolidated Edison's — but the premium they pay is less than half of Con Ed's for the same amount of insurance. Does this mean that the insurance combines have rated the Con Ed reactor, just 25 miles from New York, as twice as hazardous as Yankee Atomic's?

The problem of private participation in the atomic energy program has not improved since 1957, it has only grown worse. The Price-Anderson Act was originally to have run for only ten years. So important is this law for continued private participation in the reactor program that on May 26, 1965, Clinton Anderson and Melvin Price introduced bills in Congress which would extend the law for an additional ten years to 1977, even though it was then still a full two years from expiring. The

Joint Committee held extensive hearings on these bills in the summer of 1965 and discovered that the situation remained exactly as it was in 1957. Insurance companies did not want to take any larger slice of the reactor liability, and utilities would not buy reactors unless protection were provided.

Mr. DeRoy Thomas, of the Hartford Insurance Group, appeared as the principal spokesman for the insurance combines. At one point he referred to the "demand or suggestion" by the Joint Committee that private insurers increase their coverage beyond the token $60 million they were providing. The Joint Committee was asking the insurers to bring their insurance up to $100 million. After canvassing the few companies which were not already part of the nuclear combine, Thomas reported to the committee that 19 new members had been found and that the combines would increase their coverage — to $74 million. The Chairman of the Joint Committee pressed Thomas on this point. He testified that all available insurance capacity had been used.

Chairman Holifield: Do you have foreign participation in this?

Mr. Thomas: We do, sir.

Holifield: Lloyd's of London?

Thomas: Yes, sir. It goes past that. I think the only capacity we have refused was a small piece tendered to us from the Odessa pool.[13]

If the insurance companies were adamant about not making any substantial increase in their coverage, the numerous private utility representatives at the hearings testified over and over that they would hesitate before buying new reactors, and might even cancel contracts they had already signed, if government indemnity under Price-Anderson were not extended. Mel Frankel, a nuclear engineer appearing on behalf of the Los Angeles Department of Water and Power, one of the biggest reactor customers in the country, testified:

> Without the protection, which presently is provided by the Price-Anderson Act, it is doubtful that any utility would consider it prudent to build nuclear plants.[14]

Mr. Frankel also testified that the Department of Water and Power had inserted a clause in its contract to build the Malibu reactor that would allow it to terminate the contract in the event that government or private insurance was not available. "We understand that this provision is standard in most similar contracts," he stated.

This testimony is not reassuring about the confidence of electric utilities in the safety of the reactors they are purchasing in such great numbers. WASH-740, with its ominous projections, is apparently carefully read by utility executives. Price-Anderson shifts the burden of concern from the utilities to the Government, however, and the reactor program continues to expand.

One hundred or so reactors are now planned or are under construction; only a dozen are now in operation. This handful of power plants has a spotty record at best; nearly all of them are only a fraction of the size of the reactors planned for the coming years. The new reactors will not only be three to six times larger than anything with which there has been past experience, but they will be far closer to population centers. This

increase in size and decrease in distance from people constitutes an enormous increase in the potential hazard from the
plants, a hazard which will continue to increase as the momentum of the reactor industry gathers.

The larger a reactor is, the more economical it is. Nuclear
reactors do not begin to compete with coal-fueled plants until
their capacity is larger than 500,000 kilowatts. In low-cost coal
areas, reactors don't compete until they produce about 1,000,-
000 kilowatts — more than half the power capacity of the
Hoover Dam. Thus, to go on selling reactors, the manufacturers
(principally GE and Westinghouse, although Babcock and Wilcox, and Combustion Engineering have recently entered the
field) must build ever larger reactors.

This increase in size brings with it a host of new problems. As
we have seen, the most serious kind of reactor accident is one
in which the fuel melts — either because the flow of cooling
water has been shut off, or because there has been a failure of
the controls which keep the chain reaction within bounds (a
"runaway"). Such a "meltdown" is dangerous because it releases the enormously poisonous fission products, or radioactive
wastes, ordinarily locked in the reactor fuel. If the heating or
runaway of the reactor is sudden enough, the result could be
an explosion, or the heating may result in further chemical ex-
plosions. A sufficiently violent explosion would break open the
reactor container, with the consequent release of the radioactive wastes into the atmosphere. It is the drifting of such a
cloud of radioactive poison which is assumed to cause the kind
of damage cited in WASH-740. In that report, the worst accident postulated was one in which only half of the fission products accumulated in the reactor fuel were released.

The present approach to forestalling such an accident is to

provide all the devices which can be thought of to prevent it: to design the reactor core itself, as far as possible, so that no "runaways" can occur; and then, in case all else fails, to surround the whole reactor with a dome, generally called a "containment sphere" in the jargon of the trade. In some designs, as at Bodega, the containment sphere is replaced by a "pressure-suppression" system which acts as a safety valve to bleed off pressure before it reaches explosive proportions. The trend toward larger reactors has made this straightforward-seeming approach even more difficult than it was when WASH-740 was issued. Clifford K. Beck spoke in February 1965 at a meeting of the American Nuclear Society; he was at the time deputy director of regulation for the Atomic Energy Commission. In talking about the new problems which were appearing in the new reactors, he said,

> Let me just mention one technical fact to point up the significance of the changes that are occurring. There is a very large difference in the implications of a major meltdown in a [1,000,000-kilowatt reactor — the size which was then being planned] as contrasted to that in a [100,000 kilowatt reactor — roughly the size which was typical at the time of WASH-740]. For the small reactor, it may make good sense to surround it with a leak-proof, concrete "thermos bottle" containment, and, in the case of accident, just walk away and let everything inside settle down and cool off. For the [1,000,000-kilowatt] reactor . . . if you walk away from that "thermos-bottle," its temperature curve, after perhaps a momentary decline, will rise continuously and will simply heat up until it bursts, so a reliable cooling system must be added.[15]

In the past it had been possible to say, "No matter what happens in the reactor, even if all the safety devices fail, there is always the containment sphere to keep radiation from drifting into populated areas." Now the whole picture has changed.

Because of the greatly enlarged size of reactors, the containment is no longer sufficient in and of itself to prevent hazard to the public. *Both* the safety devices and the containment have to function. As Beck pointed out, "the necessity of other systems working, besides just the containment vessels, becomes more urgent."

The "other systems" which must work are mostly emergency cooling systems, such as high-pressure water sprays, to keep the temperatures down after an accident has happened. Because of the ever present danger of error on the part of those operating the reactor, and because reactor behavior is still not entirely understood, the potential *causes* of an accident can never be entirely eliminated, and this is well recognized. Safety measures to counteract the effects of a serious accident which results in the melting of the reactor fuel must therefore be instituted. The point of these measures is simply to protect the public, and as reactors move more and more closely to cities, the importance of these measures increases.

In the early days of the reactor program, each application to the Atomic Energy Commission for a license to build a reactor contained a "Hazards Summary" which was essentially divided into two sections. The first described the measures the applicant, an electric utility, was to take to prevent serious accidents. This section contained a number of what were called "credible accidents," each being a description of what would happen in the case of a foreseeable mishap, such as predictable operator errors or mechanical failures. In each case the safety devices which would prevent such a mishap from turning into a major accident with release of radioactivity were described. A "maximum credible accident" was then described — the worst accident believed possible should all safety devices function as expected. In all cases the "maximum" accident was described as being quite minor — resulting in little or no melting of the reactor fuel, and little or no release of radioactivity to the outside air.

Recognizing, however, that neither human error nor mechanical failures were entirely predictable, and recognizing also that reactor behavior was not entirely understood, particularly under accident conditions, a second section of the hazards summary was devoted to "hypothetical accidents." In this section the applicant would describe his estimate of what the effects would be if, despite all foresight and planning, a serious accident within the reactor were to occur.

Such a hypothetical accident would be typically either a runaway caused by operator and mechanical error combined, or a "loss of coolant" accident, in which the cooling water would be lost or driven out of the reactor core. In such an accident, temperatures in the heart of the reactor would be expected to rise into the thousands of degrees within seconds, the uranium and steel of the fuel core would melt, and the melted metals would react chemically with the water still present.

Having made his estimate of the worst conceivable accident, the reactor builder would then go on to describe the measures he proposed to prevent its effects from reaching the public. Generally, this took the form of Beck's "thermos-bottle" — some sort of containment structure designed to withstand explosive pressure of a major accident. The Enrico Fermi Plant at Lagoona Beach, Michigan, was provided with a containment structure designed to withstand the explosive force of a thousand pounds of TNT. No matter what damage was done to the reactor, it was assumed that this containment would prevent any radioactivity from reaching the public.

Even in the days of small reactors, the "thermos-bottle" approach had many weaknesses. We have already seen that natural hazards, like earthquakes and landslides, often make nonsense of the containment idea, as the same agency which causes the accident is also likely to render useless the containment structures. In some reactor designs, like the popular boiling water reactor, numerous large pipes must pass in and out of the reactor through the containment structures. In addition, all reactor designs require a number of "penetrations" of the containment, including access ports for personnel, which make explosion-proof containment a more difficult task than it seems. Yet this approach had at least theoretical simplicity, and was little subject to mechanical or human failure.

The situation today is considerably more complicated. With modern large reactors, no feasible containment structure would serve unassisted, and a host of new devices are introduced. Applications for construction permits still have the same general form, although the "hazards analysis" has now been transmuted into a "safety analysis." The two general types of accidents are still described, but discussions of the "hypothetical" accident — a loss of coolant followed by melting of the reactor fuel — are considerably more elaborate.

One recent application, for instance, describes the worst accident case, in which all safety devices fail. The applicants do not consider this to be a credible occurrence. The only comment is a laconic: "The curve shows that the system pressure rises monotonically since there is no energy rejected from the system." [16] What this means in plain English is that the pressure goes on rising indefinitely until it bursts the containment structures and releases the radioactivity of the melted fuel to the outside air.

A number of elaborate devices are described which are intended to prevent such an event. There are two spray systems for cooling the reactor fuel, and two spray systems for cooling the containment itself. These are provided with an elaborate series of interlocking valves and sensing devices, so that a malfunction in them will not itself produce an accident. In the boiling water reactors, isolation valves and other devices are needed to prevent the accident pressures from blowing out the steam lines which run directly from the reactor core out of the containment and several hundred feet to a neighboring building where the turbines are housed.

An additional complication is provided by the fact that after the fuel melts, it reacts violently with whatever water is still present in the reactor vessel. The added heat and pressure from this reaction puts more strain on the containment. The reaction of uranium or zirconium (a common fuel-container material) with water releases hydrogen. If there is air present in the system, this hydrogen can explode. Much of the damage in the Chalk River accident was caused by such a hydrogen explosion, which lifted a 4-ton structure several feet in the air. In its application for a reactor to be built at Rock Island, Illinois, on the Mississippi, the Commonwealth Edison Company notes, ". . . the capability of the containment to withstand the burning hydrogen resulting from a metal-water reaction is limited. . . ." [17]

This is again a mild way of saying that a hydrogen explosion would burst the containment and release clouds of poisonous radioactivity. In order to prevent this from happening, elaborate precautions must be taken to keep any air from entering the primary containment system.

All of these safety devices must have their own safety devices to keep *them* from failing, and the whole complex of devices must be maintained in a state of readiness, so additional devices for *testing* the safety devices must be provided. All these devices, of course, work on electric power, which would not be available from the nuclear plant itself in the case of an accident, so power must be provided from outside, and in the case of outside power failure with supplementary emergency power. This latter is important, for because of the dependence of so many of the safety devices on outside power, a power failure might itself be the cause of an accident or associated with one. But emergency power, generally provided by a diesel-fueled generator, must be available within seconds because of the speed with which accidents occur in reactors, and therefore new problems are introduced in the effort to provide such a rapid changeover.

Each of these proliferating safety devices seems to introduce new problems of its own. For instance, the AEC's Advisory Committee on Reactor Safeguards recently pointed out that the shock of emergency cooling water in an accident might crack the heavy steel of the reactor vessel and create the very breach it was to prevent.[18]

As the hazards grow, the search for preventive measures tends to produce more and more exotic techniques. The Atomic Electric Power Company announced in July of 1967 their plans to build the two largest reactors yet — 1,100,000 kilowatts each — on the western shore of Lake Michigan. For these behemoths, Westinghouse proposes to enclose the entire containment system in a refrigerated ice pack; in case of accident, insulating panels would lift and the ice would cool off the reactor before it exploded.

These elaborate and exotic safety measures are attached to

reactors which are themselves untried and in many ways badly understood. The new huge reactors expose their fuels and structural materials to high temperatures and high intensities of radiation for longer periods of time than any power plants with which we have experience. Novel effects are constantly appearing. As the reactor program progressed, for instance, it was discovered that exposure to neutron radiation in a reactor core slowly makes steel brittle. More recently it has been discovered that this effect occurs in all metals, and is due at least in part to the formation of microscopic helium bubbles within the metal. No solution for this problem has yet been found, although several proposals have been made.

Another source of damage to steel is "hydrogen embrittlement"; radiation also has more direct, long-term effects on the strength and brittleness of steel, with at least the possibility that the reactor vessel itself could fail under the pressures generated by a loss of coolant or other severe accident. All of these potential accident hazards are failures which appear only after months or years of reactor operation. The new effects which will appear after a number of large reactors have been operating for years cannot even be guessed at.

All of these problems are aggravated by the high temperatures and pressures at which coming reactors will operate. The two reactors ordered by TVA for operation at Brown's Ferry, Alabama, 1,000,000-kilowatt plants produced by General Electric, will operate at a fuel temperature of 4200°F. This is close to the melting point of the uranium oxide fuel (about 5000°F); if the reactor exceeds its normal maximum power output by as little as 20 percent, the fuel will melt.

Stepping so close to the limits of safety has brought forth expressions of concern from many quarters. In a letter to the

Chairman of the Atomic Energy Commission, the Advisory Committee on Reactor Safeguards, although provisionally approving the application for the two Brown's Ferry plants, expressed a long list of reservations. It noted that in an accident, even if all emergency systems functioned adequately, "the calculated number of fuel elements reaching undesirably high temperatures is greater" than in smaller reactors. "Also, the time margin available for actuation of [emergency] systems is less."

"In a loss-of-coolant accident," the Committee notes, "the core spray systems are required to function effectively under circumstances in which some areas of fuel clad may have attained temperatures considerably higher than the maximum at which such sprays have been tested experimentally to date."

Operation with a fuel assembly slightly out of line could also cause local melting and perhaps worse accidents, the Committee noted. "The diesel-generator sets for emergency power appear to be fully loaded with little or no margin. . . . They are required to start, synchronize and carry load within less than thirty seconds. . . .

"The Committee wishes to emphasize the importance of quality assurance in fabrication . . . and of inspection. . . . Because of the higher power level and advanced thermal conditions in the Brown's Ferry Units, these matters assume even greater importance. . . . because the Brown's Ferry Units are to operate at substantially higher power level and power density than those on which . . . experience will be obtained, an especially extensive and careful start-up program will be required." [19]

Despite its multitude of reservations, the Committee recommended approval of the application, in part because of the "favorable characteristics of the proposed site," apparently a reference to the small number of people in the area. But in a completely unprecedented move, one member of the Committee declined to go along with the recommendation:

"It is my belief that the substantial increase in power and power density of the Brown's Ferry reactors over boiling water reactors previously approved should be accompanied by increased safeguard margins for the unexpected." The lone dissenter, Dr. Stephen Hanauer, went on to repeat some of the things which had disturbed the full Committee, adding, "The dependence on immediate availability of a large amount of emergency electrical power, using diesel generators operating fully loaded in a previously untried starting mode, is of special concern, as are the high temperatures and numerous fuel-element failures predicted even for successful operation of the emergency core cooling system in a large loss-of-coolant accident." [20]

These concerns about the reliability or effectiveness of emergency systems are particularly disturbing since publication of a report from the AEC's Advisory Task Force on Power Reactor Emergency Cooling. This report, which is undated but appeared late in 1967, considered the events which might follow the accidental interruption of normal cooling in "large, light-water power reactors as currently designed and located." As we have seen, any interruption in the flow of cooling water to an operating reactor would be quickly followed by melting of the fuel; elaborate devices have been planned to see that this is not followed in turn by a release of radioactivity from the molten fuel to the outside air. Containment vessels and emergency cooling devices serve this function.

What the Task Force report does is to state finally and clearly what had for some time been widely understood — that should fuel melting occur in a large reactor, there is no assurance that any device could prevent the release of massive amounts of radioactivity to the outside air. Unless emergency measures in the first seconds following an interruption of coolant flow manage to *prevent* melting, the result would be catastrophic.

> It was concluded that the description of the events that could take place subsequent to a postulated meltdown of large portions of a [fuel] core is at present indeterminate and quite speculative. . . . Reliable and practical methods of containing the large molten masses of fuel that would probably result from such a meltdown do not exist today. . . . Accordingly, it is not considered possible to assure the integrity of the containment if meltdown of large portions of the core were to occur.[21]

The report concludes that emergency cooling methods must be available to prevent melting. Should the accident which leads to loss of ordinary coolant flow also cause some disruption of the reactor fuel core arrangement, emergency cooling systems might not work. Should the accident in some other way disrupt the effectiveness of the emergency cooling system, the fuel would melt, and once melted, would simply dissolve any material in its way. Containment would be impossible. (This has long been known in the reactor industry as the "China problem": once collected in one place, molten fuel would simply dissolve its way "clear down to China.") The AEC must have had a pretty good idea of what the conclusions of the report would be, for, late in 1966, it began putting pressure on the owners of already operating reactors to add emergency "core cooling" systems to the plants, a procedure which in some cases may run into millions of dollars.

It is probably the conclusions of this report, long known in advance or arrived at independently by others, which cause the trepidation over uncertain, over-elaborate and possibly unreliable emergency devices expressed by Dr. Hanauer and others.

Despite such scattered warnings of coming trouble, the Price-Anderson Act shifts the burden of concern to the AEC, and utilities are pressing forward. In June 1967 a news report stated, "For the 1976 nuclear plant that it wants, Con Ed is studying the possibility of an underground installation in New York City." [22] On June 20, the Administrative Vice President of Consolidated Edison, W. Donham Crawford, announced the opening of a public-relations campaign to gain public acceptance of this project. Speaking to the Health Physics Society at its meeting in Washington, D.C., Crawford said,

> With a construction permit issued by 1972, an operating nuclear plant at an in-city site should be feasible by 1976.
>
> . . . Movies, slide presentations, pamphlets and even comic books have been utilized to convey the message that the atom is here to stay. . . . The utility companies can be expected to step up their efforts to inform the public of the need to locate nuclear stations within cities. Indeed, the remarks which I am now making may be construed as part of such an effort. [23]

Although the Atomic Energy Commission has repeatedly stated that they are not yet quite ready to approve plans like Con Ed's for reactors in the heart of a major city, nevertheless nuclear plants are being planned for heavily populated areas. The New Jersey Public Service Gas and Light Company proposed a plant, the size of the Brown's Ferry reactors, to be built in Burlington, New Jersey, less than five miles from the outskirts of Philadelphia. More than five million people would have lived within 25 miles of the plant. Almost the entire city of Burlington was within one and a half miles of the proposed plant site. The application has been withdrawn, although apparently only temporarily, in the face of probable AEC refusal.

Consolidated Edison has already announced plans for a third huge nuclear plant at its Indian Point site just 25 miles north of New York City; the two giant nuclear power and desalting plants proposed for Bolsa Island are less than a mile from densely populated Orange County and 24 miles from the center of Los Angeles. Yet, in April of 1967, a representative of the AEC's Advisory Committee on Reactor Safeguards testified before the Joint Committee on Atomic Energy that "the ACRS believes that placing large nuclear reactors close to population centers will require considerabe further improvements in safety, and that none of the large power reactors now under construction are considered suitable for location in metropolitan areas." [24]

In commenting on the AEC's position, the Washington editor of the trade journal *Nucleonics* notes that rural sites, even though there may be people living quite close to the reactor, are preferable to city sites. "Rural sites have three big things going: the ability of the atmosphere to disperse any accidental release is a 'God-given engineered safeguard,' a few people could be evacuated easier than a city's inhabitants, and the fewer people living in the area means there are fewer people to intervene in public hearings." [25]

This cynical portrayal of present reactor-siting policies may not comfort rural neighbors of nuclear plants. A news story in another trade publication on June 15, 1967, was headlined "How Connecticut Yankee Met a Public Acceptance Crisis"; it described efforts of the Connecticut Yankee Light and Power Company to circumvent public opposition to its reactor, which has now gone into operation near the small town of Haddam

Neck.[26] Several local residents, and the First Selectman of the town's Board, Charles J. Wolf, had written to the AEC asking for a public hearing on Connecticut Yankee's request for an operating license. According to the report, "Connecticut Yankee sent an executive to talk with Wolf, who subsequently withdrew his application for a hearing. . . ." The story also quotes the editor of a nearby newspaper: "Not everyone is happy with the idea of the plant being there, but they're pretty well resigned to it."

As the reactor program gathers momentum, and as the investment in it by utilities both public and private, by manufacturers, suppliers, and mining companies grows into the billions, it becomes more and more difficult to consider calmly the wisdom of the way in which the program is being pursued. WASH-740's ominous warning of thousands killed and billions of dollars in property damage is submerged under mountains of comic books featuring Citizen Atom and Reddy Kilowatt. Public relations is substituted for debate.

The difficulty, of course, is that the federal agencies responsible for assuring safety in the reactor program are themselves the architects of that program, and in no position to give it an objective evaluation. Yet before the program proceeds any further such an evaluation must be made, if only because serious accidents are not the only, and perhaps not even the worst, risk which an expanded program will carry.

V

RADIATION DAMAGE

DURING THE SECOND WORLD WAR, a large area in the Tennessee mountains was acquired by the Manhattan Engineer District (the atom bomb project). This site, which became known as Oak Ridge, was chosen for its remoteness, as it was to house much of the experimentation of the project, and eventually a substantial portion of the facilities for production of bomb material. One of the world's first reactors was housed at Oak Ridge; the first plants for separation of bomb-grade uranium were established there.

From its earliest days Oak Ridge was posed with the difficulties of disposing of radioactive wastes. Operations of the reactor and uranium plants, and the wide range of experimentation carried on, all produced a bewildering variety of waste products, from contaminated clothing to the enormously radioactive reactor fuel wastes. Disposal of these wastes was an entirely new problem; the characteristics of many of the wastes were unknown, their danger to man was unknown, and their behavior, once released into the atmosphere or water supply, was unpredictable.

For the most dilute and presumably least dangerous wastes, simple discharge into air or water seemed reasonable, but caution was generally taken even then. Even when it seemed that the quantity of radiation being released was far too small to do any damage, careful watch was kept.

White Oak Creek, which flowed through the Oak Ridge area, was one logical place to dump the least harmful of the radioactive garbage produced. Liquid wastes would be diluted by the waters of the stream, which emptied into the Clinch River, which would further dilute them before reaching populated areas. In order to gain better control of the dilution process, however, White Oak Creek was dammed, to form a pond or lake of about 55 acres. Wastes were dumped into the lake, where they would be retained for about 30 days before trickling out into the creek. At its deepest point, behind the dam, White Oak Lake was 11 feet deep.

The lake quickly blended into its natural surroundings. Aquatic plants took root; migratory waterfowl began appearing, and fed on the good-sized fish which bred in the lake's quiet water. No one could have guessed from looking at it that the lake and all its living things were contaminated by man-made radioactivity.

Every chemical element of which the earth and its inhabitants are made now has at least one radioactive "twin" or isotope created by man. Natural elements are fixed and stable: the iron, copper, oxygen, carbon, hydrogen, helium, the more familiar elements — as well as the rare and unfamiliar ones, krypton, xenon, lanthanum, tellurium — of which all things are built do not change. The familiar stability of our world lies in the enormous stability of these elements.

The only exceptions to this rule are the few and rare naturally-occurring radioactive elements. The first of these to be discovered was radium; other radioactive elements, including uranium and radioactive potassium, have been identified. For unknown reasons, these elements were subject to a slow disintegration. A sort of fever of decay seemed to afflict these elements, which released heat and other radiations while slowly changing into other, lighter elements. It gradually became understood that the atoms of these elements were expelling part of their own substance in the form of particles and rays. This discharge would go on until each atom had unburdened itself and become a stable element; in the case of uranium, particles would be emitted until the atom had become stable lead.

A way of measuring this process was contrived, and gave us the term "half-life." This is a measurement of the rate at which a radioactive element is decaying. In a block of uranium, each atom is stable for a very long time. After perhaps millions of years of stable existence, it will emit a particle (an "alpha" particle, identical to the nucleus of a helium atom), lightening itself and achieving a new level of stability. Further emissions follow over long periods of time, until the atom finally achieves a completely stable weight in the form of lead.

At any given moment in time, there will be a few of the enormous numbers of atoms in the uranium block which are undergoing decay. The number of atoms emitting particles at any time determines how quickly the material will be completely changed into a block of another element. The term "half-life" describes this rate: a half-life is the period of time in which one-half of the atoms of any quantity of an element will decay into another element.

Uranium has a half-life of 4.5 billion years. This means that at any one time only a very few uranium atoms are undergoing decay, and that it takes four and a half billion years for half the atoms of a block of uranium to decay. In the uranium remaining at the end of this time, atoms are still decaying at the same rate, so it will be another 4.5 billion years before half of the remaining uranium decays; after nine billion years only a quarter of the original block will remain, and after an additional 4.5 billion years half of *that* uranium will have decayed, and so on.

These, of course, are enormously long periods of time. The half-life of uranium is roughly equal to the estimated age of the earth, which means that half of the uranium present at the earth's formation is still with us. The earth will probably not exist long enough for the greater portion of the uranium still present to disappear.

Since the "radioactivity" of radioactive elements is produced by decaying atoms, a slow rate of decay means little radioactivity. Elements which are changing more quickly, such as radium, which also occurs naturally, produce more radiation and consequently can do more harm. Yet because it decays so much more quickly, radium is a very scarce element indeed. As a result, the radiation to which mankind and other living things have been exposed from radioactive minerals in the earth's crust has been extremely mild.

Yet naturally stable elements can be made radioactive, and this process occurs to a slight extent in nature. Cosmic rays, high energy atomic particles which come from the sun or from distant space beyond our solar system, are continually crashing into the earth's atmosphere at tremendous speeds. When these particles strike the stable atoms of oxygen, nitrogen or rare gases in the atmosphere, their stability is destroyed, and either directly or indirectly, radioactive isotopes or twins of common elements are formed. Thus cosmic rays are constantly creating radioactive carbon (carbon 14) which is a chemical twin for natural carbon (carbon 12). But radioactive carbon is unstable, and decays, with the emission of radiation. The half-life of carbon 14 is more than 5,000 years; still a long time, but very much shorter than the billions of years in which the half-life of uranium is measured.

Man has discovered many means of duplicating the feat of cosmic rays, and in a variety of devices, including accelerators, reactors and atomic bombs, has succeeded in creating at least one radioactive twin for every natural element. Some of these are so unstable that they vanish in a fraction of a second; others are stable enough to remain with us for thousands or millions of years. By far the greatest volume of these radioactive elements are made in reactors; they are the fragments of the split uranium atom or the unstable forms produced by the intense radiation of the uranium chain reaction. A single 1,000,-000-kilowatt reactor installation, after a year of operation, contains more radioactive strontium, cesium and iodine than was released in all the nuclear weapons tests conducted in the world until the present.[1]

The result of this ingenuity in disrupting the stability of atoms is that all living things, including man, are now exposed to a new source of radiation, potentially many times greater than the background of radiation from earth and sky to which life has gradually accustomed itself over the billions of years of its evolution. Each of us now carries some radioactive strontium in our bones, and some radioactive cesium in our muscles, and some radioactive carbon through all our body tissues, as a result of nuclear weapons testing. As we shall see, the significance of this fact is still obscure. How much damage will this radioactivity do? When bombs were first tested, we simply did not know. Although we are learning more about the problem, we still do not know the full answer.

It is true that all living things have adapted themselves to natural radiation — the cosmic rays from outer space, the radiation from rocks, and the radioactive materials which, in small quantities, are absorbed from the normal food we eat and use in the body. Evolution itself has probably been profoundly influenced by the mutations produced by such radiations. But what can happen to a species through eons of time is something different from rashly increasing artificial radiation in the course of a few years, with our imperfect knowledge of the harm that may be done.[2]

These words were written by Ritchie Calder in 1962, in *Living with the Atom,* a far from pessimistic examination of the peaceful uses of atomic energy. He was expressing a difficulty recognized by both proponents and critics of nuclear programs, a difficulty which stems from the large lead which our understanding of physics has over the science of biology. Although we have developed great ingenuity in creating radiation, we know very little about the way in which radiation affects living things; we know less about the ways in which radioactive or other pollutants affect the complex community of living things on which people depend.

White Oak Lake is, or was, a good illustration of what we do and don't know about the biological effects of radiation. Radioactive wastes discharged into the lake followed a very complex career. Radioactive cesium, for instance, is chemically identical to stable cesium, a rare element which is quite similar to potassium. Living things make little distinction between potassium, which is quite common, and cesium; potassium is particularly important to higher animals in nerve and muscle function. It is a vital constituent of every living cell.

The radioactive forms of cesium are formed in the splitting of uranium atoms. Since cesium is almost exactly half the weight of uranium, it is a common product of fission, and hence one of the principal forms of reactor waste. The half-life of the most common form of radiocesium, cesium 137, is a little more than 30 years.

If a tiny quantity of cesium is released into White Oak Lake, it does not simply disappear. It remains dissolved in the water of the lake for a time. In this form it may be absorbed by one of the microscopic plants which exist in the billions in the lake water; one of these algae, mistaking the cesium 137 for potassium, may incorporate it into its tissues. But in doing so the cesium is concentrated. That is, the tiny plants filter a large volume of water to find the potassium they need, extracting and concentrating it in their tissues. If cesium as well as potassium is present, it too is concentrated by the algae.

Tiny plants in the lake form the food of slightly larger animals, the zooplankton; these in turn are eaten by crustaceans, which are eaten by small fish, which are eaten by larger fish. At each link in this "food chain," the cesium 137 is passed on. The algae have concentrated the originally dilute cesium; by eating a large number of algae, the zooplankton further concentrate it; tiny crustaceans eat large numbers of their smaller victims; fish eat many crustaceans. At each step, cesium is not merely passed on, it is concentrated.

This ability of living things to extract and concentrate extremely dilute substances is quite remarkable. In Par Pond, a small lake very much like White Oak Lake and used for the same purposes at another atomic energy installation, this phenomenon was studied. During several months in 1962, the concentration of radioactive cesium in the water was only 0.033 picocuries per gram (a picocurie is a very small quantity of radioactivity, equivalent to a millionth of a millionth of a gram of radium). But the flesh of bass caught in the pond contained, on the average, 35 picocuries — a thousandfold increase.[3]

For other radioactive substances, the concentration factor was even higher. The *average* concentration of radioactive zinc in the bones of bluegill was 8720 times that of the water in which they swam. The concentration of radioactive strontium had increased more than 2000 times in the bones of these same fish.[4]

A great deal has been learned about the way in which radioactive materials are concentrated by different animals, much of it through investigation of the problem of fallout from weapons testing. The testing of nuclear weapons, in fact, was probably the most massive (and unintentional) experiment in biology ever undertaken, and the results are just beginning to come in. It will be many years before we fully understand the effects of fallout; certainly they were not even guessed at when testing began. In *Living with the Atom,* Ritchie Calder quotes a statement attributed to Clement Attlee, British Prime Minister at the time the first atom bomb was dropped in Japan:

Of course, at the time we knew nothing, I certainly knew absolutely nothing, about the consequences of dropping the bomb except that it was larger than an ordinary bomb. . . . We knew nothing whatever at that time about the genetic effects of an atomic explosion. I knew nothing about fallout and all the rest of what emerged after Hiroshima. As far as I know, President Truman and Winston Churchill knew nothing of these things either, nor did Sir John Anderson, who co-ordinated research for our side. Whether the scientists directly concerned knew, or guessed, I do not know. But if they did, then as far as I am aware, they said nothing of it to those who had to make the decision.[5]

Calder comments that "it is debatable whether those scientists who were party to the decision did, in fact, know about the biological risks." In *Science and Survival,* the eminent biologist Barry Commoner points out that this ignorance persisted through the early years of bomb testing, and that in fact our knowledge of the biological effects of fallout has still not caught up with our skill in nuclear physics.

Commoner points out that in 1953, "the AEC stated that the only possible hazard to humans from strontium-90 [from fallout] would arise from 'the ingestion of bone splinters which might be intermingled with muscle tissue during butchering and cutting of the meat.' No mention was made of the simple biological fact that the milk from such an animal would also contain strontium-90. By 1956 the AEC had acknowledged that milk represented the most important source of strontium-90 in human food." [6]

Little by little, more was learned about the ways in which plants and animals concentrate chemicals in their tissues. Strontium, which resembles calcium, was concentrated in bones and milk; radioactive iodine would be concentrated by cows grazing over large areas in which fallout had settled. The iodine 131 in their milk would be further and drastically concentrated in the thyroid gland of anyone drinking the milk. Children, with their large milk consumption, were particularly vulnerable; a group of children in a particularly heavy fallout area of Utah is presently being studied by the Public Health Service, and a number of thyroid abnormalities which may be due to fallout have been discovered.

Some years ago, it was discovered that Eskimos were absorbing far more fallout radioactivity than people living in temperate zones, even though the distribution of fallout was believed to be just the reverse, with more falling in the temperate zones than at either the poles or the equator. The answer to this puzzle lay in the enormous concentrating ability of the Arctic food chain. The first link in this chain is the tough, scrubby lichen, which has the unusual characteristic of deriving its mineral nourishment from the air instead of from the soil. Ordinarily, dust and soil particles settling on the lichen provided it with needed minerals; when radioactive fallout joined the dust and soil, the lichen absorbed it too. These plants were and are extremely efficient collectors of fallout. They are also one of the principal foods of the caribou, which graze on them particularly in the winter, when other vegetation is scarce. Caribou may graze over large areas, thus effectively collecting and concentrating all the fallout which has descended in those areas. But the caribou in turn are an important — and in some areas and seasons almost the exclusive — food of Eskimos. Thus it was that the residents of Anaktavuk Pass and elsewhere received and go on receiving, as fallout continues to drift down from the stratosphere, radiation exposures which are close to, and in some cases may exceed what are considered maximum permissible exposures (we shall have more to say about radiation standards such as these later).[7]

Radioactive wastes from reactors contain the same substances that are found in fallout, which is not surprising, since both derive from the same source — atomic fission. (The fallout from hydrogen [fusion] bombs is also principally from their uranium or plutonium "trigger.") When released into the environment, they follow paths as complex and unpredictable as those of fallout components.

At White Oak Lake, the food chain did not end with fish. Birds fed on the fish, and on one occasion it was found that enormously dilute radioactive phosphorus had followed the long trail from water to algae to fish to bird; radiophosphorus was appearing in high concentration (compared to the level in the lake water) in the flight muscles of waterfowl.

The reactors for plutonium production at Hanford, near the town of Richland, Washington, empty their cooling water into the Columbia River. The discharge contains some of the fission products from the reactor fuel, as well as normal impurities which have been rendered radioactive, although this highly radioactive waste material is in small quantities and highly diluted. But in the Columbia River, as everywhere that there are living things, chemicals either stable or radioactive are picked up from the water and concentrated. Radioactivity of the Columbia River plankton — microscopic plants and animals — averages two thousand times the radioactivity of the water. Caddis fly larvae achieve concentrations 350,000 times that of the water. One survey of bird life on the river showed that the birds which feed on river insects have a high concentration of radioactivity, which is mainly radiophosphorus; first the insect and then the birds have selectively concentrated this isotope, even though it is only a tiny fraction of the total radioactivity in the water. Duck-egg yolks have 40,000 times the radioactivity of the river water; adult swallows have a concentration factor of 75,000.

At White Oak Lake, many of the birds were migratory. It is not known when it was first suggested that these birds might be carrying some radioactivity off with them when they continued their migrations. Probably this had not yet occurred to anyone when the Tennessee Valley Authority was asked to do an ecological survey of the area (the eight years which elapsed between the establishment of Oak Ridge and the making of this survey gives some idea of the nearly total ignorance of biological effects under which the early years of the atomic energy program were conducted).

The TVA scientists discovered that the thousands of water-fowl which migrated through White Oak Lake each year were picking up substantial quantities of radioactivity. The largest element in this contamination was again radiophosphorus; this isotope has a relatively short half-life of 14 days, and by the time the ducks left the lake again, was probably no more serious a problem than the longer-lived isotopes. Some of these latter, of course, would be around for a very long time. The scientists initiated a program of banding the ducks in the hope of getting back reports from hunters who shot them.

The reports, once they began coming in, showed that the radioactive ducks were being killed anywhere from the provinces of Canada to the counties of Texas. According to one report, this "winged radioactivity worried the health authorities quite a lot." [8]

What was happening in White Oak Lake was that the highly dilute wastes dumped into the water were being reconcentrated and then neatly packaged and dispatched all over the continent. When we remember that some migratory birds which stop in the United States are on their way from the Arctic to the Antarctic, the potential scope of this distribution is truly impressive.

Nor are birds the only agents by which radiation may be carried in unexpected directions. An article in the AEC's publication *Nuclear Safety* comments,

From the beginning of the atomic industry, the use of basins or other restricted aquatic environments for the disposal of radioactive wastes has prompted concern with regard to the possible avenues of escape of these materials. . . . Singularly lacking in most of this effort is research on the role of biological agents in the dispersal of radioactive contamination.[9]

The same article quotes a Russian study of possible spread of contamination from basins holding radioactive waste by aquatic insects that emerge and fly away from the basin. The authors estimate that from a typical small basin in mid-Russia, 200 million insects emerge each year (apparently caddis flies, mayflies and midges). Of these, 180 million would be eaten by predators — other insects and birds, which would presumably carry the contamination still further. The remaining 20 million insects would die and presumably be deposited in an area of radius 1.5 kilometers from the basin. The authors estimate that in this area the insect "fallout" would deposit as much radioactivity as the fallout from two hydrogen bomb tests (this refers to "stratospheric fallout" apparently, from far distant tests). The authors were pleased with these results, which indicated to them that insects could effect "a comparatively rapid and complete bioecological self-purification" of the waste basin.

Apparently no study of insect dispersal was done at White Oak Lake, nor is there any easy way of applying the Russians' figures. According to the article just quoted, "An almost complete lack of information on the numbers of individuals and population dynamics of aquatic insects makes it difficult to assess the applicability of these assumptions to other areas." But apparently the experience with the banded ducks was sufficient, for shortly after the results were in, White Oak Lake was drained.

There is literally no way of knowing what has happened to most of the radioactive chemicals which were dumped into White Oak Lake before it was drained. A given atom of radioactive cesium 137 may have passed from water to plankton to fish to bird, been transported thousands of miles; the bird may have been shot and eaten. This would not be the end of the cesium 137's career. After being retained in the muscle tissue of the man who had eaten the duck, perhaps for days or weeks, the cesium 137 atom would be excreted, picked up once again by plankton in a river, and perhaps pass again through fish, bird and man. Endless other paths might be followed. From White Oak Lake it might have been carried by an insect for a mile, and then with the death of the insect become part of the soil organic material which would cycle through plants and back to the soil for years or decades, until perhaps being ingested by another insect as part of a plant leaf and carried elsewhere, picked up by a bird and finally appearing in the human food supply a generation after its creation. Much of the lake water radioactivity may have passed to the sea before entering the biological community.

The half-life of cesium is about thirty years; even after ten half-lives, or three centuries, a fraction of any given amount of cesium will still remain. The half-life of strontium 90 is almost as long. The half-life of man-made plutonium is 24,000 years. The half-life of iodine 129, produced in small quantities in reactors, is 17,250,000 years.

All this means that every time radioactive waste is dumped into a stream, buried, dropped into the ocean, discharged into the air, or otherwise released from human control, it passes into the complex world of living things. It will pass from living thing to living thing, sometimes becoming concentrated, at other times being dispersed, with an efficiency and ingenuity which man has not yet come to understand. At unpredictable times and places, this radioactive waste will reappear in man's food, air or water. It will not go away, for decades or centuries or even millennia.

There is nothing new in this phenomenon. Nearly every

living animal on the surface of the globe, from deep-sea fish to Arctic birds, carries some DDT in its fatty tissues; the number of pesticides which are achieving such universality grows every year. Lead from gasoline additives can be found in the snows of the High Sierra. Nearly every child born on earth in the last ten years has carried some radioactive strontium in his bones. The amount of radioactive carbon in the atmosphere has been doubled, and all of us bear some of this burden in our tissues.

We are slowly coming to a realization that the thin film of life which covers the earth is a single complex web, and a chord plucked anywhere sends its vibrations worldwide. And man is a part of this web; he depends on it totally for his food, air and water.

What are the effects of radiation on man? Our ignorance of this subject is even greater than that of the means by which radiation returns to man's hand after being released into the environment.

Effects of radiation are divided into two classes by most scientists — somatic effects and genetic effects. The first refers to the effects of radiation on an exposed person's body (soma); the other refers to the effects on his progeny. Both kinds of effects are believed to be due to the same causes — the disruption by radiation of a cell's basic self-regulatory machinery. Whether this disruption eventually results in disease or in inherited malformation seems to depend simply on which of the body's cells is affected. Radiation lodged in a child's thyroid gland may produce cancer; radiation directed at the adult's gonads may, through a similar effect on germ tissue, produce mutation and malformation in later generations.

As we have seen, radioactive substances are chemically

identical to the familiar elements, except that they have been rendered unstable. In the process of changing, or decaying, from one form to another, they emit radiation. This radiation can be in the form of tiny particles, actually fragments of the atom, or as penetrating rays similar to X-rays. This radiation may pass through seemingly solid substances. Some particles, such as the heavy and slow-moving alpha rays, can penetrate only a thin sheet of paper; lighter beta rays may pass through several inches of wood or flesh; some penetrating gamma rays may pass through several feet of concrete.

When one of these particles or rays goes crashing through some material, it collides violently with atoms or molecules along the way. Such collisions are violent enough to tear away some of the electrons which form a cloud around every atom. Stripped of some of its electrons, the atom becomes a positively charged particle, or ion. Such a particle quickly undergoes violent chemical reactions with surrounding molecules as it returns to a neutral state.

Radioactive substances in food are incorporated into tissue just as their stable twins would be; imbedded deep within a cell, the radioactive atom may emit a particle which then streaks away, leaving a track of ions in its path. These ions then undergo sudden and violent chemical combination with surrounding molecules. In the delicately balanced economy of the cell, this sudden disruption can be disastrous. The individual cell may die; it may recover. But if it does recover, its self-regulatory powers may be affected in some way we do not yet understand. After the passage of weeks, months or years, it may begin to proliferate wildly in the uncontrolled growth we call cancer.

It hardly needs to be pointed out that we do not know exactly how cancers are caused; we do not know exactly what changes induced by ionizing radiation cause the cell to become cancerous. This is simply part of our greater ignorance of basic life processes, for although newspaper headlines have given the contrary impression in recent years, biologists are not at all in agreement about what makes living things tick.

For a time, following important discoveries made in the 1950's, it was believed that a single chemical, DNA (deoxyribonucleic acid), was the "master chemical" of the cell. This enormously complex molecule, which is found mainly in the cell's chromosomes, was believed to direct the activities of the living thing very much the way a punched paper tape regulates some automatic machines. Different chemical groups strung along the molecule were believed to act like the holes in a paper tape which, slowly unreeling, directed the growth, differentiation and lifelong activities of all living things; DNA was also believed able to duplicate itself and therefore embodied in itself all the characteristics of life.

While this theory held sway, it was tempting to explain the damage done by radiation in terms of DNA; if a particle smashed into one of the key DNA molecules, part of the "instructions" coded into the molecule would be obliterated. If a sufficient number of instructions were erased, the cell would simply cease to function. Smaller alterations in the DNA would produce abnormal functioning, perhaps including cancer development.[10] Since it was the DNA which was responsible for duplication and inheritance, any alterations in DNA would pass on from generation to generation — providing a simple explanation of the phenomenon of mutation.

Despite the early enthusiasm with which the theory of DNA as the "secret of life" was received by biologists, experimental evidence gathered in recent years is beginning to suggest that it is far too simple. This evidence is summarized in very readable form in *Science and Survival,* a book by the biologist Barry Commoner, himself the leading critic of what is half humorously referred to by its proponents as the "dogma" of DNA.

What the new evidence seems to suggest is that the living cell is a complex whole of which DNA is only a dependent — although important — part.

According to the newer view, self-duplication and other life processes can only be carried out by a properly functioning intact cell; damage to the DNA by radiation or other causes may result in imperfect duplication, and hence inherited defects — but damage to other parts of the cell's complex machinery may also cause such mutations.

Because the cell is a complex of interdependent processes, disturbance of one process may resonate through the whole system, causing a chain of tiny disturbances in the cell which our knowledge is simply not yet adequate to trace. On a microscopic scale, the release of radiation within the cell is very much like the release of radiation into the macroscopic human environment. Once the complex living system is disturbed, we are at a loss to predict the ultimate consequences. Under what circumstances the disturbance of a cell may result years later in the formation of a cancerous growth, we simply do not know; we are equally ignorant of the circumstances under which a cell may recover from radiation damage, or, in most cases, of those in which a mutation is induced.

Still more mysterious is another effect of radiation on most living things — life-shortening. Exposed to low doses of radiation over long periods of time, a wide range of animals and insects show no visible damage, except that their lives become shorter. Radiation has somehow accelerated the aging process. This effect is believed to occur also in man. Very little is known about how radiation shortens lives, but it is generally held that it does so by speeding up the normal process of aging. Unfortunately, once again our knowledge of biology is inadequate; Dr. Herman Blumenthal writes: "The problem of life-shortening effects [of radiation] has received only brief consideration. . . ." [11]

Dr. Blumenthal describes one likely explanation of the life-shortening effect. As a person grows older, more and more of the cells of his body show definite alterations, or mutations. These may be caused by natural radiation, or other factors. If the disturbance to a given cell is not lethal, it may cause significant alterations in the cell's proteins.

> The consequences of these alterations involve the concept of biological individuality which holds that, except in the case of identical twins, each individual's proteins differ in some subtle way from those of every other individual. The rejection of organs transplanted from one person to another, which has received so much attention in recent years, is based on this principle. The transplanted organ, which has a different "individuality" from that of the recipient, gives rise to an immune reaction from its host, and the result is its rejection. The analogy in respect to aging would be that mutations occurring in a particular organ would render the mutated cells of the organ "foreign" and thus lead to an autoimmune reaction. [12]

The process of aging is therefore seen as the body's attack on its own tissues, as these are subtly altered over the years. Since radiation is known to produce mutations in all cells, it is reasonable that constant low levels of radiation exposure simply hasten the process of change which leads to aging.

Dr. Blumenthal points out that there is gathering evidence that this attack of the body in its own tissues may be involved in a number of the diseases of the old, as well as in aging itself. He includes vascular disease, cancer, diabetes, "and several of the less frequent diseases of old people." There is a suggestion, therefore, that all of the effects of radiation — cancer, inherited malformation, and life-shortening — may all be due to the same cause, a subtle reorganization of the body's cells following a damage from radiation.

Single living things are complicated systems, no less than the communities of living things in which they may be placed. A single nuclear particle smashes into a cell; the cell, itself a highly complex assortment of interdependent processes, undergoes complex alterations to adjust itself to the damage. The changed cell, if it is a germ cell, will eventually result in offspring which are different from the parent. If it is a body cell, its alteration may set off complex responses in the larger organism which, years later, may result in cancer or other disease. Repeated damage to cells may set off the complex degenerative process of senescence.

All of what we have said gives some picture of the difficulties of estimating the damage to people from a given amount of radiation in the environment. Let us take, for instance, the problem of estimating the number of human mutations which would be induced by dumping a given amount of radioactive cesium into White Oak Lake.

This small quantity of cesium 137 may be concentrated in the food chain of the lake; it may be further dispersed by insects; it may be carried away by birds which upon dying in remote areas decompose and further disperse the radioactivity; it may be carried to the sea or enter the groundwater. Should it be concentrated in the muscles of a waterfowl, that bird might be shot by a hunter and then eaten. The cesium 137 would then be concentrated in the hunter's muscles; some of its radiation might reach his germ tissues. A single particle might crash through a germ cell, damaging without killing it; the damaged cell might, years later, produce a damaged sperm which might fertilize an egg and result in the birth of a child with some defect.

The cesium 137, whose half-life is roughly thirty years, would soon be excreted from the hunter's body, whether or not it had done any damage there, and continue its complex career through the world of living things for decades or centuries, at each passage through the human food chain creating a new risk of damage.

What then is the risk of genetic damage from a given amount of cesium 137 released into the environment? We can only say that with *any* release of radioactivity there is *some* risk of damage. This risk grows steadily with every release of radioactive waste anywhere in the world, and the risk is shared by all of us.

As the nuclear reactor program expands, its wastes will also increase, and the burden of radioactivity in our surroundings will rise, and go on rising. At some point the deleterious effects of this radiation will become unacceptable even to a nation which is able to tolerate 50,000 deaths on its roads each year. Because the effects of radiation go on making themselves felt decades after the first damage is done, it would be well to anticipate the eventual saturation of our surroundings. For the environment which supports us has only a limited capacity for radiation, and that capacity can only be used once.

VI

A NEW POLLUTION PROBLEM

IN AUGUST OF 1963, the Pacific Gas and Electric Company started up its reactor at Humboldt Bay on the Northern California coast. Late in the same year, General Electric, manufacturer of the reactor, began discovering difficulties in its design. These began showing up at the elaborate testing and research facilities GE maintained at Vallecitos, near Pleasanton, California. The stainless-steel encased fuel rods for the reactors were showing signs of cracking during reactor operation.

Uranium fuel for a reactor, as we have said, is compressed into pellets and loaded into long thin rods, about half an inch thick and several feet long. The rods are bundled together into "fuel assemblies" for ease of handling. The material from which to make the fuel tubes, or "cladding," posed an early problem for the reactor industry, which has not yet been entirely solved. This material must be thin, and yet capable of withstanding temperatures of several hundred degrees, and high pressures, for a year or more of reactor operation, while all the time being exposed to intense radiation which causes degenerative effects in most materials.

The search for a suitable fuel container led to some fairly exotic materials. An alloy called zircaloy was developed and used in the nuclear submarine program — the submarines are powered by reactors which served as the early prototypes for some present commercial power reactors.

General Electric, trying to bring the price of its reactors down, settled on stainless steel for its fuel cladding, and the Humboldt reactor was equipped with a fuel core of uranium oxide in stainless steel jackets. By late 1963, it was becoming clear that the choice of stainless steel for the Humboldt reactor was a mistake. Test fuels at Vallecitos were cracking and flaking — but the initial fuel loading for Humboldt, worth about four million dollars, had already been made, and the reactor went into operation on schedule. At that point Pacific Gas and Electric knew it would eventually run into trouble. Arrangements were made to replace the stainless steel with zircaloy-clad fuel, which seemed more reliable. But the replacement was not to be made until the first loading of stainless steel fuel had been used.

By June of 1965, the expected problems began to materialize. The radioactivity being discharged from the plant's stack began slowly to increase. In the reactor's core, the long slender fuel rods were beginning to show cracks and tiny leaks. Radioactive wastes from the fission process going on in the uranium within the rods were leaking out through the stainless steel containers and into the cooling water flowing between the rods. Some of these radioactive wastes were gases and, mingling with the steam produced in the reactor, were piped out to the turbines which drove the power generators. Passing through the turbines, both gases and steam were passed into a condenser cooled with sea water; here the steam was cooled back to water and returned to the reactor, but the radioactive gases were separated and discharged through the plant's tall stack. (This is a common and routine waste disposal procedure.)

In order to slow down the disintegration of the stainless steel fuel, P. G. & E. was operating the reactor at only a fraction of its full power. Nevertheless, radioactive discharges continued to increase, and by September, 1965, the release rate had climbed to 85,000 microcuries per second,[1] although the maximum average annual release permitted by the AEC was 50,000 microcuries per second. Testifying somewhat later before a California State Assembly Committee, P. G. & E. denied that release rates exceeded AEC limits, and pointed out that "AEC and State regulations limit these emissions to 50,000 microcuries per second on an *annual average basis* [emphasis in the original]; yet, during all of 1965 the emissions reached an annual average of only 8,300 microcuries per second, or less than one-sixth the permissible amount." [2]

Despite these protestations, it seemed likely that increasing emissions, if continued, would eventually exceed permissible limits even on a "yearly average" basis. On September 14, 1965, P. G. & E. shut down the plant for refueling and modifications. The company denied that there was any connection between the shutdown and the increasing emissions: "The schedule for the outage [shutdown] was chosen to fit refueling requirements of the reactor," said the company's spokesman.[3] The plant was out of commission until early December; during this time about one-quarter of the stainless-steel fuel elements were removed and replaced with zirconium-clad fuel. Most or all of the badly leaking fuel rods, the company announced, had been removed.

Soon after start-up, however, radioactivity in the plant's stack gases started inching up again, and in the period February to August, 1966, it was reported to be ranging upward toward 40,000 microcuries per second, close to the permitted maximum.[4] On February 18, 1966, P. G. & E. applied to the AEC for a fourfold increase in allowed releases. In proposed Change No. 20, the company asked that their operating license be changed to allow emission of 210,000 microcuries of radioactive gases per second as an annual average, with ten times that amount for the maximum rate at any one time. The latter limit would have allowed a release of as much as 181,440 *curies* per day, for as long as a month, without exceeding permissible limits. This is a staggering quantity of radioactivity, equivalent to about 400 pounds of radium each day, or six tons of radium in a month.

It should be noted here that the radioactive gases under discussion are noble gases, principally radioactive xenon and krypton; these are relatively inactive chemically and are not incorporated to any great extent by living things. Thus, while breathing radioactive krypton exposes one to external and internal radiation, and small quantities would be dissolved in body fluids, essentially none would be incorporated into tissue. Radium, on the other hand, is readily incorporated into bone, where it remains for a long time, releasing radiation. Although the noble gases of one day's permissible release, according to P. G. & E.'s request, would be equivalent, in the radioactive energy it released, to 400 pounds of radium, the biological hazard would be far less than if the release were actually radium.

Other materials than noble gases are released from the reactor's smokestack, the principal one being radioactive iodine. Iodine 131 and other radioactive isotopes of iodine are biologically active, and are concentrated by the thyroid gland of people and animals. These isotopes therefore pose a far greater hazard than the noble gases; the requested level for iodine emission was 0.8 microcurie per second annually, with a maximum at any time of 8 microcuries per second. This could result in the release of 20,000,000 microcuries, or 20 curies, during a single month without exceeding the limit; considering the potency of radioiodine, this is still a very substantial amount.

P. G. & E. did not base its request for an increase in emission rates on the difficulty it was having with its fuel, nor on the slowly rising levels of radioactivity coming from the plant. In September of 1966, P. G. & E. public relations man Hal Stroube submitted testimony to a State Assembly committee that:

> P. G. & E.'s application for the "fourfold increase" in the permissible stack release rate . . . resulted from a commitment made by P. G. & E. to the AEC in 1962. At that time the company agreed to perform a detailed meteorological study in the plant's environs to establish the correct stack release limit. . . . The meteorological study was completed in late 1965 and formed the basis for the application. There was no direct connection between the application and the alleged "alarming rise in the level of radioactive gas." [5]

Despite this protestation, however, the application itself, signed by S. L. Sibley, company president, stated, "Authorization is requested by May 1966 because operation of the unit is expected to be affected by the present limits within a few months." [6]

The P. G. & E. application was denied by the AEC in August of 1966, and in the fall another two quarters of the steel-clad fuel was replaced by zirconium-clad elements. P. G. & E. hoped that the replacement of the fuel would allow it to operate the plant at full power; the reactor had been operating at only 40 percent of its rated capacity. Had it been operated at full capacity, the radioactive emissions would of course have been far larger, but according to Mr. Stroube, this was not the reason for operating at a lower power level. With surprising frankness he commented,

> The unit currently is being operated at 40 percent of its rated power (20,000 kilowatts of its original rating of 50,000 kilowatts) in order to extend the life of the remaining stainless steel-clad fuel in the core. This is in the interest of achieving maximum fuel economy and has no relation to public health and safety.[7]

Mr. Stroube did insist, however, that emissions at full power would not exceed AEC limits. These limits would allow an average of 50,000 microcuries to be released each second for a year. If the reactor operated at this level, it would release the staggering quantity of 1.5 million curies each year — the radioactive equivalent of a ton and a half of radium.

What relation does the release of such enormous quantities of radiation have to "public health and safety"?

The Atomic Energy Commission regulations are not designed to limit the total amount of radioactivity released into air or water by any plant. Instead, their regulations seek to insure that radioactivity, in whatever amount, is released in such a way as not to harm plant employees or the nearby public. Regulations for the amount of radioactive gas which can be emitted from a reactor state that they must be such that a person spending all his time at the plant's boundary will not receive more than a specified small exposure to radioactivity. In releasing gases, therefore, the reactor operators first dilute them with large volumes of air and then discharge them through a tall stack, so that by the time they reach the outside public they have been considerably dispersed and no one person can acquire an exposure beyond the limits set.

Because, as we saw in the last chapter, any exposure to radiation, no matter how slight, may produce some damage, the setting of limits is a difficult business. A complex philosophy and elaborate techniques have been developed since the end of World War II to deal with this problem. One long-standing principle has been that large numbers of people should never be exposed to more than the equivalent of the natural or "background" radiation to which they are always exposed. This is a necessarily arbitrary standard, and seems to stem at least in part from the idea that exposures below this level would produce some damage, but not enough to be easily distinguished from the bodily and genetic damage already being done by natural radiation.

It should be pointed out that the reassuring adjective "natural" does not imply that radiation from minerals and cosmic rays is harmless. On the contrary, it does the same sorts of damage and in the same ways as artificial radiation. Radioactive potassium in sea water is just as harmful as radioactive potassium made artificially. Radium and thorium which are naturally present in small quantities in coal are released into the air when coal is burned. Coal-burning power plants therefore release measurable quantities of radioactivity from their smokestacks and pose a small hazard of their own.

In other words, man-made radioactivity once released is simply an *increase* of a hazard already present. Those considering setting radiation standards generally seem to feel that a new risk of about the same size as the old risk which has always been around is acceptable. This is one approach to standard setting, but there are clearly others.

The second widely accepted principle is that of balancing benefits against risks. This is the approach which has been taken by the Federal Radiation Council, a cabinet-level committee which advises the President on radiation standards. The FRC's standards are not binding unless adopted by a governmental agency. The principal two federal agencies dealing with atomic energy are the AEC and the Defense Department; the AEC sets its own standards and regulations, many of which predate the FRC (which was formed in 1959) — and the Defense Department apparently just ignores FRC standards. According to one source,[8] Defense had insisted from the first that they be exempted from any standards set outside the Department, and finally extracted an explicit statement in an FRC memorandum dated May 13, 1960, regarding radiation "guides" established by the FRC. The memorandum said, "The guides may be exceeded only after the Federal agency having jurisdiction over the matter has carefully considered the reason for doing so in the light of the recommendations of this paper."

Despite the fact that its recommendations were binding on no one, the Federal Radiation Council issued a number of standards or guides. These were at first called Radiation Protection Guides, or RPG's. Since at the time of their issuance the principal source of radioactivity was fallout from nuclear weapons testing, the RPG's were universally treated by the press as safe limits below which fallout was harmless. Numerous reassuring statements, that exposures to fallout were only a small fraction of those considered safe, were generally based on these RPG's.

Treating the guides as safety standards was simply misleading, as they were nothing of the sort. We have already seen that there is no "safe" level of radiation exposure. What the Federal Radiation Council had done was to strike a balance between the benefits and risks, as they saw them, of the then principal source of radiation exposure, weapons testing. Rough estimates of the damage which would be done by fallout in terms of increased numbers of thyroid cancers, cases of leukemia, mutations and other forms of damage were made, although not at first released. Benefits of weapons testing were presumably estimated in some fashion, although how this was done or could be done is unclear. A balance was then struck — the radiation protection guide represented the greatest exposure to radiation which the whole population might receive for which the benefits to the population outweighed the damage done.

This is a far cry from a safety standard, of course. Nor is it easy to see how any group, even a committee of cabinet officers, could carry out the procedure just described. For neither the benefits nor the risks of bomb testing could really be put into numbers easily, and even if they could be, the result would not necessarily be very useful. How many dollars saved in the weapons program, or how many new bombs, are justified by how many cases of leukemia?

What actually seems to have happened is that estimates of radiation damage were made from experiments on animals and past exposures of people to X-rays and radium in medical treatment. From these estimates, a guess was made of the amount of exposure of a large number of people which would clearly show damage to the population above and beyond that already being done by natural factors. Thus, estimates of leukemia or thyroid cancer production by artificial means were constantly compared, in FRC reports, with the natural incidence of these diseases.

When this exposure had been estimated, it was reduced by a substantial margin of safety, and then the reduced figure was issued as a "radiation protection guide." In short, despite the FRC trappings of balancing benefit against risk, they were following precisely the philosophy of the AEC in simply assuming that damage which could not be differentiated from natural causes was acceptable.

There are a number of other agencies which issue radiation standards. The International Commission for Radiation Protection, successor to the International Congress of Radiologists, is affiliated with the World Health Organization, and issued the first recommendations for limits of exposure to the general population from artificial radioactivity; these recommendations became the basis of many later standards. The National Committee on Radiation Protection and measurements is the successor to the United States radiologists' organization; this remains a private organization although it is closely associated with the Bureau of Standards of the U.S. Department of Commerce. Its recommendations have force only if adopted by government agencies.

The AEC has regulations for its own activities and those of its licensees; the Defense Department has its own regulations. Not all radiation is under the jurisdiction of the Federal Government: the states regulate uses of X-rays, radium, and, under agreements with the AEC, a number of other activities. The operations of uranium mines are under a number of overlapping federal, state and local jurisdictions, as are transportation of radioactive materials, waste disposal, and operation of atomic-powered ships, rockets and other devices.

There is a growing proliferation of agencies which in some way are responsible for regulating activities which do or might result in exposure of the general public to radiation. On the other hand, there is no agency with overall responsibility for finding out what total exposures to the population are and setting standards or limits. The result has been the almost universal adoption of the AEC's — and in present circumstances the only feasible — approach. This is simply to make sure that in every activity or device which exposes people to radiation, there is no release which would cause noticeable harm to the people directly exposed. Generally speaking, it seems safe to say that radiation exposures about equal to natural background will produce damage which is not noticeable, and emissions are kept to this level.

There is clearly a great deal wrong with the current state of affairs. First off, there is a world of difference between "no damage" and "no noticeable damage." Reactors, X-ray machines and even coal-burning plants are doing *some* damage; because so many people throughout the world ordinarily die from cancer, many thousands of additional cases could go by without notice. The fact that our biological knowledge or statistical techniques do not allow us to identify the small boy whose leukemia is a result of bomb testing does not mean that he does not exist.

The principle of keeping radiation exposures below the limit of noticeable damage is therefore perfectly arbitrary, and gains its appeal from the false reassurance derived from not actually seeing the damage being done. Whether in fact the benefits from reactors or other atomic energy devices justify the damage being done is a question which remains unresolved as long as the damages do not obtrude themselves into the public consciousness.

Secondly, the "no measurable damage" principle is based on a simplistic and inaccurate picture of the living world. It is possible to ignore the absolute quantity of radioactive wastes being discharged into our air and water only when it is assumed that, once sufficiently diluted, the wastes have ceased to be a problem. In the last chapter we have seen that this is emphatically not the case. Many of the radioactive wastes produced by reactors are long-lived and biologically active; iodine 129, which is selectively absorbed by the thyroid gland, and hence poses a special threat through concentration in that organ, has a half-life of more than 17 million years; although this isotope is produced in very small quantities by reactors, the amount of iodine 129 in the environment must steadily increase as the reactor program expands.

One of the radioactive gases being released by reactors poses a similar and perhaps more immediate problem. A recently published study estimates that radioactive krypton 85 will be produced in such enormous quantities by the reactor program that in less than a hundred years man's exposure to radiation may be nearly doubled.[9] This is a profoundly disturbing prospect, for, of course, krypton 85 is only one of the many radioactive wastes to which we are to be exposed.

Another source of exposure which may someday become serious is tritium, the radioactive form of hydrogen. Two or three thousand curies of this material, which is almost impossible to separate from the water of which it becomes a part, are discharged each year from each of the larger reactors planned.

What will be the effect of increasing radiation exposure for all living things? We have very little idea. Our understanding of life is too primitive for us to know. The rate of mutation will certainly increase — and a beneficial mutation in man has never been recorded. Subtle effects are more likely to predominate than dramatic ones — slightly increased disease rates, slightly shortened life spans, subtle readjustments in the balance of species.

We can see that the present approach to radiation limits is inadequate, and sooner or later will lead to serious trouble. What we have been doing, quite simply, is to avoid killing or injuring anyone directly by spreading the damage thin over the whole environment. But that damage will not disappear, it will accumulate, slowly and inevitably, until the level of "no noticeable damage" is passed not for a single isolated area, but for the earth as a whole.

At present, saltwater fish caught far from land contain some DDT, washed from fields to streams and to the ocean, being concentrated by microscopic plants and animals, and then by the fish themselves. Nearly every bite of food each of us in this country takes adds another dose of pesticide to our bodies. Rainwater throughout the country contains a bewildering variety of chemicals, ranging from nitrates from agricultural fertilizer to gasoline additives.

Radioactive wastes are now beginning to repeat this pattern, and in the coming years our food and water will be increasingly burdened with radiation. The first step in this new assault on the environment was taken with atomic bomb testing, in secrecy and in almost complete ignorance. That first step having been taken, we are continuing with nuclear power plants. In other forms of air and water pollution, we had to reach the point of real disaster before beginning to think of control. This must not be allowed to happen with radioactive wastes; once released into the atmosphere, there is no conceivable way of retrieving radioactive gases; once entered on their winding course through the environment, radioactive isotopes are out of reach of man's control. The damage, once done, is irremediable. There is a real danger that such damage may be quite extensive before it is brought home to us, for the effects of radiation are so often far removed in time and place from their cause.

It is not only the nearby neighbors of reactors, therefore, who should be concerned with the radioactive poisons they release. Those releases are contributing to the slow degeneration of the environment in which we all live; radiation is the most serious of the many stresses we are putting on the fabric of life. Rachel Carson quotes in *Silent Spring* the ecologist Paul Shepard, who sees us stumbling toward a "life with only its head out of water, inches above the limits of toleration of the corruption of its own environment . . . Why should we tolerate a diet of weak poisons, a home in insipid surroundings, a circle of acquaintances who are not quite our enemies, the noise of motors with just enough relief to prevent insanity? Who would want to live in a world which is just not quite fatal?"

It is long past time that we realized that in radiation "no measurable damage" eventually means "just not quite fatal" for everyone. The haste with which the commercial reactor program is being pursued at present simply does not allow reasonable consideration of this problem. The Humboldt reactor is an excellent example of the kind of difficulty which is in store for us. The reactor was built, and its fuel core fabricated, before the difficulties of the fuel became apparent. This happened in 1963. By 1966, the reactor boom was on, and twenty power plants were ordered in that year; yet by mid-1967 a whole new series of fuel problems were beginning to appear.

There are only two types of fuel cladding tubes in widespread use in this country or planned for the near future — stainless steel and zirconium alloy (zircaloy). A hot debate rages in the industry as to the relative merits of the two fuel jackets, for both have suffered difficulties. (At present, zircaloy seems to have triumphed.) In hearings before the Joint Committee on Atomic Energy early in 1967, these problems were discussed, briefly. Congressman Craig Hosmer quizzed members of the AEC and its staff:

Representative Hosmer: We had some cracks out at Dresden No. 1 in the zirc cladding to begin with.

Mr. Shaw: In the boiling water reactor?

Mr. Ramey: They took care of those.

Representative Hosmer: They put stainless steel in, did they not? . . .

Mr. Johnson: I think they started with zircaloy and changed over to stainless and then back to zircaloy later. That is my recollection.[10]

Hosmer was also interested in more recent fuel problems, particularly at the Big Rock Point reactor at Charlevoix, Michigan, and the Carolinas–Virginia Tube Reactor (CVTR) at Parr, South Carolina. The Big Rock Point plant, operated by the Consumers Power Company, had been suffering problems with its stainless steel clad fuel for over a year. The Consumers

Power Company reported that "the stainless steel seems to have been subjected to some sort of stress corrosion attack. . . ." The stainless steel fuel elements, like those at Humboldt, were being replaced by zircaloy-clad fuel; all the fuel was expected to be replaced by the end of 1967.

At Parr, South Carolina, however, the trouble was with zircaloy-clad fuel. The Carolinas–Virginia Tube Reactor is owned by four Southern utilities. In response to Representative Hosmer's question, Milton Shaw, Director of the AEC Division of Reactor Development and Technology testified:

> We had four test fuel samples in the reactor. Of these four development samples, three have failed long before achieving the design exposure levels.

> We are quite concerned about the implications of the failure of these fuel assemblies. As a result, we have gone ahead and removed the fourth assembly. . . .

> In addition, the CVTR has also experienced failures in two of the normal fuel assemblies clad with zircaloy 4 — the same material being planned for other commercial plants. . . .

> The first part of your question was related to the situation at the Consumers of Michigan Plant at Big Rock Point. This is a boiling water plant. They have been experiencing fuel cladding failures in both stainless steel and Incaloy bundles over a longer period of time. These failures, too, are being examined to determine the exact cause of the problem.

> Representative Hosmer: Is this the kind of fuel that is being sold commercially for other reactors, too?

> Mr. Shaw: Yes sir, stainless steel, zircaloy 4, and Incaloy 800 clad fuel has been sold for commercial reactors.

Representative Hosmer: How serious should we regard this, or can we make a judgment at this point?

Mr. Shaw: Although there is serious concern, I don't believe we can make a judgment at this time in the absence of determinations as to what caused the failures, sir. The failure could have been caused by defective manufacturing techniques or by something not understood about the design of the fuel.[11]

At the time Mr. Shaw was speaking, March 15, 1967, sixteen large new power reactors were under construction, and, by the first of July, orders had been placed for thirty-six more; utilities across the country had indicated plans for about two dozen further plants which had not yet been ordered. Seventy or eighty large reactors were being planned, then, or were already under construction, representing an investment of capital of several billion dollars. Roughly one-quarter of the initial investment in a reactor is its first batch of fuel; over the plant's life, the cost of fuel and fuel services is roughly equal to the initial cost of the plant itself.

In the face of this enormous investment, it is almost certain that presently available fuel tube materials will be used: the story of Humboldt Bay is about to be repeated on a massive scale. There, despite early signs of trouble with stainless steel, the first fuel loading was used and the reactor operated with some defective elements. At this writing, it is not known whether the difficulties with the three fuel cladding types reported by Mr. Shaw were due to faulty manufacture or "something not understood about the design of the fuel."

What is disturbing here is that there will be a number of reactors going into operation, as well as the dozen or so already in commercial use, which will necessarily rely on fuel which is presently available, not prohibitively expensive, but liable to failure and radioactivity release. Still more disturbing is the pattern which has been established and which will apparently continue. The rest of Mr. Shaw's testimony is illuminating:

> The general information available on water plant fuel, such as burnup and power densities, is sufficient that we know a safe and reliable fuel can be designed for the water reactor plants, if one doesn't extrapolate too far.
>
> However, there is no question but that the fuel warranties being provided right now [by manufacturers] far exceed the meaningful information which is available to us through the research and development programs.[12]

Translated, this means simply that we have now acquired enough information to design fuel for the plants which are presently in operation — that is, plants which were being built ten years ago. We do *not* have enough information yet to design safe and reliable fuel for the reactors now being built and planned, which are many times larger, and which expose their fuel to higher temperatures, higher radiation intensities and higher pressures for longer periods of time. The result will be operation of the plants with some faulty fuel elements for several years; but by then the industry hopes to have under construction the *next* generation of reactors (described in the next chapter) which have a whole new set of problems, many of them still more severe than those now being faced.

We seem to be permanently committed to a program, then, which is just a little bit ahead of the state of technology. This has been a long-standing state of affairs. In its 1962 report to the President, the Atomic Energy Commission stated:

Attempts to optimize economies by working on the outer fringes
of technical experience, together with the difficulties always experienced in a new and rapidly advancing technology, have led
to many disappointments and frustrations. . . . Such difficulties
led to considerable diminution of the earlier optimism regarding
the early utilization of nuclear power, which in turn contributed
to the withdrawal of some equipment and component manufacturers from the field.[13]

The industry continues to work at the outer fringes of technical experience, as Mr. Shaw pointed out. In earlier chapters
we considered the possible damages from a severe reactor
accident; in view of those possibilities, this willingness to take
risks with reactors is not encouraging. In terms of dispersal of
radioactive wastes, however, we are dealing with what, in the
light of past years' experience, we can consider a virtual certainty. The problems of Humboldt will be repeated, and reactors will continue to function just barely within AEC limits.
This means an enormously increased discharge of radiation
to air and water in the next few years. Most of the reactors
presently planned are ten to twelve times as large as Humboldt.
Total discharges of waste will be proportionately greater. More
than seventy of these mammoth plants are scheduled to go into
operation within the next seven years, and dozens more will
follow.

Nor are reactors themselves the only — or even the worst —
source of radioactive pollution in the atomic power industry.

The fuel for reactors undergoes a complex series of extractions and transformations over a course of years. Uranium ore
is mined, and the uranium is extracted and shipped to a chemical plant, where the extracted ore, called "yellow-cake" from
its appearance, is converted into uranium hexafluoride, which

is then shipped to one of the government's huge gas diffusion plants at Oak Ridge, Tennessee; Portsmouth, Ohio; or Paducah, Kentucky. Here the content of fissionable uranium 235 is increased, or "enriched." The product is then shipped to a series of other plants, where it is converted to uranium oxide, compacted into small pellets, packed into long tubes which are assembled into finished fuel elements. The finished fuel is shipped to a reactor where it is used; but this is by no means the end of its travels. After wastes, or fission products, have accumulated in the fuel to the point where it is no longer usable, it is stored for a while, and then shipped to a reprocessing plant. Here the radioactive wastes are extracted, and the depleted uranium and small amounts of plutonium are recovered. The reclaimed uranium may be shipped to a chemical plant to rebegin the fuel cycle. The plutonium is sold to the government; the extracted wastes are either discharged to the air and water, or packaged and shipped to a storage or burial site.

At every step in this long path, there is some release of radiation to the environment. Some of the releases are known and controlled; some are unforeseen or, in some cases, ignored.

Radiation problems in the reactor industry therefore begin in the shafts of uranium mines. Uranium ore also contains radium and other radioactive substances; radium, in the process of slow decomposition, releases radon, which is a gas. When the ore is mined, radon gas and its own decomposition products accumulate in the mine shaft and pose a severe hazard to miners. The first disastrous effects of radon gas were observed in the 1930's in mining communities in the Erzgebirge Mountains; the mining area is called Schneeberg in Germany and Joachimstal in Czechoslovakia. A study performed between

1935 and 1939 revealed that approximately half the deaths among miners were due to lung cancer, and that 80 percent of the remaining deaths were due to other lung diseases.[14]

Shortly after the Second World War, great efforts were made by the Atomic Energy Commission to encourage exploration and uranium mining in the United States; by the early 1950's vast deposits in the West and Southwest had been uncovered. The United States Public Health Service, aware of the studies of European mines, surveyed the domestic situation. Four hundred air samples were taken from 75 mines; most samples showed radioactivity which far exceeded standards set by the International and National Commissions on Radiation Protection. These results were reported in 1955, and the International Labor Organization commented that they "give cause for considerable disquiet." [15]

Nothing, however, was done. By 1960, there were 1,000 active underground mines, but the AEC had no jurisdiction over them and the state and federal agencies which did seemed unaware of the problem. The problem was not brought to national attention until the summer of 1967. On April 26, 1967, Leo Goodman of the Industrial Union Department of the AFL-CIO, who has for many years been watchdog of the nuclear industry, addressed a meeting of the American Public Health Association. Goodman recounted the long history of evidence of hazards and complete inaction in uranium mining, and stated that the Colorado Industrial Mining Commission had paid a number of claims to the families of miners who had died of lung cancer. He pointed out that, in 1956, the Public Health Service had issued a report which concluded that "Surveys of the Colorado Plateau uranium mines have shown that 65 percent of the miners were exposed to concentrations of radon and its daughters [decay products] comparable to those reported to exist earlier in European mines." [16] Some of the mines surveyed had as much as 59 times the permissible level of radiation.

Following Goodman's speech and a number of newspaper stories which appeared at about the same time, the Department of Labor suddenly exercised its authority to set protective standards. Protests from the Joint Committee on Atomic Energy and uranium mining companies that the standards were too stringent and perhaps unenforceable resulted in a series of congressional hearings and a certain amount of acrimonious debate. After some weeks, a standard (the more lenient one recommended by the Federal Radiation Council) was finally accepted. Evidence adduced by Joint Committee hearings showed that the standard adopted would result in some increase in the rate of lung cancer among miners, beyond that in the general population; the additional cancer deaths would not be so many as to be easily distinguishable from those of other causes, but that there would be some additional deaths seemed generally accepted.[17]

Although the AEC published its first price schedule for uranium in 1948, it was not until July of 1967 that a safety standard of any sort for uranium miners was enforceable. All this despite the record of disastrous experience in European uranium mines. A very similar pattern can be seen in the history of radioactive water pollution from uranium mines.

Twelve million tons of radioactive sand, the refuse of uranium mining in the Colorado River Basin, is heaped in largely untended piles in an area affecting at least seven states in the Southwest. For nearly twenty years these sands have been accumulating, being blown by the wind into neighboring communities, and being washed by the rain into the tributaries of the Colorado River and eventually into Lake Mead: a water system which provides water for drinking and irrigation to parts of California, Nevada, Utah, Wyoming, Colorado, New Mexico and Arizona.

In the late 1950's the magnitude of the pollution hazard from uranium mining was discovered by the Public Health Service. Concentrations of radium 226 in algae in one river were as high as 3560 picocuries per kilogram. Alfalfa harvested in the area showed a high of 1160 picocuries per kilogram. Water in the San Miguel River reached 88 picocuries per liter during 1955. We can compare these figures to the maximum permissible concentration established by the Public Health Service of three picocuries per liter for drinking water. The Federal Water Pollution Control Administration estimated that up to 1959, people drinking water from the Animas River received three times the maximum permissible exposure from radium 226 and strontium 90 (from fallout).[18]

Once alerted to the hazard, the PHS began pressing for control of wastes from the uranium mills in the area, and much progress was made. Wastes are no longer dumped directly into neighboring streams and certain of the discharges of the mills have been halted, but the huge quantities of refuse produced by the processing of uranium ore remain a problem. For every ton of uranium ore passing through the mills, only about five pounds of salable uranium oxide is produced. The remainder, which resembles sand, is called "tailings" and is heaped near the mills.

In the early 1960's the Atomic Energy Commission cut back considerably its requirements for uranium, and a number of mills in the Colorado Basin were closed down. At the mills which closed, the radioactive tailings produced during their operation were simply abandoned. About three million tons of such abandoned tailings have been slowly blowing and washing away, producing further contamination of the Colorado River watershed. Some of the enormous heaps of tailings are directly on the banks of rivers and are being slowly washed away and deposited in the reservoirs of Lake Mead and Lake Powell, which supply water to a large part of the Southwest.

On May 6, 1966, the Subcommittee on Air and Water Pollution of the Committee on Public Works of the United States Senate held hearings on "Radioactive Water Pollution in the Colorado River Basin." The chairman of the Subcommittee was Senator Edmund S. Muskie of Maine, who has a continuing interest in problems of water pollution. The day's hearing was based on a report in March of 1965 by the Federal Water Pollution Control Administration, which has maintained a continuing effort to curtail pollution in this area.

Two thousands grams of radium 226 are present in the abandoned tailings piles. (Hazardous quantities of radium are usually measured in trillionths of a gram.) A larger amount of radium is presumably present in the tailings at operating mill sites. There is, in addition, an unknown quantity of radioactive thorium and lead, but the radium is considered the most serious problem. It is probably the most damaging of all radioactive isotopes, accumulating in the bone where it causes cancer and other diseases. The maximum permissible concentration established for radium is the lowest of any isotope. The FWPCA estimates that if ten tons from one of the tailings piles slips into an adjacent river (a not unlikely event), the concentration of radium 226 in the river water might go as high as 70 picograms per liter within the first hour. This compares to a maximum permissible concentration of three picograms per liter. If a larger slippage occurred in the abandoned piles — an event which has occurred in the past at operating mills, dumping as much as 120 tons of tailings into the river — levels of radium in the river water would remain above the maximum permissible concentration for days afterward.

Testifying before Senator Muskie's subcommittee, Dr. Peter Morris, Director, Division of Operational Safety, AEC, stated that "there is currently no significant hazard associated with uranium milling activities in the Colorado River Basin." He also stated that "we do not think that data available at this time support the conclusion that there is longterm radiological hazard." [19] This statement contradicted the FWPCA report which found "the Federal Water Pollution Control Administration is concerned with the potential problems that appear to be associated with the tailings because of their extremely long-lived radioactivity." [20] The half-life of radium 226 is 1620 years; the half-life of thorium 230, also present in the tailings, is 80,000 years.

Much of the area affected by contamination from the mills is also an area of high fallout from the Nevada test site. Murray Stein, chief of the enforcement program of FWPCA, testified as follows: "We found, when we first got into the area of the Colorado River Basin, that people were being exposed to several times the maximum permissible limit of radioactivity. The source at that time was, or course, fallout."

In other words, the same population which in the past has been exposed to high levels of radioactivity from fallout and from dumping of wastes from uranium mills continues to be subjected to exposure from erosion of the tailings piles. There has been no attempt to determine what total exposure people have actually received. About 25,000 people on the Animas River in New Mexico probably have received the most severe exposures.

While maintaining that the radiation hazard did not warrant control measures, the AEC had not opposed the proposal from the FWPCA for reducing erosion in the abandoned tailings piles by covering them with gravel and establishing vegetation. No plant life will grow in the uncovered tailings. The FWPCA considers that reduction of erosion is an interim measure of control to allow the government and the mill owners to agree on the methods and the responsibility for permanent disposal of the wastes. This is liable to be a difficult problem. About 30 million tons of tailings have accumulated in various parts of the country, and the total, of course, is growing. A single mill processes several thousand tons of uranium ore each day, the vast bulk of which is returned to the environment as radioactive waste.

In the summer of 1967, a conference was held among the concerned parties at Denver, Colorado, and some interim control measures, including erosion control, were agreed to. A study is presently under way to determine the extent of release of radioactive gases (radon and its products) from the tailings piles. As in the case of the miners, the remedy, partial in any case, was proposed 20 years after the problem had been created.

Similar problems occur at every point along the long uranium fuel cycle. Potentially the most serious by far of these occurs at the fuel-processing plant.

The fragments of fissioned atoms, radioactive wastes, slowly accumulate in reactor fuel. After a period of time, enough wastes accumulate to extinguish the chain reaction going on in the fuel, as ashes may smother a fire. Before this point is reached, the fuel must be removed from the reactor and the radioactive "ashes" extracted. This is a more difficult and dangerous operation than it seems. It must be borne in mind that it is precisely these radioactive wastes which constitute the radiation hazard in the civilian atomic energy program. Uranium fuel elements, before they have been placed in a reactor, are nearly harmless, and may be held in a bare hand. After undergoing a slow, controlled chain reaction in the reactor for several months, however, the same fuel element becomes the most hazardous object, short of an atomic bomb, known to man. It can only be transported in enormous lead and steel casks weighing many tons, and contains within it enough radioactivity, if distributed, to poison whole cities.

This enormous hazard derives from the violently radioactive fragments of split atoms, fission products. These are a bewildering array of radioactive twins of common elements, and range from a form of radioactive nitrogen with a half-life of just over seven seconds to iodine 129 with a half-life of more than 17 million years.

When a fuel assembly has been in a reactor for its allotted time, it is lifted out of the reactor core with remote-control equipment and lowered into a pool of water within the reactor building itself. Here it is stored for several weeks, to allow the shorter-lived radioactive elements to decay. This reduces the hazard in handling, and also lowers the temperature of the fuel element (even when removed from the reactor, the fuel assembly is so hot, and remains so for months, that it would melt unless artificially cooled). Two of the fission products have become familiar to the public, as they are also (and for the same reasons) among the principal hazards in fallout from bomb testing: strontium 90 and cesium 137. Both have half-lives near 30 years, and hence will not decay appreciably over any feasible period of storage. Tritium, a radioactive relative of hydrogen with a half-life of 12 years, is also present, although in far smaller amounts; like radioactive cesium and strontium, tritium is readily taken up by living things. Iodine 131 is still more biologically active but shorter-lived. Its close relative, iodine 129, lasts a far longer time, although present in far smaller quantities. The other fission product of concern is one we have already encountered, krypton 85, the noble gas which was being released in such surprising quantities from the Humboldt Bay reactor.

After a period of storage, the fuel assembly is loaded, again by remote control, into a massive lead-and-steel "shipping cask." This enormous cylinder, ten feet or more high, contains its own cooling system. The shipping cask is loaded onto a truck and shipped to a fuel-reprocessing plant which may be hundreds of miles from the reactor itself. Until very recently, the AEC did all fuel reprocessing at its own plants at Savannah River, near Aiken, South Carolina, and at the National Reactor Testing Station, near Idaho Falls, Idaho. In 1966, the first private fuel-reprocessing facility was dedicated at West Valley, about 30 miles south of Buffalo, New York. It is owned by Nuclear Fuel Services, Inc., which in turn is owned (principally) by W. R. Grace and Company. Several other such private plants are planned for the near future, principally by the reactor manufacturers. Construction will soon begin on such a plant in Marion, Illinois, to be owned by General Electric.

Having traveled perhaps halfway across the country, the fuel assembly is again stored for a time in a deep pool of water, along with other fuel elements which are waiting their turn for processing. In storage, shipping, and storage again, great care must be taken that fuel assemblies are not bunched together in a critical mass — one which could sustain a chain reaction. Once out of the reactor, no control of the fission process is possible, and such an event could lead to melting of the fuel and release of radioactivity. Since the neutrons which sustain a chain reaction can travel a considerable distance through air or water, fuel assemblies must be well separated.

The fuel processing is carried out entirely automatically or by remote control, in massive concrete chambers, because of the intense radioactivity of the fuel. First, the assembly is transferred from the storage pool to a chamber in which its external fittings are removed, leaving only a bundle of fuel rods, each less than an inch thick and several feet long. These rods are then chopped into sections a few inches long, and dumped into a nitric acid bath which dissolves the uranium and fission products, but leaves the steel jackets intact. The acid solution containing the fuel and wastes is then piped into a series of chambers in which the complex process of chemical separations is carried out. These in essence consist of passing the water-and-acid solution of fuel and wastes past a flow of organic solvent moving in the opposite direction; by delicately adjusting conditions, different substances may be forced to pass from one fluid to the other, and are thereby separated.

Uranium and plutonium are extracted, and separated from each other, and further purified. The uranium may eventually find its way back into reactor fuel, after passing through a series of chemical, enrichment and fabrication plants; the plutonium will be turned over to the government for storage, against the time that it may be used as reactor fuel in future designs.

The nitric acid solution which remains contains most of the

fission wastes and, hence, is intensely radioactive; this liquid is concentrated to reduce its volume, and then pumped into huge underground storage tanks. These tanks must be cooled, for the heat produced by the radioactivity in the wastes raises the temperature of the liquid far past the boiling point, and if allowed to accumulate would soon rupture the tanks. Cooling is accomplished by passing steam from the tanks into a condenser above ground. The tanks themselves are huge, holding 750,000 gallons each, and are stirred continuously with compressed air to keep radioactive solids from settling to the bottom.

The wastes in these tanks pose a singularly difficult problem. The quantities of radioactivity in them are simply staggering. For instance, the maximum permissible concentration of strontium 90 in drinking water is a few billionths of a curie per gallon, yet the wastes in storage contain on average about 100 curies per gallon. There are now something like 65 million gallons of hot waste in storage in the AEC's "tank farms" or atomic graveyards, more than enough to poison all the water on earth. The half-life of strontium 90 is a little over 27 years: it will be many centuries, therefore, before the wastes in storage will have decayed to tolerable levels.

These boiling hot wastes must therefore be stirred and cooled for generations. This is clearly an unsatisfactory method of operation, to put it mildly, and was recognized as such from the earliest days of the atomic program. Weapon production needs in the forties and fifties, which created most of the wastes now in storage, could not be delayed while a satisfactory solution to the waste-disposal problem was found. Now, twenty years after the fact, the AEC is experimenting with a process which gives promise of being a feasible disposal method. In project Salt Vault, the liquid wastes are reduced to a relatively inert solid form which is not easily dissolved in water; the most promising method is to produce a kind of glass, which is then encased in a sealed steel container. This container is stored for a time, and is then transported to a large abandoned salt mine, or natural or artificial cavern in a deep salt deposit. The point of using salt caverns is that they are quite impervious to water, and have been dry for millennia and can be expected to remain so for a comparable period of time. Once disposed of in salt caverns, therefore, radioactive wastes could be expected to stay put.

This seems to be a reasonable disposal method for the most highly radioactive wastes which will be formed in the future; it rather aggravates another, and in the long run perhaps more serious, problem, however.

At the fuel reprocessing plant, the stainless steel jackets of the fuel elements are broken open, and the fuel itself dissolved in nitric acid. Radioactive gases which had until then been trapped in the fuel are released. These include large volumes of noble gases, especially krypton 85, and radioactive iodine. Within the sealed air-circulation system of the reprocessing plant, these gases are scrubbed and filtered, to remove any solid particles and to capture as much of the highly dangerous radioactive iodine as possible. The remaining gases are then discharged to the outside, being mixed with large volumes of air at the same time.

This is essentially the same procedure used for discharging controlled amounts of radioactivity from reactors, and in fact the reprocessing plant in this respect resembles a reactor in which all the fuel elements have ruptured and released their radioactive contents. The krypton 85 which was not released from the Humboldt reactor itself is eventually released at a fuel reprocessing plant.

The same standards which apply to reactors apply to fuel processing plants: they may release unlimited quantities of radioactivity as long as it is sufficiently diluted and poses no *direct* hazard to people in the surrounding area. It is estimated that by the year 2000 more than one billion curies of krypton will have accumulated,[21] and all of this staggering quantity of radioactivity will be released into the air, permanently beyond control. Eventually, it is likely that all of the presently allowable exposure of the general population to radioactivity from whatever source will be exhausted by exposure to krypton 85 in the air.

A similar problem exists with radioactive tritium, which is a twin of hydrogen. This is a weakly radioactive substance with a half-life of about 12 years and is produced in small quantities in reactor fuel. Nearly all the tritium in fuel is presently discharged from reprocessing plants in waste water, along with a number of other dilute radioactive substances. By the year 2000, there will be an accumulation of something like 36 million curies of this substance knocking around.[22] Unlike the noble gases, tritium is easily incorporated into living tissue.

Other isotopes will follow similar patterns of buildup in the environment. This burden will be increased by the disposal methods proposed for higher-level wastes. If the hot liquid wastes from reprocessing plants are to be solidified, they will be heated and treated chemically in yet another plant, and the result will be a new series of releases of low-level liquid and gaseous wastes which, if present methods continue, will be released to the environment.

Although mines, reactors and chemical plants are the most visible sources of radioactive pollution, they are by no means the only ones.

At every stage of the fuel cycle, radioactive materials are being shipped from one place to another — from mine to processing plant to enrichment plant to reactor to fuel reprocessing, and so on. Soon it seems likely that a new step will be added: the transportation of high-level liquid wastes from reprocessing plants to other plants, like the pilot installation now in operation at Hanford, for converting the radioactive liquid wastes into more easily stored solids. Particularly in some stages, this transportation process is quite hazardous.

The most ticklish problem to date has been the shipment of irradiated fuel elements — fuel after it has been in a reactor for some time, and has been removed for the extraction of wastes. Such fuel is generally shipped by truck or railroad. Only one or two fuel assemblies are generally shipped at any one time — which is understandable enough, since the shipping "cask" for one element may weigh as much as 70 tons. A typical cask will be a cylinder three feet in diameter and ten feet high, with a foot-thick inner wall of lead shielding. As mentioned earlier, the cask typically has its own cooling system to keep the temperature of the fuel assembly below the melting point.

A truck or train accident which would breach the shipping cask could be a disaster, and therefore the cask is carefully designed to withstand severe impacts and high temperatures. A really severe accident, perhaps followed by a sustained fire, could conceivably lead to breaking open the container and exposing the fuel, and this might happen in a populous area. More likely, however, is the release of radioactivity from such an accident into surface water which eventually finds its way into human use.

The prospects of such a catastrophic shipping accident have

been discussed for years within the AEC. In 1958, Dr. Harold Knapp, then of the AEC, delivered a paper in which he noted that the Safety and Fire Protection Branch of the AEC believed that for some transportation accidents "costs of several million dollars would be credible." [23] Using available statistics for truck and train accidents, Dr. Knapp went on to calculate the likelihood of serious radioactivity accidents, and conclude that, "Very roughly one might expect a serious accident every 100 million vehicle miles of shipment for ordinary methods of transport." In 1962, it was estimated that shipments of reactor fuel wastes to burial grounds already totaled 2 million miles per year; this figure is probably larger now and will continue to grow.[24]

It should be emphasized that radioactive materials are shipped on common carriers — that is, the same railway, barge and truck concerns which handle other commercial shipping, and are transported according to rules for hazardous materials such as explosives, where the radiation level seems to warrant this. Packages containing small amounts of radioactivity, as for instance isotope packages for research or medical use, are simply shipped or sent through the mails like any other parcel.

The risk of catastrophic accident in transportation, as in reactor operation, is low. Dr. Knapp points out that "One hundred shipments per year of 1000 miles each with present rail accident rates would mean a serious accident as defined here every 800 years, on the average. Should the rate of shipment go as high as 10,000 shipments per year, the average time between serious accidents would come down to 8 years." [25] The number of shipments of irradiated fuel elements is expected to be at the lower end of this range for several years, but will obviously increase as the reactor program enlarges. Dr. J. W. Morgan commented, at a conference on this subject in 1962:

"It is quite possible that some time in the future there will be an accident that could be described as catastrophic. Whether we describe it as catastrophic on a dollar basis or on the basis of persons involved who may be injured, that is something else, but I think it would be interesting to look at this whole thing on a task force basis." [26]

Truck and train accidents happen regularly and predictably. As the volume of shipments goes up, the risk of serious accidents actually happening increases steadily each year. Most accidents, of course, are far short of catastrophe, and result only in the release of relatively small quantities of radioactivity. At the same conference in 1962 at which Dr. Morgan was expressing the above trepidations, another report recounted the 47 accidents which the AEC had had to date; only 17 were considered "serious." [27]

Radioactivity releases within the AEC's operations are not always so easily identified, as much of the Commission's work is highly classified. The operations of the Hanford and Savannah River reactors, used for producing plutonium for weapons, are not public knowledge, although some items are released from time to time. It is known that several thousand curies of radioactive zinc, chromium and other "activated corrosion products" are released to the Columbia River each year. Other releases at Hanford are less well known. For instance, a recent authoritative and exhaustive compilation of public information regarding radiation accidents lists the following incident:

45. *Location:* Hanford, Washington
   Date: 21 December, 1959
   Nature of Incident: Fuel element rupture in a reactor resulting in contamination of desert. Such ruptures are considered routine and minor releases of radioactivity occur perhaps once or twice a year.[28]

No explanation of the term "minor" is given. Entry no. 69 gives even less information:

Location: Hanford, Washington
Date: 7 June, 1957
Nature of Incident: Uranium dissolver explosion.

or item 70 also at Hanford, the following year:

Nature of Incident: Purex plant explosion.

These were apparently both accidents in fuel-reprocessing plants, and therefore could conceivably have resulted in considerable release of radioactivity, but no further details are given. These examples could be multiplied almost indefinitely.

Although a detailed picture is almost impossible to draw, it is clear that the sources of radioactivity being added to our environment are growing rapidly in number and size. As twenty years ago it was quite clear that there would eventually be a problem of radioactive wastes from uranium mines, and severe risks to miners, so at present we can see that eventually there will be serious problems with the disposal of radioactive wastes. In mining, in transportation, in reactor operation, fuel reprocessing and storage, there will be small losses or intentional releases of radiation, in each case designed to avoid killing anyone nearby. But the radioactivity will not go away. It is in our surroundings, and will accumulate in living things until the point of severe damage is reached; nothing in the present reactor program indicates that there will be a way of halting releases before that point.

VII

THE COMING THING

AT THE TIME OF THIS WRITING, plans are being made to re-activate the $120 million Enrico Fermi atomic power plant, on the shore of Lake Erie between Detroit and Toledo. Built in spite of bitter opposition and plagued by a series of technical failures, this nuclear plant, in 1966, suffered an accident that might have just missed being a disaster. Designed to produce electric power and plutonium for nuclear weapons, the plant has never produced usable amounts of either; as a prototype of the next generation of atomic power plants, its failure may have serious implications for the future of civilian nuclear power. Plans to start it up again may mean further accidents which might endanger nearby cities.

In 1956, when the Power Reactor Development Corporation first proposed building the Fermi reactor at Lagoona Beach, Michigan, atomic electric power was still a new idea. The first nuclear plant to produce commercial electric power — at Shippingport, Pennsylvania — was a year away from its opening. A dozen years later, and after far wider acceptance of atomic energy, the Fermi reactor continues to be a controversial facility, and a source of grave concern. The debate has a history as old as the reactor itself; in 1957, Senator Clinton Anderson of New Mexico made the following remarks toward the end of an ad-

dress to the Second Annual Convention of the New Mexico
AFL-CIO:

> Yes, I have found it necessary to urge labor unions to intervene
> against the action of the Atomic Energy Commission in granting
> a permit for the construction of the Lagoona Beach reactor next
> to the City of Detroit. . . . I telephoned not only the Governor
> of the State of Michigan, but I called labor unions and said to them
> that here was a reactor being built next to a metropolitan area
> where workers in other factories would be subjected to the harm-
> ful radiation effects if there should be a breakdown in the La-
> goona reactor. I felt that we should not permit the reactor to be
> constructed until we knew it to be safe.[1]

Senator Anderson apparently was concerned because the
Atomic Energy Commission, in going ahead with the Fermi
reactor, acted despite a report from its own Advisory Committee on Reactor Safeguards, which was at best noncommittal
about the safety of proceeding. Several unions responded to
Anderson's plea, and extended litigation began. A federal court
voided the license which the AEC had granted for construction
of the reactor, but the Supreme Court, in a divided decision,
reversed the lower court's action — and construction resumed.
Justice Douglas, with Justice Black concurring, worded a very
strong dissent, called the AEC's interpretation of the Atomic
Energy Act "a light-hearted approach to the most awesome, the
most deadly, the most dangerous process that man has ever
conceived." [2]

Why so much controversy over this particular reactor? Fermi
was to be the prototype of what industry still feels is going to
be the coming thing in reactors, the "sodium-cooled fast
breeder," in the jargon of the trade. And in spite of Fermi's

near disastrous failure, all reactor manufacturers hope to begin construction on new fast breeder prototypes by about 1970. By 1980, some firms hope to have full-scale commercial power plants under construction; eventually, it is believed, this and other advanced reactor types will completely replace the current form of reactor.

This optimism is based chiefly on the hope of lowered fuel costs in the fast breeder. Fuel costs in the present commercial atomic plants may be as much as or more than the cost of the reactor itself; the fast breeder, on the other hand, may eventually burn plutonium it has itself produced instead of the very expensive uranium 235 used in other commercial reactors.

Most modern reactors use a design very different from that of the Fermi plant. In a typical reactor, such as the Quad-Cities plant in Illinois on the Mississippi River, uranium 235 and uranium 238 are mixed in tiny pellets which are packed into metal tubes about a half-inch thick and several feet long. These long, delicate rods are then arranged in rectangular packages about five inches wide and fourteen feet long; 724 of these "subassemblies" are put together to form the core of the reactor. Such a core contains 362,000 pounds of uranium oxide.

This enormous mass of uranium is at a temperature of 1000°F. Millions of gallons of water flow through the core, between the long, thin fuel elements, cooling it; the water boils immediately and steam is drawn off from the core to turn a turbine, which can produce 715,000 kilowatts of electricity, enough power to supply a city of one million.

Within the core of the reactor, the nuclei of uranium 235 atoms are fissioning; when a nucleus shatters, it produces typically two or three neutrons. Some neutrons may collide repeatedly with the atoms of water flowing through the core until their speed is slowed by a factor of thousands. The slowed neutrons may then be absorbed by other nuclei of uranium 235, which absorb slow neutrons much more easily than the fast ones.

Other neutrons may escape from the reactor entirely or may be absorbed unproductively by uranium 238, uranium 235, the cooling water, the metal walls of the fuel element, or any of the many impurities present in the fuel and the reactor materials.

Still other neutrons may be absorbed by the nucleus of uranium 238 in such a fashion that it is then converted to plutonium.

After months of operation, the fuel is removed from the reactor and transported to a processing plant, where it is dissolved in acid and the plutonium and impurities are removed. Ideally, the recovered plutonium can be used to make new reactor fuel; this is what happens in a "breeder" reactor. Unfortunately, in the kind of reactor just described, typical of those now being built, far less fuel is made than is burned.

This is because only two or three neutrons are produced in each uranium fission. One must be used to keep the chain reaction going. If one escapes or is captured unproductively, then there are simply not enough neutrons available to convert uranium 238 to plutonium at the desired rate. The Fermi reactor is an attempt to solve this problem.

In the Quad-Cities reactor, the cooling water will act also as a moderator, slowing down the neutrons. In Fermi, the moderator is removed and the neutrons are not slowed. At higher neutron speeds, "unproductive" capture by U-235 and plutonium is reduced. More neutrons are available for transforming U-238 into plutonium, so that more plutonium is produced than the uranium 235 that has been burned. The reactor has then been able to "breed" fuel and is called a breeder reactor. In theory, one and one half pounds of fuel could be produced for each pound burned.

Fermi achieves further conservation of neutrons by making the core highly compact, with a very high percentage of fissionable material (uranium 235 or plutonium) in the fuel. This further acts to maintain the high energy of the neutrons. The compact core is surrounded by a "blanket" of uranium 238 which is slowly converted to plutonium. A "fast breeder" reactor core which produced as much power as the Quad-Cities plant might be only four or five feet high, instead of fourteen or fifteen.

Because it is so much more compact, the fast reactor must be cooled by a more efficient cooling medium than water; liquid sodium is usually used, although this is very difficult and hazardous material to handle, as it burns in air or water.

When fast breeders were first designed, it was thought that uranium was a scarce element, and this was an added factor in making them attractive. Subsequent explorations have uncovered vast reserves of uranium in this country, in Canada, and elsewhere. For a time, in fact, uranium exploration ran far ahead of the demand, and in the early years of this decade a number of mines had to be closed, and the AEC accumulated stockpiles far in excess of its needs in order to prevent complete collapse of the uranium mining industry which had developed. The present rash of reactor orders, coming unexpectedly, has created a sudden new demand which may strain the present supply, but new exploration is again being conducted with something of the heat of the earlier uranium rush, and supplies will probably keep pace with demand, whether or not fast breeders are developed to conserve uranium. Some predict a

rise in uranium prices, as reactor expansion outstrips new mining of high-grade ores, but this could easily be offset by an eas-
ing of import restrictions, by release of the AEC's stockpile, or
by advances in mining or extraction technology which would
make lower-grade ores available. A recent industry-sponsored
study concludes: "Sufficient uranium is available in known deposits to permit electric power companies to proceed with plans
for additional (water-moderated) power reactors for a number
of years ahead. The results of current exploration efforts should
become apparent well before 1971. . . ." [3]

With these vast new reserves, it was possible to give emphasis to the presently popular water-moderated reactors which
burn much more fuel than they produce; despite their uneco-
nomical use of fuel, water cooled and moderated reactors are
far more easy to build and operate safely and reliably — and
are far cheaper in terms of initial cost.

Revenue from the sale of plutonium for weapons had originally been expected to offset the high building and design costs
of the Fermi plant; eventually, if the design succeeded, plutonium would also be sold for fuel in other reactors. But the government's demand for plutonium has slackened considerably,
as the arms race has slowed, and can be met at government
plants in Richland, Washington, and Aiken, South Carolina.

Despite the apparent abundance of uranium to fuel water-
cooled reactors and the absence of the expected demand for
plutonium, and in the face of the dramatic failure of the Fermi
reactor, fast reactors are again being proposed. At a meeting
of the American Nuclear Society in San Francisco, April 10–12,
1967, several firms in this country, Great Britain, France, Italy
and Germany unveiled plans for various types of fast reactors;
the British seem to have the lead in this field, and their proto-

type is already being built and is expected to be operating by 1970. The U.S.S.R. is also building a prototype, and Russian scientists were expected at the meeting but did not appear.

The reason for this resurgent interest is economic; fast breeders may burn the plutonium they themselves produce, obviating the need for enriched uranium 235 fuel which contributes so much to the cost of present commercial reactors. An additional factor is that only the United States, the U.S.S.R., China, Britain and France have the capability to separate the uranium isotopes; other countries wishing to develop nuclear power are therefore dependent on foreign supplies of fuel unless they can develop plutonium producing and burning reactors. This is probably an important factor in the German and Italian programs.

Yet, despite their possible economic advantage over the presently used water reactors, fast reactors pose serious safety problems. In November 1954, a conference was held in the offices of the Detroit Edison Company, attended by some of the most prominent physicists in the country. The proceedings of this conference were classified by the AEC. It was devoted in part to a discussion of the problems which had arisen in the operation of the Experimental Breeder Reactor I, the prototype of the Enrico Fermi reactor. There was considerable discussion during the conference of the possibility that an accident would cause the highly dangerous uranium 235 core to reassemble in a "prompt critical" configuration — one which would undergo rapid and uncontrolled chain reaction like that in a nuclear weapon. At one point, Dr. Zinn, who headed the design of EBR-I, said:

> If you do melt the central section of the reactor and it runs down the tubes as Dr. Bethe suggested, does this give you an increase

in reactivity which is greater than the amount that you can subtract with your control rods? . . . If you couldn't do it with your
rods, you would be in bad shape.

Chairman Bethe: Right. I suppose it would increase the reactivity
some.[4]

At another point in the conference, the question of fuel melting
or warping to create a more critical configuration was brought
up again, and the chairman of the conference, Dr. Hans Bethe,
asked,

Suppose that it did. What would happen?

Dr. Zinn: It is very probable, when it does that, it will disassemble the machine.[5]

"Disassemble the machine" was a euphemism for a small nuclear explosion. By the end of the conference everyone was
agreed that such an event, particularly if for some reason the
fuel melted, and subsequently ran together in a more dangerous configuration, was possible, and that the fast reactor was
so new and complex that all the possible causes of such an accident could not be foreseen.

Some at the conference expressed the opinion that a prototype fast reactor should be built in a remote location before a
commercial plant was attempted. This point of view was also
put forward by AEC Commissioner Willard Libby at the 1955
"Section 202" hearings before the Joint Committee. Commissioner Libby said that the construction of a fast breeder in a
populated zone "requires that the safety of this type of reactor

be determined experimentally . . . by construction of a reasonably similar prototype in an isolated area."

This approach was opposed by another at the conference, which eventually won out: The way to build fast reactors would be to provide them with containment structures which could resist the force of an explosion and so keep radiation, in the event of an accident, from reaching the outside and the public.

The fears as to the possibility of a serious accident in a fast reactor were partly justified a year after this secret conference. In November of 1955, an experiment was conducted in the AEC's experimental breeder reactor (EBR-I), to identify the source of an unsafe characteristic: a "positive temperature co-efficient." The reactor was to be run briefly with the coolant (an alloy of sodium and potassium) shut off. The operator was instructed to shut off the reactor with the fast shut-down rods, but instead used the slower control rods. The reactor did not shut down, but instead the power went on increasing. Safety measures were instituted, but despite these procedures, the temperature within the core rose within seconds to more than 2000°F. The fuel and its steel cladding in the center of the core melted:

> . . . contact with coolant eventually chilled and froze the mass [of molten uranium 235], blocking further downward movement. . . . The melted and refrozen material . . . formed a pot of sorts which tended to hold and collect the materials [fuel and cladding] falling from the upper part of the core. . . . Partially melted rods from above apparently dropped into the eutectic mass below.[6]

Fortunately, no serious damage to persons resulted from this accident; the reactor core was damaged beyond repair. It was demonstrated quite clearly, however, that when an accident in a fast reactor caused a meltdown of fuel, the U-235 could collect in fairly large quantities in one place. In a very large reactor, this could have catastrophic implications. In 1965, a conference on fast breeder technology was again held at Argonne Laboratories, and the record of those discussions shows that there was still no agreement on how serious the resultant explosion might be in a given reactor, nor were the participants sure that the possible causes of such an accident were all known. Yet in January of 1966, the Enrico Fermi reactor, the only commercial fast breeder ever built, after years of malfunction, was run up to full power for the first time; by October of that year, it had suffered a serious accident.[7]

In October of 1966, preparations were made to restart the Fermi plant, which had been shut down because of the latest in a long series of difficulties. The difficulty this time had been in the steam generator, where the heat carried by the sodium from the reactor is used to make steam. On the evening of October 4, 1966, the technicians in the control room in a separate building adjusted their controls, and control rods withdrew slightly from the faraway reactor core, hidden by tons of steel and concrete shielding.

By 11 P.M., the reactor was operating at a low power level; it was maintained at this level while the tons of sodium flowing through the core slowly heated to a temperature of 550°F. Instruments in the control room indicated that the reactor was operating normally. At eight o'clock the following morning, October 5, the operators of the reactor began the long and complex procedures which must precede operating the reactor at a higher power. The plan was to increase the heat being generated by the reactor, in order to test the newly-repaired steam generator and steam system.

A minor malfunction was found in a valve in the steam generator, and the program was delayed. At 1:45 P.M., the slow withdrawal of control rods to increase reactor power began again; within fifteen minutes, another small malfunction had appeared in a pump, and the reactor was damped again. A replacement pump was switched on, the slow increase in power began again. By 3 P.M., the reactor was producing 20,000 kilowatts of heat energy, still only a small fraction of its maximum capacity of 200,000 kilowatts.

At this point, the reactor operator noticed an abnormality in one of his instruments measuring the change in neutron production in the reactor core; the signal from the instrument became erratic. Reactors have their own personalities — the operator had observed this particular fluctuation in his instruments many times before, and often at the same time of day — 3 P.M. He ended automatic control of the reactor and switched to manual control for a while. The erratic signal disappeared, and automatic increase of reactor power began again.

Five minutes later, when the power level had reached 34,000 kilowatts, the erratic signal appeared again. A staff member present noticed that the control rods seemed to have been drawn farther out than was normal. Stepping to the back of the control panel, he examined the recorders which registered temperature at different points in the distant reactor core. At two points the temperature seemed higher than normal.

At almost the same moment, radiation alarms sounded from the reactor building and from detectors elsewhere in the plant. Automatic devices immediately sealed off the buildings in which the alarms had sounded; no personnel were present at the time.

By this time the power increase had halted; at 3:20 P.M., almost half an hour after the first abnormalities had been noticed, the reactor was scrammed — six safety rods were inserted their full distance, completely halting the chain reaction because of their absorption of neutrons.

The only visible signs of the accident were the abnormal meter readings in the control room and the automatic radiation alarms. High radiation levels were occurring in the plant buildings, but their cause was not known.

A meeting was held at the plant immediately. In order to try to determine what had happened, automatic samples of the liquid sodium coolant and of the argon gas in the sodium system were made (sodium reacts violently with air, and therefore the sodium system is filled with the inert gas, argon). Large amounts of radioactive fission products in these samples made it clear that a portion of the reactor fuel had melted. Once this had been established, there was great concern, for the possibility of further, and far more serious, accidents existed. Walter J. McCarthy, Jr., Assistant General Manager of the Power Reactor Development Corporation, who was present at this meeting, later stated that the possibility of such a secondary accident was "a terrifying thought." [8]

The long, thin fuel rods of the Fermi core contained about half a ton of uranium 235 — enough to make forty Hiroshima-sized atom bombs. These pins are arranged in 105 subassemblies, each composed of 140 pins. The sodium coolant must be pumped through the narrow gaps between fuel pins.

The cause of the accident was thought to be some interference with the flow of coolant among the fuel pins, and this has

proved to be the case. In September of 1967, a specially designed forty-foot flexible periscope was wormed down through
the reactor's innards and was used to sight, and then to photograph, a small object lying at the very bottom of the reactor.
This object, which in early blurred photographs looked like a
flattened beer can, has now been identified as a piece of crumpled sheet metal pulled loose from the reactor itself. On October 5, 1966, this object probably blocked one or two of the
openings which admit cooling sodium to the reactor core.
Within minutes, a large portion of the fuel in two subassemblies melted, and the assemblies themselves buckled, forcing
nearby elements out of line. The reactor was apparently shut
down in time to prevent severe damage to other portions of
the fuel.[9]

It took more than a year to identify the cause of the accident.
The presence of a crumpled bit of metal inside the delicate
mechanism of the reactor seemed inexplicable. The mystery
of its presence, and the difficulty of solving it, were not fully
explained until February 5, 1968. Milton Shaw, Director of the
AEC's reactor division, was testifying before the Joint Committee on Atomic Energy, explaining that within the previous
week, the culpable piece of metal had been identified as a portion of the reactor itself. Congressman Craig Hosmer interrupted:

Now, there is more to the story, is there not?

Let me put it this way, then. I understand that late in the construction of the reactor, around 1959, the designers decided to
cover the bottom of the vessel with a zirconium sheet as an added
safeguard to prevent fuel melt from going through the bottom of
the vessel, anticipating this Chinese syndrome. . . .

As we have seen, in case of an accident, the molten fuel might dissolve its way right through the reactor vessel, and anything beneath it, presumably "right down to China." The bottom of the Fermi reactor vessel was therefore coated with zirconium which, it was hoped, would hold the molten fuel. Projecting upward from the center of the zirconium sheet laid at the vessel's bottom was a cone about a foot high. During normal operation, the function of this cone was to direct the flow of coolant upward into the reactor core. During an accident, it was hoped, reactor fuel falling on this cone might be dispersed. The question arose of whether this cone should not also be covered with zirconium.

Representative Hosmer: Now, I understand that APDA (Atomic Power Development Associates), received from Al Amorosi a memo which said, in effect, that it would be easier to put zirc shrouds over the cone than to have to justify not doing so to the ACRS [Advisory Committee on Reactor Safeguards] when it came time for an operating license.

Is there such a memorandum in existence, to your knowledge?

Mr. Shaw: I understand there is, Mr. Hosmer, but your research staff seems to be much ahead of mine.

Representative Hosmer: Based on that, I understand that they hurriedly rounded up some zirconium sheet and fabricated these six triangular pieces, and they were bolted on the cone, maybe tack welded, I don't know, at least three bolts were used in each, and that the total cost of these sheets was about a hundred bucks.

Mr. Shaw: We understand that this was a last minute decision, hurriedly made, to put the zirconium pieces in.

We also understand that these additions were not shown on the final construction "as built" drawings. This became one of the problems related to identifying whether the object was part of the reactor or an object foreign to the reactor.

This again gets to the point that when you take shortcuts like this you must be prepared for the consequences.

In this case, the consequences were the accident of October 5, 1966, when one of the six triangular sheets of zirconium, less than a foot long, broke free of the flow-guide cone, and blocked the flow of coolant to a portion of the core.

In concluding this exchange, Mr. Hosmer put a final question:

One other thing I want to ask you, Mr. Shaw. In your judgment, was this cover on the flow regulator really needed, in the first place?

Mr. Shaw: I cannot answer that, Mr. Hosmer. . . . I think these are the kinds of engineering decisions that can go either way and still come out right.

Or wrong, one is tempted to add. The fast reactor seems to be the sort of mechanism in which the devices employed to forestall one sort of accident simply precipitate another. In any case, the Fermi reactor is now out of operation until at least the end of 1968, while its owners try to decide what to do about the remaining five triangles of zirconium, any one of which could break free and cause another, and perhaps more severe accident. Removing them will be inordinately difficult. And are they needed or not? The melting of fuel in a fast reactor is a disturbing risk.

The possibility that Walter McCarthy called a "terrifying thought" and that preoccupied the meeting after the accident was that a large quantity of fuel had melted and then recongealed when the reactor was shut down. Those at the meeting feared that enough uranium had recongealed so that a disturbance of the core — by an attempt to remove the damaged fuel, for example — would jar it into a critical mass too great to be controlled by the control rods, which were already at their maximum.

The result could have been an explosion — nowhere near as great as that of a nuclear weapon, but perhaps great enough to rupture the steel and concrete containment structure of the reactor. A large portion of the radioactive gases held within the core would then have been released to the atmosphere, and would have drifted uncontrolled with the wind. The huge quantities of radioactivity involved, and the proximity of Detroit, made such a prospect terrifying indeed.

No attempt was made to investigate the reactor core for a month, for fear of a second and more terrible accident. "It's one of those accidents the consequences [of which] are so terrible the probability has to be very very small," Walter McCarthy later said, describing the intensive study and calculation which went on during that month. When the operators of the reactor and the AEC felt assured that no further damage would occur, attempts to retrieve the damaged fuel were begun. To everyone's enormous relief, nothing did happen.

Some idea of the size of that relief can be gained by reading a report dated July, 1957, titled "A Report on the Possible Effects on the Surrounding Population of an Assumed Release of Fission Products into the Atmosphere from a 300 Megawatt [300,000 kilowatt] Nuclear Reactor Located at Lagoona Beach,

Michigan." This report was prepared at the Engineering Research Institute of the University of Michigan, for the Atomic Power Development Associates. APDA was the research, design and development organization established by the prospective owners and operators of the Enrico Fermi reactor; the membership of the latter (Power Reactor Development Corporation) and APDA were almost identical.

The report produced by APDA was very much like the AEC's WASH-740 report on the "Theoretical Consequences of Hypothetical Accidents." The two reports appeared at the same time, although each was prepared independently of the other. As in WASH-740, the APDA report did not delve very much into possible causes of an accident, but simply tried to ascertain the maximum possible damage to the surrounding population if a drastic accident were to occur. Unlike WASH-740, the APDA report considered a reactor in a specific location — the site of the Fermi plant. And unlike WASH-740, the APDA staff was willing to consider the worst conceivable circumstance, rather than those which seemed most likely. Thus the APDA report includes consideration of the case in which all of the radioactive wastes contained in the reactor fuel are released to the air, presumably after an explosion has burst the reactor's containment structures. WASH-740's worst case was the release of only 50 percent of fission products.

APDA also considered a range of weather conditions including the most highly unfavorable, a thermal inversion lasting for many hours, with a slow steady wind blowing radioactivity in the direction of the most populous areas of Detroit. These weather conditions were estimated to occur during about 5.4 days in each year. Assuming that these weather conditions prevailed at the time of the accident, and that the radioactive cloud released from the reactor lost none of its virulence by depositing fallout while it drifted, the report estimated these damages:

One hundred and thirty-three thousand people would receive fatal doses of radiation (450 roentgens or more); 181,000 would receive immediate injuries (150 roentgens or more); 245,000 would receive doses which could result in long-term injury, such as increased incidence of cancer, shortened lifetimes or hereditary defects (25 roentgens or more). No attempt was made to estimate property damage.[10]

It is constantly, and rightly, emphasized that the probability of such a disastrous accident is low. This does not mean that such an accident will not happen. Even one a hundred times less severe — releasing only one percent of the reactor's accumulated wastes — could result in 420 deaths, according to the APDA study. Accidents do happen, and it is in their nature that their causes and consequences may not be entirely foreseen.

The accident which did happen at Fermi in 1966 is particularly disturbing when we examine the portion of the application to construct the Fermi reactor called the "Hazards Summary Report," prepared by the Power Reactor Development Company (PRDC), the consortium of public utilities and equipment manufacturers which built and operates the Fermi reactor.[11]

As is required by the AEC, the Hazards Summary Report contains a section describing the "maximum credible accident." This is an attempt to specify an accident which is not expected to occur, but which is the worst which the designers feel could occur. Page 603.15 of the Hazards Summary states:

The maximum credible accident in the Fermi reactor is the melting of some or all of the fuel in one core subassembly, due to either complete or partial plugging of the nozzle of that subassembly, or to a flow restriction within the subassembly. . . .

As a result of the October 5 accident, fuel in at least two subassemblies melted. Some damage was done to at least two other subassemblies.

The reactor would probably be shut down automatically as a result of the reactivity loss due to the melting of the fuel. . . .

This did not occur on October 5; the reactor was shut down manually.

. . . fission products . . . would have been released to the primary coolant system, and . . . the inert gas system. Since these systems are normally radioactive and sealed, there would be *no additional outward effect* caused by the addition of fission products from melted fuel [emphasis added].

In fact, there were outward effects, including high radiation levels in the reactor containment and fission product detection buildings. It is fortunate that there was leakage of radioactivity, for it was the sounding of radiation alarms which prompted the shutdown of the reactor. Had there been "no additional outward effect," the reactor operators might not have shut down the reactor until more serious damage had been done.

In short, the accident that happened was a bit worse than the "maximum credible accident," and the results worse than foreseen by its designers. More than one subassembly was damaged, the reactor did not shut down, and there was some release of radioactivity. It should be emphasized that the "maximum credible accident" was assumed to occur at a power level fifteen times that at which the actual accident occurred. In other words, the actual accident was not only "incredible," it might have been far worse.

Whether a disastrous accident like that described in the 1957 report could have happened remains a matter for speculation. Despite the confidence of its designers, the Fermi reactor is surrounded with a steel and concrete containment which is designed to withstand the force of an explosion of 600 pounds of TNT. The question of whether a core meltdown could produce an explosion greater than this, and whether the containment would in fact completely contain such an explosion, is the subject of a great deal of detailed calculation and educated guesswork. Since an experimental test of these calculations would require the destruction of at least one extremely expensive reactor, they are likely to remain unconfirmed unless and until a still more "incredible" accident happens.

Fermi, in any case, is out of commission for some time, and perhaps for good. But, at the same American Nuclear Society meeting in April of 1967 at which the Fermi accident was first described in detail,[12] four major American firms announced plans to build new prototype fast breeder reactors. General Electric, Westinghouse, Atomics International and General Dynamics Corporation all presented different designs; (Babcock and Wilcox have since made public their fast reactor plans); GE is farther down the road than the other firms, and intends to build sodium-cooled fast breeders, of the same general type as the Fermi reactor. The companies plan construction of prototypes roughly the size of Fermi's original design in two or three years, and aim toward commercial plants in the 1980's. These would be 1,000,000-kilowatt plants.

Plans for operating plants five times Fermi's size only fifteen years from now may seem a little precipitous (even a proved reactor type requires seven years from the time of the order to the manufacturer to the date of operation). Despite complaints of foot-dragging from industry, however, the AEC has accepted this schedule in rough outline. The official program for fast breeder development is at present being circulated for comment, and will appear late in 1968. The 1967 AEC report[13] to the President stated: "It does not appear that a prudent commitment to build the first U.S. demonstration plant can be made before 1969. . . ." Members of the Joint Congressional Committee on Atomic Energy seem to feel the program is not being pushed vigorously enough, however, and this position is apparently prompted by the same fear that spurs industry — the threat of foreign competition in the growing nuclear reactor market. In a guest editorial in *Nucleonics,* a trade journal, Craig Hosmer, ranking Republican House member of the Joint Committee on Atomic Energy asks:

"In the 1980's will U.S. utilities order fast breeder reactors from the U.K.?" He goes on to criticize severely the AEC's program in this field, and concludes, "Our fast breeder commercialization schedule must be telescoped to 1980 or earlier if the AEC is to serve the nation's nuclear needs on time and preserve our lead in nuclear technology." [14]

There is enormous pressure on the AEC from both industry and Congress to accelerate the fast breeder program. Several reactor manufacturers have already formed joint agreements with groups of private utilities (Detroit Edison, principal architect of the Fermi project, is prominent among these) to finance design and construction of prototypes, presumably with federal assistance. In 1968 or 1969, applications will probably be made to the AEC for construction permits and for funds.

This schedule has not been set back noticeably by the accident at Fermi, yet the fact that severity of the October 5 accident somewhat exceeded expectations diminishes confidence in the assurances of the safety of fast breeders given by reactor engineers and by the AEC. The potential economic benefits of breeders, and the threat of foreign competition, seem to outweigh the potential hazards, at least for the AEC and Joint Committee.

In a recent address Wilfred E. Johnson, a member of the AEC, commented on the economic benefits of fast reactors in terms of lowered electric bills. A saving of a tenth of a cent per kilowatt hour, Johnson said, "which seems entirely feasible, will by the year 2000, mean a saving to the public each year of four billion dollars." He estimated the cost of developing the program at two billion dollars, to be borne largely by the Federal Government.[15]

There is a large question mark in the economic equation, however, which perhaps accounts more than anything else for the AEC's present comparatively conservative policy on fast breeders. This is the question of reliability.

Commercial power plants are being built ever larger; the first commercial fast breeders will have a capacity of a million kilowatts of electricity or more, enough to supply a good-sized city. The construction of such large central plants is made possible by the increasing connectedness of power systems, which means that when power from a large plant is not needed locally (as for instance late at night) it can be shipped to far distant points. By the 1980's, perhaps all of this country and even most of the North American continent will be interconnected in a single huge power grid.

The failure of a very large generating plant and its removal from service for an extended period of time, however, could cause a severe and extended power shortage.

There is, therefore, an increasing emphasis on power plant reliability, and so far the sodium-cooled reactor has shown itself to be singularly unreliable. This stems largely from the difficulty of handling molten sodium at high temperatures — typically at about 1000°F. This material reacts explosively with air and water, and yet in a power plant, the heat from the sodium must somehow be transferred to water to produce the steam needed to run turbines which in turn drive the electric generators. The difficulty of achieving this feat has plagued Fermi and other plants like it. The reactor at Hallam, Nebraska, intended to improve sodium-cooling technology, has finally been abandoned, after years of difficulties. Hallam and Fermi were the only two sodium-cooled reactors to be placed in commercial power grids in this country, and both were out of operation during most of their lifetimes because of difficulties with the sodium systems.

Only time and expensive experimentation will tell whether these difficulties can be overcome. The Experimental Breeder Reactor II at Arco, Idaho, is the only remaining sodium-cooled fast reactor in this country; other test facilities are under construction or are being planned. Whether on industry's short schedule, or on the AEC's slightly longer one, this country seems firmly committed to a $2 billion fast breeder development program. In its 1967 report to the President, the AEC stated:

> Emphasis is being placed on the high gain breeders as recommended in the 1962 report. In particular, the program for development of the liquid metal-cooled [sodium] fast breeder has been substantially augmented. . . .[16]

. . . The sodium-cooled fast breeder choice is based on potential economies, industrial and worldwide interest, technological experience, and its capability to conserve uranium resources.[17]

. . . Plans are being developed for the introduction of a number of sodium-cooled fast breeder demonstration plants to be built during the 1970's.[18]

The AEC's fiscal 1968 budget includes $71,350,000 for development of fast breeder reactors.

The growing commitment to fast breeder reactors as "the next step" in the reactor program may be premature, as the real first step — commercial water-moderated plants — has not yet really been taken. The first of these which are expected to be commercially feasible (at San Onofre, California, and Nine Mile Point in New York) went into operation early in 1968. It will be some time before enough experience has been gained to judge whether or not their predicted economic advantages are to materialize. For most of the country, even more advanced (and larger) plants will be required to compete economically with coal-burning plants, and the first of these 800,-000- to 1,000,000-kilowatt plants will not go into operation until around 1970. All reactors which are presently in operation are considered experimental, and are far from being economically competitive with conventional plants.

Fast breeders will, therefore, have to compete, not with current electric power plants, but with the 1,000,000-kilowatt plants of the future, and to do so, they will have to be at least as large. This fivefold increase over the size of the Fermi plant brings with it a similar increase in hazard. In an article which appeared in August, 1967, Dr. Edward Teller wrote:

In order for [a fast breeder reactor to] work economically in a sufficiently big power-producing unit, it probably needs quite a bit more than one ton of plutonium. I do not like the hazard involved. . . .

If you put together two tons of plutonium in a breeder, one-tenth of one percent of this material could become critical. . . .

In an accident involving a plutonium reactor, a couple of tons of plutonium can melt. I don't think anybody can foresee where 1 or 2 or 5 percent of this plutonium will find itself and how it will get mixed with some of the other material. A small fraction of the original charge can become a great hazard.[19]

When fast breeder reactors grow to the size which Dr. Teller discusses, a whole new class of hazards appears. Dr. Teller touched on these. Writing in 1964, Walter J. McCarthy, whom we have already met, and Dr. David Okrent, past chairman of the Advisory Committee on Reactor Safeguards, describe another possibility:

Under a number of circumstances, one part of a large reactor core may heat, even to the melting point, while other areas are relatively unaffected, as seems to have happened in the Fermi accident. As in that case, blockage of a liquid coolant nozzle might cause a temperature increase in one portion of the reactor so great that the fuel in that area would melt; local melting, in one portion of the core, could be followed by the collecting and refreezing of the fuel in a prompt critical configuration and a mild explosion equal perhaps to several hundred pounds of TNT, which could be contained by the reactor structures.

The possibility that only a portion of such a reactor melts, undergoes a relatively mild explosion which acts to compress other parts of the core extremely rapidly, thus instigating a very much larger energy release, needs further investigation.[20]

Compressing large amounts of fissionable material by means of an explosion is precisely what happens in an atomic bomb. This possibility does indeed seem to call for further study. A "very much larger energy release" could be a full-scale nuclear explosion.

VIII

WHY REACTORS?

SOMEDAY COAL, OIL AND NATURAL GAS will be in short supply. The amount of these fossil fuels present in the earth's crust is limited; our consumption of them increases at an ever-growing rate. At some point we must face the need to replace this source of energy on which all of industrial society depends. How soon will that time come?

> . . . we cannot long maintain our present rate of increase of [coal] consumption . . . the check to our progress must become perceptible within a century from the present time . . . the cost of fuel must rise, perhaps within a lifetime, to a rate injurious to our commercial and manufacturing supremacy. . . ." [1]

> . . . the United States may be able for the next few years (five or ten) to meet the increased demands for petroleum and . . . thereafter the production may remain stationary for another short period, following which there will be a period of twenty or more years during which production will decrease from year to year, while consumption increases, causing greater and greater imports from foreign fields and higher prices, culminating in acute shortage.[2]

> Reserves of such "low-cost" . . . fossil fuels are small by comparison with the maximum plausible demands. . . . new sources

of low-cost energy must begin to carry some of the load by A.D.
1975 or sooner, and much of it by A.D. 2000, if we are not to run
the risk of seeing economic systems throughout the non-Commu-
nist world falter in the face of steeply rising costs of energy.[3]

The first of the quoted paragraphs was written in 1865, the
second in 1916. The third quotation is from an Atomic Energy
Commission study published in 1953. All three of these prophecies have proved incorrect. Prophecies of doom have a long
history: the earliest scholarly warning that coal was about to
be exhausted (that the author has been able to find) dates from
the late eighteenth century. Yet coal prices at present are dropping, and current estimates are that they will remain stable or
drop further for the rest of this century. Domestic United
States oil is heavily protected from competition from foreign
imports; natural gas sales continue to expand. Despite the
many warnings of scarcity which we continue to hear, there
seems to be an abundance of fossil fuel.

How much coal, oil and gas do we really have? Estimates
vary widely and, oddly enough, seem to increase with time. In
1953, Palmer Putnam, acting as consultant to the AEC, estimated that the United States had reserves of fuel recoverable at
"substantially present costs" of 4 Q. ("Q" is the usual unit for
estimating such large quantities of fuel; it is a measure of the
energy content of fuel equal to a quintillion British Thermal
Units.) Putnam quotes another estimate made in 1952 by Ayres
and Scarlott which gives the "minimum plausible ultimate" reserves of coal, oil and gas, in the United States, as "about 5.2
Q." These figures were alarming, for Putnam estimated that
the United States economy would require at least 4.3 Q by the
year 2000. Unless other sources of energy were found, all of

the country's economical fuels would be exhausted in this century.[4]

By 1962, things looked a little brighter. Putnam had predicted: "peak production of oil-gas may be reached between 1955 and 1960.

"Peak production of good coking bituminous coal may be reached before 1960."

In 1962, ten years after those words were written, coal prices were still dropping, and coal, oil and gas production were all increasing. The Atomic Energy Commission issued its report to the President on civilian nuclear power, in which it summarized some more recent estimates of fuel reserves. These ranged from 26 Q (U.S. Geological Survey) to 130 Q (Department of the Interior).[5] The lower figure indicated that fuel resources would be exhausted in a hundred years; 130 Q, on the other hand, would not be exhausted for two centuries despite rapidly increasing rates of consumption.

Shortly after this report appeared, President Kennedy requested the heads of nine federal departments to undertake a comprehensive study of "the development and utilization of our total energy resources." A steering committee was formed, and it in turn established an Energy Study Group under the leadership of Dr. Ali Bulent Cambel. A year later this Group produced the exhaustive "Energy R&D and National Progress," the most thorough and authoritative examination of the nation's energy resources and prospects ever undertaken.[6]

Basing its recommendations on the detailed findings of the Cambel report, the Steering Committee issued its own report in 1966.[7] They estimated total United States fuel resources as between 1,040 and 1,064 Q.[8] Consumption was expected to rise to slightly less than one-seventh Q per year by the end of this century. At that rate, fuel resources in this country would be adequate for something over seven thousand years.

What accounts for the discrepancies among the various estimates of fuel resources? Putnam and other writers, even today, see the almost immediate exhaustion of our coal, oil and gas; the federal interdepartmental study shows resources adequate for thousands of years. Most of these authors, nevertheless, work with the same basic knowledge of geology and with the reported reserves of mining companies and their estimates of future discoveries.

The reason for the differences among estimates is simply a matter of fuel cost. In 1865, W. Stanley Jevons, M.A., L.L.D., F.R.S., first published *The Coal Question: An Inquiry Concerning the Progress of the Nation, and the Probable Exhaustion of our Coal-mines,* a book, quoted earlier, which has become a minor classic of economics. Mr. Jevons, who, among other honors held the Stanley Jevons Chair at Owens College, Manchester, feared not the actual exhaustion of coal, but its increasing price:

> It is shown that in all probability there is no precise physical limit of deep mining, but that the growing difficulties of management and extraction of coal in a very deep mine must greatly enhance its price. . . .
>
> Should the consumption multiply for rather more than a century at the same rate, the average depth of our coal-mines would be 4,000 feet, and the average price of coal much higher than the highest price now paid for the finest kinds of coal.
>
> It is thence simply inferred that we cannot long continue our present rate of progress.[9]

This is precisely the same argument made by Putnam one hundred years later, in his report to the AEC which has influenced so much rhetoric about the need for atomic energy. Putnam made what are still reasonably accurate estimates of fuel resources which were "recoverable substantially at present costs by present methods." "Present" refers to 1950. The booby trap here, as it was in Mr. Jevons' prophecies of doom a century before, is in the phrase "present methods." Jevons could not foresee the great advances in coal-mining technology which made it possible to mine cheaply coal seams which were simply inaccessible to mid-nineteenth-century technology. Putnam similarly writes off this country's huge reserves of oil shale (as much as 1600 Q in the Cambel report), because in 1950 there was no cheap way of mining this resource. "If we are to avoid the risk of seriously increased real unit costs of energy in the United States, then new low-cost sources should be ready to pick up much of the load by 1975 or sooner." Putnam could write these words in 1953 because the great advances in coal-mining and transportation techniques which have brought coal prices down over the last fifteen years were not yet making themselves evident. If coal and oil costs had not remained low, however, only a slight increase would have spurred the development of the oil shale mining technology, tapping the greatest supply of fuel in this country or in the world.

Oil shale is a sedimentary rock whose polished surface is reminiscent of mahogany. Trapped between the twin layers of the rock is a hydrocarbon, kerogen, which can be converted to oil plus a solid residue, coke, by heating; rich ores may be as much as 65 percent hydrocarbon. The richest presently-known deposit is the Green River Shale, which extends over 16,000 square miles in Wyoming, Colorado and Utah. In order to release the oil, shale must be crushed and then heated; the liquid released is petroleum much like that which comes from wells.

Present mining methods (oil shale is used in a few parts of the world, and a recent Canadian project is mining the similar Athabasca tar sands) involve digging the rock out of the ground, crushing it and then heating or "retorting" it to extract the oil. This is an expensive process, and furthermore produces huge quantities of crushed-rock waste which must somehow be disposed of. A potentially more promising method is "in situ retorting." This involves detonating explosives in the oil shale underground, accomplishing the crushing of a large volume of rock. A zone of controlled burning, regulated by compressed air, could be driven through the zone of fractured rock. The kerogen, heated by the advancing front, would decompose into oil and coke. The oil would drain to the bottom of the region of the crushed rock, and be pumped to the surface. The coke remaining in the rock would provide fuel to continue the retorting. This process would avoid the scarring of the landscape and the problem of disposing of the crushed-rock wastes, which remain underground.

The Department of the Interior has recently begun doing research on in situ retorting, and so has the Atomic Energy Commission. An explosion of a small nuclear weapon underground might release huge quantities of oil from shale. According to a recent news story, "One Atomic Energy Commission official has predicted that when this happens the [oil] companies will be able to produce oil from shale at a cost of only 29 cents per barrel. Crude oil now costs roughly $2.50 a barrel." [10]

To be sure, the oil produced in this way might be radioactive and therefore unusable or costly to use. Conventional explosives may provide more promise. No matter what the eventual process used, however, it is clear that oil shale represents a huge untapped reserve of potentially cheap fuel; the Green

River Shale alone is estimated to contain about 2 trillion barrels of oil. Should other fuel become more expensive, this reserve will certainly be drawn upon.

It is easy to see, therefore, how Putnam and Cambel could come to such differing conclusions using the same basic facts; with only the then-available technology, Putnam was right in saying that resources would soon be exhausted. Cambel and the interdepartmental study group were more foresighted, and reckoned up all the potential resources which might be tapped in future, including low-grade oil shale at depths down to 20,000 feet.

Putnam perpetuates a venerable position, one which economist Harold Barnett calls the "myth of our vanishing resources." The interdepartmental study group, on the other hand, may be too optimistic. At some point short of total exhaustion, the energy required to extract fuels from the earth becomes as great as the energy contained in them.

All we can say with any degree of certainty is that some time in the future, probably centuries hence, we will be confronted with a shortage of fuel, if industrial civilizations continue on the course of the last two hundred years. Probably at some point before that, fossil fuels will become more valuable as raw materials for manufacturing synthetic chemicals than as fuel (a change which is already being felt in the oil industry), and our heat and power will be derived from other sources. If present economic and social patterns persist, then atomic energy should certainly be examined as a possible replacement for coal, oil and gas. Other alternatives, such as fusion and solar power, should also be explored.

A prudent man would therefore likely recommend that in the next century or two we try to develop an economical and safe source of atomic power. There does not seem to be any urgency about this, however; the fuel shortage can hardly explain the present pace of the atomic energy program. What does account for the present rush to atomic power? The following are the principal stated justifications for nuclear reactors. With one exception, these all derive from the supposed cheapness or prospective cheapness of electric power generated by the atom.

The stated virtues of a program are not always identical with the personal motives of those who propound it. Although the program must be judged on explicit benefits and risks, these do not often give us any real idea of the reason for the program's existence, or of the circumstances which have created the need to make a judgment. Thus the shortages of fuels, uranium as well as coal, which seemed to face this country in the 1940's and which prompted so much of the early interest in fast breeder reactors, have now withdrawn into the distant future — yet the pace of the reactor program expands. On the other hand, many of the reasons now given for building reactors were simply not considered when the development of these plants was undertaken. To a certain extent, all enterprises have inertia and once set in motion tend to proceed, generating ever new justifications, even though their original purpose has long ago disappeared.

The magnitude and speed of the present reactor program indicate that much more than simple inertia is operating, however. In earlier chapters, we have tried to show two factors which have contributed to the present program. Both are consequences of military development of atomic energy. On the one hand, a number of large manufacturing firms made considerable investments of capital and talent in military-contract projects, investments on which they were reasonably anxious to find new sources of return. On the other hand, civilian customers for reactors were created through the fears felt both by private utilities and by members of the government, in both the Congress and the Executive, regarding federal investment in military reactors. It was felt that this was a step toward federally-owned civilian power plants, and advocates of privately owned power wished to preempt the field. These two pressures, acting on the Atomic Energy Commission and the Congress, as well as more directly on manufacturers and utilities, accounted, I believe, for much of the urgency of the effort to develop economical atomic power, and are acting as strongly now as they ever did.

A third, and more subtle, pressure was created by this country's investment in military nuclear programs. Particularly in its early days, the atomic energy program was operated by civilians. To the thousands of scientists and engineers engaged on the Manhattan Project, the development — and then the use — of a major scientific discovery for simple destruction was repugnant. The arms race which followed so quickly after the war was also highly disturbing to many within and outside the new Atomic Energy Commission. The thought of peaceful blessings from the atom to counterbalance its destructiveness gave a good deal of comfort to those whose responsibility was the development of nuclear weapons. David Lilienthal, first chairman of the Atomic Energy Commission, tells in his journal of the pleasure which both he and President Truman felt at the medical and research advances which radioactive isotopes made possible.[11]

The wish that atomic energy not be simply an unmitigated curse of weapons is felt by most of us in this country. It accounts in large part, I think, for the strenuous advocacy of reactors by many who have participated in one way or another in military atomic development. It is a more creditable motive than the strictly economic arguments generally advanced by such advocates. Reactors must be judged on their merits, however, and aside from fuel conservation and one further exception, all the claims are economic.

The other exception is the argument that reactors avoid the serious air pollution problems created by plants which burn coal, oil or gas. This argument can be made only because we have not yet had to confront the problems which will be created by radioactive pollution of air, water and soil by reactors and their associated industry. Unfortunately, we have already experienced the enormous discomforts and damages of pollution from fossil fuel burning. There are always, it seems, many who are ready to exchange a present danger for one which is still securely in the future. Yet it does seem that, if the reactor program continues on the course it has begun, the problems of radioactive pollution, ten, twenty or more years ahead, will make present difficulties seem trivial. Our descendants may wonder how, in the face of past mistakes, we could go on to make such another terrible one.

It is not going to be possible to exchange one set of problems for another in any real way. By all estimates, most of the electric power in this country will be produced by fossil-fuel burning plants for some years to come. The Atomic Energy Commission estimates that the major portion of power will be generated by fossil plants until the year 2,000. With the steady growth of our population and the more rapid growth of power needs, this means that not only will present coal, oil, and gas consumption continue, but that it will increase drastically in the next thirty years. A coal industry source gives the estimate of 829 million tons of coal to be supplied to electric utilities in the year 2000 compared to 242 million tons sold in 1965.[12]

Nuclear power is, therefore, no cure for air pollution problems, even if it did not create a more serious problem of its own. Sanguine announcements by utilities that they are "going nuclear" to combat air pollution are simply ways of trying to avoid a problem which will not go away. Air pollution from coal, oil, and gas must be dealt with; reliance on atomic power is both dangerous and misleading.

These are not, however, the only factors weighed when a power company is deciding whether its next plant will be fired by coal or atomic energy. Dollars and cents must also have been important in deciding the rush to reactors of the past three years. For nuclear reactors do seem to be, at some times and places, the cheapest way to produce power. And their economy is due to the fact that, to an extent unprecedented in American history, their costs are passed on to the taxpayer and the general public.

The costs of reactors are passed on to the public in two ways: by avoiding the necessary steps to limit radioactive pollution, the nuclear industry allows the public to pay in health damages what the industry should be preventing with dollars; by hiding behind the protection of the Price-Anderson Act, the nuclear industry is avoiding the cost of necessary safety measures and passing it on to the taxpayer and the general public, who provide the insurance for and suffer the physical risk of nuclear power plants.

In Chapter IV we saw that neither power companies nor reactor manufacturers would be interested in atomic electricity if it were not for the Price-Anderson Act, which excuses them from assuming the responsibility for the risk inherent in their industry. The federal insurance provided under this act makes nuclear power economically attractive; without that support and subsidy it would not be. What has happened is that the Federal Government, largely through the prodding of the Joint Committee on Atomic Energy, has exempted nuclear power from the normal competitive restraints of the marketplace. Freed from economic restraint, it has grown at a pace which endangers us all.

Used properly, atomic energy might be a valuable force in the civilian as well as the military economy. Reactors can be safe and clean; further research might make them so, at a price which would still allow their use in a competitive economy. The passage of Price-Anderson has removed the incentive to do the needed research, however, and instead we are developing, not safer, but more dangerous reactors, the fast breeders discussed in the last chapter, the hazards of which make even the present plans for huge reactors in the hearts of cities seem tame.

One of the ways in which reactors might be made more safe would obviously be to put them in unpopulated areas. Recent advances in transmitting electric power long distances over extra high voltage (EHV) transmission lines allow a plant to be quite far from its customers; with EHV transmission, a reactor could be hundreds of miles from any city. This would, of course, increase the cost of nuclear power, but further advances in transmission technology will probably reduce the penalty. A more serious difficulty is the requirement for large amounts of cooling water for reactors; sites with the needed water which are also sufficiently isolated are rare, and becoming more scarce each year.

There are a number of conceivable ways out of this impasse. We might restrict reactors to only the few remote locations suitable; we might develop reactors which are economical, and yet small enough to be housed in an impenetrable containment; or new reactor designs which did not require so much — or any — cooling water could be developed. The latter two possibilities have received some attention, but research on new reactor types has all but halted in this country, with the exception of fast breeder development.

Small reactors are attractive for a number of reasons, the greatest being that containing the radioactivity released in an accident becomes possible with small reactors. Under 100,000 kilowatts is a size we have some experience with, and as indicated earlier, it seems possible to enclose them in a "thermos-bottle" containment which will not be breached in an accident — although again possibility is not certainty. Such small plants would be highly attractive to the many small rural cooperative and municipal electric power companies which are themselves too small to invest in the mammoth reactors which are now being marketed.

The whole trend of the country's economy and technology is away from small power plants and toward ever-larger ones in increasingly interconnected power systems; the economic incentives for small plants seem small. And, too, distributing many small reactors over the landscape increases the chance of small accidents, negligence and the increasing load of accidental radioactive release during transportation of wastes. Another difficulty with the small plant is that the pollution controls which will be increasingly needed for reactor operation will probably not be much cheaper for a small plant than for a larger one, putting a very heavy burden on the former.

A large reactor, which requires little or no cooling water, and which is in a remote location with its own waste-disposal system, seems a distinct possibility, and by far the most attractive one. All that would go into such a plant would be relatively innocuous uranium fuel; all that would come out would be electricity. The reactor and waste-disposal systems would be designed to prevent emissions of radioactivity; the wastes of irradiated fuel would be buried in impermeable formations deep underground. Such a completely self-contained reactor installation could be in desert or mountainous country, tied into the nation's power grid through EHV transmission lines. Far from any center of population, even an accident disastrous to the reactor itself would not be a disaster to any nearby city. Underground construction may be an important safety device. It is already in use in Sweden.

There is no reason, in principle, why such a remote, underground, self-contained large reactor cannot be developed to the point where it is competitive with other forms of power generation. There are a number of ways in which large power stations could economically do away with most of their requirements for cooling water; cooling towers and ponds are already in use in areas where heat poses a hazard to water quality or to fishing. Commonwealth Associates, nuclear consultants, have recently proposed an economically competitive design for use in Iowa which would rely on well water.[13]

A more difficult task would be removing all the radioactive waste releases from the reactor and fuel-processing cycle. One step toward this goal could be made quite easily, however, and that is to avoid all transportation losses by locating the plant for processing spent nuclear fuel on the same site as the reactor, and by burying the wastes extracted from the spent fuel at the same location. This is already feasible for large plants — in fact, is already being done with one government-owned reactor, Experimental Breeder Reactor II. If the reactor fuel were also manufactured at the reactor, as it is at the EBR-II site, then all the hazards of transporting radioactive materials would be wiped out. Only unirradiated and therefore relatively harmless uranium (unused fuel can be safely held in the hand) would be shipped to the plant; nothing would be shipped out except electricity. In 1966, Cyril M. Slansky of the Phillips Petroleum Company, Atomic Energy Division, presented a paper before an AEC waste-disposal symposium which showed that at least for some kinds of reactors and fuels, such a completely self-contained system would be as cheap as the present method, which involves the expensive and hazardous transportation of nuclear wastes from the reactor to a distant processing plant.[14]

The principal objection to this scheme raised at the symposium was the fact that present regulations require wastes to be buried on government-owned land. The requirement stems from the extremely long times, ranging into centuries, that the waste will remain dangerous. It is felt that only on government-owned land is continuity of surveillance properly assured. This would not be an insurmountable problem if reactors were restricted to remote locations, for there are probably many such sites on government-owned land. Alternatively, provisions might be made to have ownership of a reactor site pass to the Federal Government in case its private owner is unwilling or unable to continue management.

A more difficult problem would be that of reducing and eventually eliminating the radioactive pollutants released by reactors and fuel-reprocessing plants. The problem is clearly soluble, however. Reactors, even in their current form, could be operated so that, with few exceptions, no pollutants would be released. For it should be remembered that even when the fuel elements are leaking, the radioactive wastes can be retained within the coolant water (at least in pressurized water reactors). All present releases from reactors are intentional, in the sense that the released contaminants could be retained and packaged for burial like the more highly concentrated wastes from the fuel. All that is required is the extra expense of retaining and concentrating the lower-level wastes.

One exception is the noble gas produced in reactor fuel. Noble gases, especially krypton and xenon, are extremely difficult to capture, partly because they are gases, and partly because they do not enter into chemical reactions very easily (hence, the appellation "noble"). Although laboratory methods for trapping these gases into solid compounds are available, commercial-scale techniques have not been developed. There is no reason in principle why this could not be done.

Another exception is tritium (radioactive hydrogen), which physically becomes a part of the cooling water. This is a serious problem even now, and will not be easily solved.

In principle, then, it is possible to end all intentional releases of radioactivity to the environment. Accidental releases would be much reduced by housing all the elements of fuel fabrication and processing at the reactor site. Disposal of radioactive wastes by dumping them in rivers or in the ocean, or by releasing them into the air, or by burying them in shallow graves near the surface could be entirely ended simply by concentrating all wastes, reducing them to solid form or packing them into unbreakable containers, and burying them deep underground in salt caves or granite formations which would not be disturbed for thousands of years.

Although present reactors could, at least in principle, be made safe and clean, it is hard to see how the far greater difficulties of the fast breeder are to be solved. Yet, fast breeders are being justified in exactly the same terms that water-cooled reactors have been justified. We *must* have them, because uranium is in short supply. Soon it will start going up in price, and the reactors we have built will become ever more expensive to operate, until the irreplaceable uranium is all exhausted. Breeder reactors, which make more fuel than they burn, are an inexhaustible energy source.

It is not likely that this argument will prove to be true of uranium, where it has proved false of coal and oil. Uranium is a plentiful element. The present seeming shortage is caused by lack of demand for uranium in recent years; very little prospecting has been done since the AEC stopped enlarging its military requirements for the metal. Since the reactor boom began to take hold, prospecting has revived, and it seems almost certain that vast new reserves will soon be uncovered.

Even if this should not be so, however, low-grade ores are already known which are more than adequate for our energy needs for quite some time to come. The Cambel report points out that even if all the electric power in this country were to be generated by nuclear fuel, which is very far from being the case, there is sufficient uranium for many years. The interdepartmental study group concludes, "All the estimates indicate that *either* coal or uranium resources *alone* are adequate to take us through the year 2000 and longer."

In the August 1967 issue of *Nuclear News*, Dr. Edward Teller said, "There probably is enough uranium, and breeders will not be needed in the foreseeable future, such as a hundred years or 300 years, or longer. . . . I wonder, if we were to resume the needed research in mining and chemical engineering to obtain improved methods of uranium extraction, how greatly we would then increase our uranium reserves."

As in the past, the principal virtues claimed for fast breeder reactors, as for their predecessors, will be economic. What reactors really represent is a choice between higher electric bills and greater risk to life and health. The public bears the full costs in either case.

In all this we are rather charitably assuming that reactors would, in fact, produce cheaper power. This is simply an assumption, for none of the reactors which presumably will do this have yet been built. The costs of reactor power are estimated on the basis of information provided by their manufacturers. In many cases the estimates may be less than reliable. In his authoritative study of the atomic energy program, *Contracting for Atoms*, Harold Orlans discusses the calculations, down to several decimal places, of projected costs of atomic power and notes. "Some of the assumptions upon which these calculations are based are so gross, the decimal places are 'a joke in the fraternity,' one reader observes." [15] Baltimore Gas and Electric recently *opposed* a reduction in its rates in part because of "the company's plans to expand in the nuclear field." [16]

Somewhere along the line, in any case, a decision has been made that the benefits of nuclear reactors outweigh their hazard. It is difficult to see just where this determination was made (if indeed such decisions are made at a single time and place). One point at which it could at least have been challenged was that at which the Price-Anderson Act was proposed.

For here was a straightforward statement of the judgment: The benefits of the reactor program, as it presently exists, are great enough for the public, through the Federal Government, to assume its risks.

There was little debate of this bill in Congress, in the newspapers or elsewhere in the country outside the nuclear establishment itself. Except for the opposition of insurance companies and among parties to the debate over the Fermi reactor, the bill, like the reactor program as a whole, passed almost unchallenged. This was all the more surprising for, aside from the enormous potential dangers of the reactor program, the bill empowered the Federal Government to intervene in private industry to an unprecedented extent.

Why has there been, and why does there continue to be, such nearly complete lack of criticism of the Price-Anderson Act and of the nuclear power program as a whole? Although there has been sporadic opposition to nuclear plants from their prospective neighbors, and general concern has been growing, both remain to a large degree helpless or inarticulate. This helplessness derives from two sources, both of which are common to many modern technological enterprises which affect the public at large.

First, the question of reactor safety and usefulness involves a number of extremely complex and difficult scientific questions. Most people who are not professionally engaged in the nuclear field tend to feel that these questions are beyond their grasp. Believing themselves incapable of forming an independent judgment, many feel that the government experts must know what they're doing. Yet, more and more, we are beginning to find that the attitude of "leave it to the experts" often produces unwelcome results. A growing proportion of the national resources and manpower are being devoted to large technological projects, like the space program and the construction of a supersonic transport, which few of us understand. The benefits and dangers of these programs are not always clear; yet, if only through our tax bill, they affect us all.

It was only with the publication of *Silent Spring* that the public at large discovered they were being exposed to potentially grave hazards from the use of pesticides. It was only after years of testing of nuclear weapons that many of us discovered the real hazards of radioactive fallout.

It was not until billions of pounds of detergents were disseminated in our water supplies that we discovered the nuisance and the pollution hazard this would pose. This relatively minor problem exemplifies the pattern of modern uses of science and technology. The drawbacks to a particular program never seem to be discovered until too late.

In the case of the reactor program, we are in a position to anticipate many of the difficulties which will soon be encountered. Warnings of what is to come have been seen at Bodega, at Humboldt Bay, at Fermi and elsewhere. It is long past time for a broader understanding of the risk from accident and radioactive pollution that present reactors pose, and the far greater risks of the fast breeder reactor which we are about to assume. The relevant information must be made available, and debate within Congress and outside it must begin. Only a very much broadened base of discussion will allow us to judge wisely whether in the reactor program, as it now stands, the benefits outweigh the hazards; only such a national discussion will enable us to judge among the various alternative ways of generating cheap and safe electrical power in the future.

Which brings us to the second reason that critics of the

reactor program have found themselves helpless. Modern science is profoundly affecting our political and legal system; traditional governmental organizations have not been adequate, and new forms, like the Joint Committee on Atomic Energy, and the Atomic Energy Commission, are appearing.

In *The Government of the Atom,* a study sponsored by the National Law Center, Harold Green and Alan Rosenthal say:

> The Joint Committee on Atomic Energy (JCAE), since its creation in 1946, has played an unusually influential role in the conduct of the nation's atomic enterprise. Although originally a part of the legislature, the Joint Committee's behavior uniquely resembles that of the higher echelons of the executive branch. In this respect, the JCAE represents a significant innovation in a governmental system of separated powers.
>
> Members of the Committee itself, other congressmen, and officials of the executive branch have long recognized the JCAE as an extraordinary Congressional institution. Despite its unique structure as the only joint committee with legislative powers, its broad statutory authority, and its unprecedented role in the formulation of national policy, the Committee has largely escaped the attention of scholars.[17]

We might add, and the attention of the general public, for surprisingly few have any real knowledge of the most powerful Congressional institution ever established, a major force in national policy formation over a wide range of foreign, domestic and military matters.

No less remarkable is the Atomic Energy Commission, the agency which has sole responsibility for the development and use of atomic energy. The AEC is also the agency with sole responsibility for regulation in this field. In fact, it is responsible for regulating its own activities, a situation which has been strongly criticized by its first chairman, David Lilienthal, among others.

The AEC has broader powers than have ever been given to a single federal agency. Among other things, the Atomic Energy Act of 1954 apparently gives the AEC power (according to its own contention) to impose security restrictions on any activities, whether conducted with or without government support, which bear on atomic energy, however tangentially. Regulations proposed by the AEC at the time of this writing, but not yet enacted, would allow the AEC to prohibit any research, whether undertaken by private individuals, private companies, universities or anyone else, which the AEC felt impinged on certain sensitive areas. The AEC has made clear its intention to broaden the areas coming under such control at any time it deems such action in the interest of national security or defense.

With sole authority in its area of activity, extremely broad powers, and with much of its activity cloaked by security restrictions on information, the AEC is a singularly difficult body to influence. It is subject only to the restraints of the Joint Committee, designated by law its "watchdog." Yet over the years, the two bodies have drawn together until they are almost indistinguishable. There has been considerable exchange of staff between the two bodies. The former Executive Director of the Joint Committee is now one of the five Commissioners who head the AEC, and, according to most observers, the most influential of the five. Although the senior members of the Joint Committee have been active in atomic energy affairs for twenty years or more, the Commissioners generally change with each Administration or, in most cases, even more frequently. Some remain on the Commission for only a single

IX

INFORMATION AND ACTION

FROM THE PRECEDING CHAPTER it will be seen that altering the present course of atomic energy development in this country would be no easy task. There are many billions of dollars invested or committed to present plans. The process of decision-making is thoroughly insulated from outside criticism and debate.

Yet we can see that many substantial improvements can be made in the reactor program, without abandoning its present basis. Reactors currently being manufactured are capable of being modified for suitability at remote locations and for self-contained operation. It may be too late to reconsider the national decision to invest in the development of atomic power, but it is certainly not too late to decide how that investment may best be used for the benefit of the nation's welfare and health.

In the preceding chapters we have suggested some of the reasons for the present shape of the reactor program. Whatever its history, that program is now clearly aimed toward the accomplishment of narrow economic objectives, at a cost of safety and pollution hazards which seems steep. The various alternative routes to atomic power — and the even larger number of alternative means to reach cheaper electricity in general year. As a result, the Joint Committee dominates the AEC; at least in terms of the civilian reactor program, the two bodies have become one.

To compound this concentration of power, most scientists and engineers with experience of atomic energy are directly associated with the AEC or its contractors, or have received their training through the AEC. It is therefore not surprising that hearings before the Joint Committee show such little basic disagreement among expert witnesses, or that it is so difficult to contest the expert judgments produced by industry, the Joint Committee or the AEC.

In short, decision making in atomic energy programs has largely been removed from the normal process of open debate. There is no question but that the Joint Committee and the AEC are conscientious and acutely aware of the need for safety. Yet it is too much to ask them to make decisions unassisted which have such sweeping importance for society. It is too much to ask them to judge the safety and advisability of programs in the development of which they have themselves invested many years and great efforts.

— are not being considered. The single reason this state of affairs is permitted is simple. The public does not know about the risks the present course runs, nor that there are alternative actions, each with its own sets of benefits and risks, which might be considered.

This is a state of affairs which often holds true in social and political issues which derive from, or depend on, technology. These issues are effectively screened from outside examination by the public's — and in most cases, the Congress's — lack of facts. Whether it is an antiballistic missile system, or whether it is the nuclear power program, the supersonic transport, or a pointless race to the moon, we have been given not information, but judgments propounded by experts.

This is not a necessary state of affairs. In most cases, the pertinent facts can be made clear to a layman. This book is an attempt to demonstrate that belief. A far more important demonstration has been carried on for ten years by the Committee for Environmental Information, in St. Louis, Missouri.

In the middle 1950's, the American public became aware that their government was conducting a vast experiment, the testing of nuclear weapons, and that the results of that experiment had not been entirely foreseen. Beginning in 1954, the AEC began lifting the cover of secrecy from the fallout question, and a heated debate began. Official government statements, and scientists working in the weapon program, assured the public over and over that there was no hazard to health; many outside the government, and some within, were not so sure. But in fact, no one within or without the government really knew. The testing program had begun, and continued, in almost complete ignorance of the biological hazard from fallout. Violent disputes broke out among scientists, each proclaiming from the authority of his position his own opinion.

The public was naturally confused. When scientists of equal prominence took diametrically opposed stands, most people felt unable to resolve the dispute in their own minds. Not in possession of the basic facts himself, the layman could not choose among differing opinions.

The difficulty was acutely felt in St. Louis, which was a high-fallout area during most of the period of weapon testing. Radioactive strontium in St. Louis milk reached record highs. Government pronouncements assured that the levels were harmless — yet they continued to creep upward. Scientists from St. Louis universities were increasingly called upon to render their own judgments; doctors, especially pediatricians, were increasingly asked, "What should we do about the milk?" Dr. Barry Commoner, a St. Louis biologist, recalls being called upon to explain over and over again that the white spots on the lawn were mold, and not fallout.

Responding to the increasing demands for facts about fallout, St. Louis scientists and physicians joined with a group of concerned laymen to form the Committee for Nuclear Information. Although the founders of this group held varying moral and political judgments of the merits of bomb testing, the purpose of CNI was simply to provide the scientific evidence regarding the effects of fallout, to the extent that it was available. Where no real evidence existed, the group said so.

One of the founders of CNI described its early days this way: "About 200 people joined the group as soon as it was organized (about 30 being physicians and scientists) and contributed sufficient funds to permit a start. The technical members agreed to fill speaking engagements on nuclear problems, and in August 1958 a form letter offering this service was sent

out to about 1,000 St. Louis civic organizations." Between
October 1958 and December 1960, the group filled about 160
engagements. "The audiences [were] quite varied; about 50
church groups, about 45 PTA's and other school groups, about
30 fraternal, civic and professional organizations, and the remainder medical and scientific associations. A total estimated
audience of 15–20,000 people [were] reached in this way." [1]

From its earliest days, CNI began publishing a monthly
bulletin, *Nuclear Information*; in the ten years since its first
issue, this has grown from four mimeographed pages to a national magazine with a professional staff. Although the CNI
Speakers Bureau continues, the group's various publications
have become its principal means of reaching a greatly enlarged
audience. The first step toward this new role was taken in
September of 1959, with the publication of "Nuclear War in
St. Louis."

In May, 1959, the Joint Committee on Atomic Energy held
extensive hearings to ascertain the extent of our knowledge of
what might be the effects of a nuclear attack on the United
States. Days of highly technical testimony were taken, detailed
reports were submitted for the record. CNI arranged with the
Joint Committee to obtain copies of the testimony as it was
delivered; a team consisting of two physicists, two biologists
and a physician prepared summaries of the physical, ecological
and medical effects of the two nuclear bombs that the Joint
Committee's assumed attack had assigned to St. Louis. A biologist who was also a talented writer, Dr. Florence Moog,
translated these summaries into a fictional account of the supposed survivors of the hypothetical bombing of St. Louis.

The result was an accurate and moving account of what was
known about nuclear warfare, and reached far more members

of the public than the technical hearings on which it was based. "Nuclear War in St. Louis" was reprinted in 16 newspapers and magazines in six countries. CNI answered requests for 50,000 reprints of the publication, from church groups, schools, labor organizations; 2500 copies were ordered by state and federal civil defense organizations. Permission was granted to the War College, Air University of the United States Air Force, to reprint the bulletin for the use, within the War College, of each graduating class.

This was the first of a series of successes which were to confirm the judgment on which CNI was founded, that the public wanted, and could handle, the technical facts underlying political issues. In 1961, CNI published an analysis of the AEC's proposed Project Chariot, a plan to blast a harbor in the northern Alaskan shoreline, using nuclear explosives. The CNI article showed the peculiar biological risks from fallout in the region. In 1963, a detailed analysis of the difficulties involved in the planned reactor for Bodega Head in California was published.

In both cases, the CNI magazine reached large numbers of those most directly affected by the project; in Alaska, these were the inhabitants of scattered Eskimo villages along the coast, who have no written language of their own. The CNI bulletin, recorded on tape, "literally swept the Arctic coast, from Kakhtovik all the way down to Nome and below . . . ," according to one report. Both in California and in Alaska, it was the pressure of an informed citizenry which led eventually to abandonment of both projects; CNI was a large factor in providing the needed facts.

By 1964, it had become clear that the uses of atomic energy were only a few of the many political issues born from scientific progress. More and more large technological enterprises were making their effects felt in the environment, through growing pollution of air, water and soil, through the assaults of sonic booms and through the rapid degradation of the quality of life. Realizing that its experience in bringing information on atomic energy to the public would be invaluable in the wider range of science-based issues, CNI slowly began enlarging its scope, until in 1967 it formally became the Committee for Environmental Information; its monthly magazine is now *Scientist and Citizen.*

At about the same time, similar groups began appearing in other cities; the oldest of these is the Scientists' Committee for Public Information, in New York City. Similar groups in Washington, D.C., Denver, Colorado, Berkeley, California, Rochester, New York, Missoula, Montana, Minneapolis, Minnesota, and elsewhere began to form. A national coordinating body, the Scientists' Institute for Public Information, serves as a central organizing body for the dozen or so groups now active across the country. *Scientist and Citizen* has become the publication of this growing national "information movement."

The growing success of this movement gives considerable hope that the barrier between the atomic energy program and the general public is being breached, and that more than one voice will be heard when atomic energy is talked of; that the moral and political decisions regarding reactors will be made, at least in part, by those who will bear the consequences of the decisions. In short, we can hope that advancing science has not left democracy behind.

NOTES

INDEX

NOTES

The abbreviations AEC and JCAE used throughout represent the United States Atomic Energy Commission and the Joint Committee on Atomic Energy of the United States Congress, respectively. The abbreviation "Wash-740" represents a study done by the AEC entitled, "Theoretical Possibilities and Consequences of Major Accidents in Large Nuclear Power Plants."

CHAPTER I

1. The account of the accident at the NRX reactor is drawn principally from Lewis, W. B., "Accident to the NRX Reactor on December 12, 1952," Canadian Report AECL-232, Atomic Energy of Canada, Ltd. 1953, quoted in *The Technology of Reactor Safety*, Vol. 1, "Reactor Physics and Control," T. J. Thompson and J. G. Beckerley, eds. (Cambridge, M.I.T. Press, 1964), pp. 619–622.
2. The account of the Windscale Accident is drawn in part from "Accident of Windscale No. 1 Pile on 10th October, 1957," British Report Cmnd. 302 (London, November 1957), quoted in *The Technology of Reactor Safety*, pp. 633–635.
3. McCullough, C. Rogers, AEC, "The Windscale Accident," in *Proceedings, 1958 AEC and Contractor Safety and Fire Protection Conference, June 24–25, 1958*, TID-7591 AEC Technical Information Service, Oak Ridge, May 15, 1959, p. 76.
4. *Ibid.*, p. 78.
5. Thompson, T. J., in *The Technology of Reactor Safety*, Vol. 1, p. 699.

CHAPTER II

1. Quoted in Samuel Glasstone, *Sourcebook on Atomic Energy*, Second Edition (Princeton, D. Van Nostrand Co., Inc., 1958), p. 387.

2. Hahn, Otto, *New Atoms* (New York, Elsevier Publishing Co., Inc., 1950).
3. Quoted by Glasstone, *op. cit.*, p. 386.
4. Laurence, William, *Men and Atoms* (New York, Simon and Schuster, 1959).
5. *Ibid.*
6. Compton, Arthur Holly, *Atomic Quest* (New York, Oxford University Press, 1956).
7. Mullenbach, Philip, *Civilian Nuclear Power* (New York, the Twentieth Century Fund, 1963), p. 140.

CHAPTER III

1. San Francisco *Chronicle,* October 30, 1964.
2. Santa Rosa *Press Democrat,* March 19, 1963, p. 7.
3. Teller, Edward, "Energy From Oil and From the Nucleus," *Journal of Petroleum Technology,* May 1965, p. 506.
4. Saint-Amand, Pierre, "Geologic and Seismologic Study of Bodega Head," Northern California Association to Preserve Bodega Head and Harbor, 1963, p. 19.
5. Schlocker, Julius, and Manuel Bonilla, U.S. Department of the Interior, Geological Survey, "Engineering Geology of the Proposed Nuclear Power Plant Site on Bodega Head, Sonoma County, California," TEI-884, December 1963.
6. "Earthquakes, the Atom, and Bodega Head," Northern California Association to Preserve Bodega Head and Harbor, Berkeley, 1964.
7. *Ibid.,* p. 15.
8. *Ibid.*
9. *Ibid.,* p. 18.
10. Mattison, Lindsay, and Richard Daly, "Bodega, The Reactor, The Site, The Hazard," *Nuclear Information,* April 1964, available from the Committee for Environmental Information, 438 N. Skinker Blvd., St. Louis, Mo.
11. *Ibid.*
12. "The Proposed Malibu Nuclear Power Station," undated.
13. "Geology of Malibu Coastal Belt in Vicinity of Proposed Nuclear Reactor Site in Corral Canyon," Ventura, California, February 12, 1964, p. 7.

14. Quoted by Frank A. Morgan, Consulting Geologist, in "Review of Geological Work at the Proposed Corral Canyon Nuclear Reactor Site, Malibu," Los Angeles, January 21, 1965 (mimeographed), p. 2.
15. *Ibid.*
16. *Ibid.*, p. 3.
17. *Ibid.*
18. *Nucleonics Week*, April 30, 1967.
19. "An Assessment of Large Nuclear Powered Sea Water Distillation Plants," a Report of an Interagency Task Group, March, 1964, Office of Science and Technology, Executive Office of the President, TID-19267 UNC (revised).
20. Wyant, William K., Jr., "Proposed California Desalinization Plant," St. Louis *Post-Dispatch*, September 11, 1966.
21. *Nucleonics*, December 1966.
22. *Ibid.*
23. *Ibid.*
24. "The Ravenswood Reactor — a Preliminary Report to the Public," Citizens' Committee for Radiation Information, New York, undated (mimeographed).
25. March 21, 1963.

CHAPTER IV

1. "Wash-740," p. vii.
2. *Ibid.*, p. viii.
3. "Proposed Extension of AEC Indemnity Legislation," *Hearings*, Subcommittee on Legislation, JCAE, June 22–24, 1965, p. 348.
4. Commissioner John G. Palfrey, at a meeting of the Atomic Industrial Forum, quoted by David Pesonen in *The Nation*, October 18, 1965. Palfrey reportedly opened his talk by saying, "My assignment today was to review with you the updating of the Brookhaven report [Wash-740] . . . . Well, the Brookhaven study is not ready yet. . . . my guesses on what it will say or should say would be irresponsible chatter on a ticklish subject. . . ."
5. Wash-740, p. 3.
6. See "Nuclear Reactors Built, Being Built, or Planned," Appendix, TID-8200, revised annually by the Office of the Assistant General Manager for Reactors, AEC. The only reactors with which there had been extensive experience at the time of the report aside from

small experiments, were the military plutonium production reactors. The reliability of these is unknown, as details of their operations are classified.

7. WASH-740, p. 5.

8. Strauss, Lewis L., *Men and Decisions* (New York, Popular Library Inc., 1963).

9. Groves, Leslie R., Lt. Gen. USA Ret. *Now It Can Be Told* (New York, Harper and Bros., 1962).

10. Subcommittee on Legislation, JCAE, *Selected Materials on Atomic Energy Indemnity Legislation* (June 1965), p. 96.

11. Yount, Hubert W., Vice President, Liberty Mutual Insurance Co., appearing on behalf of the American Mutual Alliance, *Hearings*, on Governmental Indemnity before the JCAE, 84th Congress, second session, pp. 248–250.

12. *Selected Materials*, p. 66.

13. "Proposed Extensions of AEC Indemnity Legislation" *Hearings*, Subcommittee on Legislation, JCAE, June 22–24, 1965, p. 192.

14. *Ibid.*, p. 46.

15. Quoted by David Pesonen in *The Nation*, October 18, 1965.

16. Quad-Cities Station, Unit 1, Plant Design Analysis, Vol. I, Commonwealth Edison Company, Chicago, Illinois, p. V–1–20.

17. *Ibid.*, p. V–1–16.

18. *Nucleonics Week*, July 20, 1967, p. 3.

19. AEC Docket Number 50 — 259 & 260: letter dated March 14, 1967, from N. J. Palladino, Chairman ACRS to Honorable Glenn T. Seaborg, Chairman, AEC.

20. *Ibid.*

21. "Emergency Core Cooling: Report of Advisory Task Force on Power Reactor Emergency Cooling," AEC Division of Technical Information, Oak Ridge (undated), p. 6.

22. *Nucleonics*, June, 1967, p. 6.

23. Crawford, W. Donham, Remarks before Health Physics Society, Twelfth Annual Meeting, Washington, D.C., June 20, 1967 (mimeographed).

24. "Licensing and Regulation of Nuclear Reactors," *Hearings*, JCAE, April 4, 5, 6, and 20, and May 3, 1967, p. 129.

25. Hanchett, James, "Letter from Washington," *Nucleonics*, May, 1967, p. 11.

26. *Nucleonics Week*, June 15, 1967.

CHAPTER V

1. Slansky, Cyril M., "Waste Management in Close-Coupled Nuclear Fuel Cycles," *Proceedings,* Symposium on the Solidification and Long-Term Storage of Highly Radioactive Wastes, February 1966, CONF-660208, AEC, Oak Ridge. Slansky gives equilibrium values for a 1,000,000-kilowatt (electrical) reactor on a 1-year fuel cycle as 13,500 megacuries, including about 760 megacuries of cesium. Roughly 140 megacuries of cesium were released by the 140 megatons exploded through 1963. Other radionuclides are presumably in similar proportion. (See Federal Radiation Council Report 4, 1963).

2. Calder, Ritchie, *Living With the Atom* (Chicago, University of Chicago Press, 1962), p. 31.

3. Data from *Health Physics* 9:83 (1963) and 10:243 (1964), quoted in *Scientist and Citizen,* November, 1965, p. 8.

4. *Ibid.*

5. Calder, *op. cit.,* p. 37.

6. Commoner, Barry, *Science and Survival* (New York, Viking Press, 1966), p. 17.

7. Palmer, H. E., W. C. Hanson, B. I. Griffin, L. A. Braby, *Science,* Vol. 147 (1965), p. 620. See also Letters, *ibid.,* p. 1598.

8. Calder, *op. cit.,* p. 215.

9. Olson, J. S. and S. I. Auerbach, "Biological Contamination of Vegetation and Dispersal of Radioactive Wastes by Insects," *Nuclear Safety,* Vol. I, No. 3, p. 62.

10. This is a somewhat simplified account. Cellular mutations may appear as the result of errors in the repair of damage done to DNA rather than as a result of the damage itself, and it is quite possible that the damage is mediated by other substances and need not require a direct "hit" on a DNA molecule.

11. Blumenthal, Herman T., "Radiation and Aging," *Scientist and Citizen,* February 1957, p. 21.

12. *Ibid.*

CHAPTER VI

1. Engdahl, Don, in Santa Rosa *Press Democrat,* May 1, 1966.

2. Letter from Hal Stroube, Coordinator of Atomic Information to Hon. Mervyn M. Dymally, Chairman of the California State Assembly Committee on Industrial Relations, dated September 29, 1966, enclosing comments on the testimony of David Pesonen before the Committee.

3. *Ibid.*

4. Report to the AEC on operations during the period February to August, 1965, quoted by Don Engdahl in personal communication to author, dated May 26, 1966.

5. Stroube letter, *op. cit.*

6. In "Proposed Change No. 20" to the Humboldt operating license.

7. Stroube letter, *op. cit.*

8. Goodman, Leo, "Radiation Hazard in Modern Industry," Address to the American Public Health Association and the D.C. Public Health Association, April 26, 1967, Washington, D.C. (mimeographed), p. 4.

9. Coleman, J. R. and R. Liberace, *Radiological Health Data and Reports*, November 1966. They estimate exposures to the general population from reactor-produced krypton 85 dissolved in body fluids, at 20 to 100 millirads per year by the year 2060. Natural background radiation averages about 150 millirads; the NCRP guideline for exposure to the general population, from *all sources* is 170 millirads per year.

10. AEC Authorizing Legislation — 1968, *Hearings*, JCAE, March 14 and 15, 1967, Part 2, p. 883.

11. *Ibid.*, pp. 882–883.

12. *Ibid.*

13. *Civilian Nuclear Power: A Report to the President*, AEC Division of Technical Information, Oak Ridge, 1962, p. 4.

14. Goodman, Leo, *op. cit.*, p. 12.

15. *Proceedings*, First United Nations Conference on Peaceful Uses of Atomic Energy, Geneva, 1955, Vol. 13, p. 168.

16. Goodman, *op. cit.*, p. 14.

17. Gardner, John W., Secretary of Health, Education and Welfare, "Report on a Review and Evaluation of the Public Health Service Epidemiological Study," August 1967, submitted for the record, "Radiation Exposure of Uranium Miners," *Hearings*, Subcommittee on Research Development and Radiation, JCAE, May 9 to August 10, 1967, Part 2, p. 1261. This review corrected earlier Public

Health Service evidence that the standard recommended by the Federal Radiation Council would result in a doubling of lung cancer rates in miners. The review concluded, however, that "association of excess mortality from lung cancer . . . with estimated exposure of 800 CWLM [cumulative working level months] and above is evident. A demonstrable relationship can be inferred to exist as low as an exposure range of 100 to 400 CWLM." The standard adopted, 1 WL (working level) could be expected to result in exposures of 100 to 400 CWLM. See p. 1269.

18. "Disposition and Control of Uranium Mill Tailings Piles in the Colorado River Basin," U.S. Department of Health, Education and Welfare, Federal Water Pollution Control Administration, Region VIII, Denver, Colorado, March, 1966.
19. "Radioactive Water Pollution in the Colorado River Basin," *Hearing*, Subcommittee on Air and Water Pollution, U.S. Senate, May 5, 1966.
20. FWPCA, March 1966, *op. cit.* ,
21. Lieberman, Joseph A. and Walter G. Belter, "Waste Management and Environmental Aspects of Nuclear Power," *Environmental Science and Technology*, Vol. 1, No. 6 (June 1967), p. 474.
22. *Ibid.*
23. Knapp, Harold A., "Cost and Safety Considerations in the Transport of Radioactive Materials," *Proceedings*, AEC and Contractor Safety and Fire Protection Conference, Germantown, Md., June 24–25, 1958, AEC Technical Information Service TID-7569, p. 54.
24. Calder, Ritchie, *Living With The Atom* (Chicago, University of Chicago Press, 1962), p. 230.
25. Knapp, *op. cit.*, p. 62.
26. Morgan, J. M., Jr., informal remarks in *Summary Report*, AEC Symposium on Packaging and Regulatory Standards for Shipping Radioactive Material, Germantown, Md., December 3–5, 1962, TID-7651, AEC Division of Technical Information Extension.
27. Patterson, D. E., "Types and Quantities of Materials Being Shipped and AEC Accident Experience," *Summary Report*, p. 3.
28. Smets, Henri B., "Review of Nuclear Accidents," *Progress in Nuclear Energy*, Series X, Law and Administration, Vol. 3, Jerry L. Weinstein (ed.), *Nuclear Liability* (New York, Pergamon Press Inc., the MacMillan Company, 1962), p. 118.

CHAPTER VII

1. Second Annual Convention, New Mexico State AFL-CIO, October 26, 1957 (mimeographed), p. 9.

2. Power Reactor Development Company v. International Union of Electrical Radio and Machine Workers, AFL-CIO, et al., 367 U.S. 396.

3. *U.S. Uranium Reserves — A Report by the Committee on Mining and Milling,* Atomic Industrial Forum, Inc., New York, August, 1966, p. 7.

4. *AEC Research Development Report, Fast Reactor Control and Safety Meeting,* November 10, 1954, AEC Technical Service. Extension, APDA-105 (declassified), 1956, p. 109.

5. *Ibid.,* p. 169.

6. *The Technology of Nuclear Reactor Safety,* Vol. I, "Reactor Physics and Control," T. J. Thompson and J. G. Beckerley (eds.), p. 631.

7. The account given of the October 5 accident is based on AEC Docket No. 50-16 "Preliminary Report on Fuel Damage in Fermi Reactor," October 11, 1966; "Investigation of the Fuel Melting Accident at the Enrico Fermi Atomic Power Plant," J. G. Duffy, W. H. Jens, J. G. Feldes, K. P. Johnson, and W. J. McCarthy, Jr., National Topical Meeting, American Nuclear Society, San Francisco, April 1967; and on additional remarks made by W. J. McCarthy, Jr., while delivering the latter paper.

8. At the April American Nuclear Society meeting.

9. McCarthy, Walter J., Jr. and Wayne H. Jens, "Enrico Fermi Fast Breeder Reactor," *Nuclear News,* November, 1967, p. 54.

10. *A Report on the Possible Effects on the Surrounding Population of an Assumed Release of Fission Products into the Atmosphere from a 300 Megawatt Nuclear Reactor Located at Lagoona Beach, Michigan,* Engineering Research Institute, University of Michigan, AEC Document number APDA-120, July 1957.

11. AEC Docket No. 50-16, Revised License Application, Enrico Fermi Atomic Power Plant, *Technical Information and Hazards Summary Report,* Vol. 7, Section VI, September 13, 1961, AEC Public Document Room, Washington, D.C.

12. National Topical Meeting, Fast Reactors, American Nuclear Society, San Francisco, April 1967.

13. "The 1967 Supplement to the 1962 Report to the President on Civilian Nuclear Power," AEC, February, 1967, p. 49.

14. Congressman Craig Hosmer, "Running with the Breeder Ball," *Nucleonics,* January 1967, p. 5.
15. Johnson, Wilfred E., Commissioner, USAEC, "Some Implications of the Fast Reactor Program in the United States," April 10, 1967, AEC Press Release No. 5-12-67.
16. "1967 Supplement," p. v.
17. *Ibid.,* p. xvi.
18. *Ibid.,* p. xvii.
19. Teller, Edward, "Fast Reactors: Maybe," *Nuclear News,* August 1967, p. 21.
20. *The Technology of Reactor Safety,* p. 600.

CHAPTER VIII

1. Jevons, W. Stanley, *The Coal Question,* first edition 1865, reprinted by Augustus M. Kelley, New York, 1965, p. 274 (quotation italicized in original).
2. Requa, M. L., 1916, quoted in Raybrawls, Arthur L., *The Energy Resources of the United States* (Washington, D.C., Catholic University of America, 1932), p. 75.
3. Putnam, Palmer Cosslett, *Energy in the Future* (New York, D. Van Nostrand Co., Inc., 1953), p. 252.
4. *Ibid.*
5. AEC, *Civilian Nuclear Power, a Report to the President — 1962,* Oak Ridge, 1962, p. 18.
6. U.S. Gov. Printing Office, Washington, D.C., 1964.
7. *Energy R&D and National Progress: Findings and Conclusions,* an Inderdepartmental Study, U.S. Gov. Printing Office, September, 1966.
8. *Ibid.,* table on p. 5
9. Jevons, *op. cit.,* p. 11 (italicized in original).
10. Hochschild, Adam, "Teapot Dome 1967?" *Ramparts,* May 1967, p. 10.
11. Lilienthal, David E., *The Journals of David E. Lilienthal,* Vol. II, *The Atomic Energy Years 1945–1950,* (New York, Harper and Row, 1964).
12. O'Brien, Brice, National Coal Association, memorandum dated August 7, 1967, Washington, D.C.
13. *Nucleonics Week,* January 18, 1968.
14. Slansky, Cyril M., "Waste Management in Close-Coupled Nuclear Fuel Cycles," *Proceedings,* Symposium on the Solidification and Long-Term Storage of Highly Radioactive Wastes, February 14–18, 1966, Richland, Washington. AEC, CONF-660208, November, 1966.

15. Orlans, Harold, *Contracting for Atoms*, Brookings Institution, Washington, D.C., 1967, p. 47.
16. *Electrical World*, August 14, 1967, p. 12.
17. Green, Harold and Alan Rosenthal, *The Government of the Atom*, (New York, Atherton Press, 1967), pp. viii-ix.

CHAPTER IX

1. Commoner, Barry, unpublished speech, 1962.

INDEX

Amazing
Insider Secrets

Outsmart the Experts
with *the* Consumer Guide
for Getting the Best Deals—
from Skin Care to Home Repairs

Jeff Bredenberg

Reader's Digest

The Reader's Digest Association, Inc.
Pleasantville, New York | Montreal

Project Staff

PROJECT EDITOR Don Earnest

PROJECT DESIGNER Michele Laseau

COVER DESIGNER George McKeon

EDITOR Daryna Tobey

COPY EDITOR Jeanette Gingold

INDEXER Cohen Carruth Indexers

ILLUSTRATOR Travis Foster

Contributors

EDITOR AND LEAD WRITER Jeff Bredenberg

WRITERS Mary Beausoleil, Jeff Edelstein, Kelly Garrett, Debra Gordon, Dougald MacDonald, Eric Metcalf, Elizabeth Shimer, Logan Ward

HEALTH AND FITNESS ADVISORS
Mary Hardy, M.D., Jeff Novick

Reader's Digest Books

EDITOR IN CHIEF Neil Wertheimer

EXECUTIVE MANAGING EDITOR
Donna Ruvituso

CREATIVE DIRECTOR Michele Laseau

ASSOCIATE DIRECTOR, NORTH AMERICAN PREPRESS Douglas A. Croll

MANUFACTURING MANAGER John L. Cassidy

MARKETING DIRECTOR Dawn Nelson

PRESIDENT AND PUBLISHER,
TRADE PUBLISHING Harold Clarke

PRESIDENT, U.S. BOOKS & HOME ENTERTAINMENT Dawn Zier

The Reader's Digest Association, Inc.

PRESIDENT & CHIEF EXECUTIVE OFFICER
Mary Berner

First printing in paperback 2008

ISBN: 978-0-0761-0983-8
Amazing Insider Secrets was originally published as *Forbidden Advice* (ISBN: 978-0-7621-0777-3)

Address any comments about *Amazing Insider Secrets* to:
The Reader's Digest Association, Inc.
Editor in Chief, Books and Music
Reader's Digest Road
Pleasantville, NY 10570-7000

For more Reader's Digest products and information, visit our website: **www.rd.com**

Printed in U.S.A.
1 3 5 7 9 10 8 6 4 2 (hardcover)
 9 10 8 (paperback)

Note to Our Readers

The information in this book has been carefully researched, and all efforts have been made to ensure its accuracy and safety. The Reader's Digest Association, Inc., and the author do not assume any responsibility for any injuries suffered or damages or losses incurred as a result of following the instructions in this book. Before taking any action based on information in this book, study the information carefully and make sure that you understand it fully. The mention of any brand or product in this book does not imply an endorsement. All prices and product names mentioned are subject to change and should be considered general examples rather than specific recommendations.

1,703 **Ways to Win!**

You've thought it a thousand times: If I'd only known the full story ... the hidden facts ... the way the system really works ... the inside dope. I could have saved my hard-earned cash. I could have made a lot better use of my time. I could have used my energy for something much more important or enjoyable.

The fact is, we've all been victims of either misinformation or withheld information that ultimately cost us precious resources of money, time, and energy. Call it the silence of the experts. It's not that they are outright lying, or even consciously being deceptive. But sometimes they know information that could help you—and they just don't tell it to you. They're bored, they're lazy, they assume you know, or worse, they don't want to jeopardize a sale. And yes, sometimes experts withhold information for the worst of reasons—to make a quick buck off you. Whatever the reason, withheld expert advice is rampant, touching every aspect of our lives.

Oh, to be a mind reader! Wouldn't you love to know what's *really* going through the mechanic's mind when he peruses your engine? The dark secret your banker is hiding from you when you sign up for a checking account? The few words you need to murmur to your pharmacist before you save a bundle on your prescription?

A Boatload of Insider Secrets

If the answers to those questions are "yes," then you are about to be quite delighted. For much of a year, we have searched out as many expert insider secrets as we could find. Tips that are not only guaranteed to preserve your valuable resources but will make you feel like a genius to boot. And here they are!

In the pages ahead you'll find hush-hush hints and tips from pros, experts, and other insiders that will give you the upper hand at home, at work, in stores, on the road and on vacation, anywhere, anytime, even in casinos. They range from food industry secrets that can magically slash your food costs and health risks from food to crucial appliance care instructions that should be in every owner's manual. Our inside secrets tell you what corporations and marketers don't want you to know, from the drug company that wants you to ignore perfectly effective home remedies to the established, well-reputed website that slides hidden software onto your home computer.

Amazing Insider Secrets gives you the facts that will make you the smartest, sharpest consumer on the block. Over and over again, we found shockingly effective ways to outsmart the sneaky pros and beat them at their own game. Each of the 1,703 pieces of "forbidden advice" in this book come straight from the mouth of knowledgeable insiders (reluctant though they were to give it up). Here are just some of the things that you'll discover:

- games that supermarkets play to get you to buy the priciest product
- inexpensive home treatments that your doctor and drugmakers don't want to you know about
- unspoken rules that HR and office bigwigs actually follow
- sneaky ways the slim-and-trim get their edge
- rarely revealed info that will make the steely car salesman blush
- tricks that insurance companies are hiding up their sleeves
- corner-cutting tricks of seasoned travelers
- $95-an-hour subterfuges that repair people use
- expiration dates that are just a ploy to steal your money

You'll be amazed at how surprisingly enlightening and simple many of these expert remedies and professional solutions are. You'll discover the secrets for navigating a health food store … the pitfalls of travel websites … the gadgets that clever home-makers use … a notorious tightwad's negotiating tips. You'll find out when you can safely ignore that oil-change sticker, why you should skip the expensive sports drink, how a simple squirt bottle can cut the need for expensive on-the-road dry cleaning, and why you should always get a player's card when you go to casino. You'll even discover that yogurt may be your best bet for avoiding a cold this winter.

Unrigging the Game

Of course, you're no bumpkin. You probably already knew—or at least strongly suspected—that the game is rigged. And by "the game" we mean absolutely everything around you—repair people, credit cards, supermarkets, clothing stores, car dealers, hotels, airlines, restaurants, medical care, insurance, your job, the educational system. It's a fact: Mixed in undetected among the many well-intentioned professionals is the occasional sneaky glad-hander who has laid a trap that's ready to snap closed on your money. It's a complex world, getting more and more confounding all the time, and no matter how hard the average person tries, it seems at times to be almost impossible to keep up with all of the distorted information and all the smooth talkers who are out to make a fast buck at your expense.

That's why we wrote *Amazing Insider Secrets*. It's the book that all the penny-pinching companies, scheming marketers, and sneaky bigwigs didn't want published. Anywhere your finances or well-being is at risk, we hounded expert insiders until they surrendered their secrets. Oh, scores of our informants provided the inside dope openly—because they believe in giving us regular folks an even break. But many more experts, fearing for their jobs and their professional reputations, insisted on anonymity. Picture these experts testifying in shadow behind a screen, while their less reputable colleagues squirm and squeal when their underhanded tricks come to light.

What's Inside

In this book, you will learn the times when you're most likely to get a rookie doctor at the hospital. About the heart-damaging sweetener you find in just about every processed food on the market. About the scary chemicals that sneak into your home in household products and building materials. Not only do we reveal these health threats, but we also tell you what to do about them. (While we're on the subject of health, we'd like to give special thanks to two professionals who helped ensure the accuracy of our health advice—Dr. Mary Hardy, an integrative medicine expert at the University of California, Los Angeles, and Jeff Novick, director of nutrition for the Pritikin Longevity Center & Spa in Aventura, Florida.)

You also will find out how manufacturers gouge extra money out of your wallet every day. Learn the inexpensive dandruff cure that you keep in a bottle by the sink—but it's not shampoo! Get the over-the-counter sleep aid you need—without that hefty price tag. Revive the musty air in your house without those pricey air fresheners. Buy cosmetics for pennies on the dollar. And learn about the secret clothing codes that will lead you to enormous discounts.

You'll discover easy, low-cost solutions to problems around the house—annoyances that you have been throwing big money at. Learn the most common, simple fixes that you could easily do yourself, but that instead keep repair people laughing all the way to the bank. Find out the common lawn care mistake that will kill your trees. Read about the common kitchen item that will keep your icemaker running smoothly and prevent huge repair bills.

Speaking of fixes, this book was written for both U.S. and Canadian readers, so we've included metric measurements as well as traditional "pound-foot" ones. But even in metricized Canada, traditional units are commonly used for some products and materials such as lumber. When in doubt about a size, consult a knowledgeable staffer at your local harware store, home center, or lumberyard.

As this book hits the streets, you can just about hear the collective howl from all the schemers and other sneaks who have been getting a free ride up to now off your goodwill and trusting nature. No more. We've turned a big, bright spotlight onto those closely guarded secrets, and now all of us everyday Janes and Joes can fight back!

—Jeff Bredenberg

Contents

when you head to the great outdoors. If you get stung, spray with the vinegar first. If the sting persists, slather on a paste of baking soda (just mix a tiny amount with some water or even your spit). If the stinger is still in your skin, gently rub it with a wet bar of soap—the stinger will come right out, she says.

Use yogurt to dry up cold sores. Why is it that a cold sore seems to pop out just as you have an important event coming up, like your daughter's wedding? Probably because most cold sores are caused by the common herpes virus. It lives quietly in your body until some kind of stress (aforementioned wedding) wakes it up. To quickly get rid of the ugly cold sore, do what Dr. Schlachter does: Put a teaspoon of cultured yogurt on the area several times a day. The active microorganisms in the yogurt "attack" the virus, she says, reducing the itching and helping the sore heal faster.

Use an onion to remove a splinter. So your grandkid was playing on your back deck barefoot and now he's got a 1/4-inch (6.35-mm) splinter stuck deep in his foot. When you pull out the needle and matches, he begins screaming like you've suggested cutting off the foot. No need for those tears. Just take a 1/4-inch-thick piece of onion, place it over the splinter site, and wrap a bandage around it to keep it close to the skin. Leave overnight. In the morning, the splinter will have worked its way out of the skin with no pain, thanks to chemicals in the onion that shrink the skin.

Put an onion on that bruise. If you bruise so easily that your coworkers have begun leaving brochures about domestic abuse on your desk, try this folk remedy. Place a slice of yellow onion on the bruise for 15 minutes. The same compound in onions that makes your eyes water—allicin—stimulates the lymphatic flow in your body, helping flush away the excess blood in the tissue that creates the bruise. This only works, however, if you apply the onion *immediately* after the injury.

Treat a bruise with witch hazel. If the onion remedy just isn't doing it for you, try rubbing the bruise with witch hazel (available in health food stores and drugstores) and covering with ice for five minutes. The two together constrict blood vessels, reducing bleeding into the tissue and speeding healing, says Dr. Schlachter.

Use baking soda to prevent athlete's foot. Snatch that box of baking soda out of the fridge and sprinkle it on your feet and between your toes. By absorbing moisture, it can help prevent itchy, unsightly athlete's foot. Need the baking soda for biscuits? No problem. Just crush six garlic cloves in two tablespoons olive oil and let it sit for a few days, then strain and apply the oil to the area once a day. The active ingredient in garlic, ajoene, is a powerful antifungal substance, says Dr. Schlachter.

Prevent contact irritation with nail polish. Your husband just bought you a set of gorgeous (and expensive) diamond stud earrings (and he didn't even do anything wrong!). Problem is, you're having an allergic reaction to the metal. Before getting your doctor to write a prescription for a steroid cream, try coating the backs with clear nail polish to provide a barrier between the metal and your skin. ◁

Hair and Nail Care
4 Secrets for Keeping Your Hair Healthy and Your Nails Strong

Wash your hair in Listerine. Why? Because your hair stinks. No, not really. Turns out that Listerine is an effective cure for dandruff, says Dr. Schlachter. Mix your own dandruff rinse by combining one part mouthwash with nine parts water. After shampooing with your regular shampoo, apply the mixture to your scalp and leave it on. Your dandruff will improve, your hair won't be sticky, and you can be assured people won't accuse your hair of having bad breath. You don't actually have to use Listerine. Most drug chains carry a much cheaper house-brand antiseptic mouthwash that has the same active ingredients as Listerine. Just compare labels.

Give your hair a mint rinse. Okay, the Listerine remedy works, but if you'd rather not have your hair smelling like mouthwash, try this other remedy from Dr. Schlachter: Mash a handful of fresh or dry peppermint leaves and cover them with vodka (sounds good already, doesn't it?) Let it steep for a full day (no tasting), then strain. Add 1/4 teaspoon water at a time to the mix until it becomes cloudy. After shampooing, apply the mix to your scalp and leave it on. You should see results by the second shampoo, and if not, you can always drink the stuff (the vodka mix, not the shampoo).

Take B vitamins for strong nails. Nails as strong as horses' hoofs, to be exact. It's a secret veterinarians have long known—that the B vitamin biotin strengthens horses' hoofs. The hoofs are made from keratin, the same substance that makes up fingernails (the natural ones, at least). Several studies find it works just as well in humans. One from Swiss researchers found that patients with brittle nails who supplement with 2,500 micrograms of biotin for six months increased their nail thickness 25 percent. Take 300 micrograms of the vitamin four to six times a day.

Skip the quick-drying nail polish. Most quick-drying polishes contain more formaldehyde and alcohol than regular polishes, and those fluids can dry and split your nails. The best way to fast-dry your nails is by freezing them. Dump a tray of ice cubes into your bathroom sink, add enough cold water to cover them, then dip your wet nails into the cold water for a minute or two after each coat. ◁

Stifling the Sniffles

6 Secrets for Dealing with Colds, Allergies, and Other Respiratory Difficulties

Eat raw honey to prevent hay fever. It's spring, and while everyone else is outside enjoying the warmth, you're a prisoner in your air-conditioned house, not even an open window to bring the season inside. That's because you're allergic to some form of pollen. Well, start eating raw honey. Since it contains grains of pollen, it helps to gradually accustom your overactive immune system to the pollen so it doesn't go nuts when it encounters the grains every spring. Aim for 3 or 4 tablespoons a day. You can lick it right off the spoon, mix it into your tea, or drizzle it onto your toast or corn muffin. Make sure you're using *raw* honey, and use local honey so it contains pollens from your local region. You can usually find this type of honey at roadside vegetable stands and farmers' markets.

Try algae for allergies. Here's another trick for controlling those seasonal sniffles: Try sucking down green drinks or supplements that contain spirulina, a blue-green algae. This strong anti-inflammatory can quell the overreactive immune response to allergy triggers that leads to your miserable symptoms. That's what University of California, Davis, researchers found when they gave 24 people with allergies either 2,000 milligrams a day of spirulina or a placebo. The algae group produced 32 percent fewer inflammatory chemicals that trigger those symptoms—the placebo group saw no change. Now, just

---

WHAT YOUR **DOCTOR** DOESN'T WANT YOU TO KNOW ABOUT Homeopathy

Homeopathy, a 19th-century form of medicine in which you take a highly diluted form of a component capable of causing the symptoms you're exhibiting to cure your condition, has some serious scientific backing behind it. In 1991 a review of 107 studies on homeopathy published in the *British Medical Journal* found 81 trials whose positive results couldn't be attributed to placebo. In 1997 the renowned British journal *Lancet* published another well-done analysis of 89 placebo-controlled clinical studies on homeopathy, concluding the treatment provided twice the therapeutic benefit of a placebo. Another study published in the *Annals of Internal Medicine* in 2003 concluded that while more and better research is needed, "it is important that physicians be open-minded about homeopathy's possible value and maintain communication with patients who use it." The therapy seems to work best for treating the flu (*Oscillococcinum*), hay fever (*Galphimia glauca*), and pain and bruising (*arnica*).

For other conditions, seek out someone trained in homeopathy to develop individually mixed preparations for you.

imagine your allergist's face when you cancel your next six appointments!

Prevent colds with yogurt. If the thought of downing live bacteria turns your stomach, stop reading now. But if, like the rest of us, you'd like to avoid the sneezing, sniffling annoyance of colds this winter, then this tip is for you—and we're pretty sure your doctor never heard of it. Two six-ounce servings of Stonyfield Farm yogurt, or any other yogurt that contains the healthy live bacteria *Lactobacillus reuteri,* can cut your sick days in half. That's what researchers in Sweden (capital of yogurt) found when they had factory workers drink a concoction with 100 million units of the little bugs or a placebo for 2 1/2 months. Just 11 percent of the bacteria guzzlers took a sick day during the study compared to 23 percent of those taking a placebo. Why? These little guys help your immune system work better.

Actually, the yogurt itself may also help fend off colds. In another study from researchers at the University of California, Davis, people who eat a cup of yogurt a day have 25 percent fewer colds than non-yogurt eaters. And it didn't matter whether the yogurt was live culture or pasteurized. Start your yogurt eating in the summer to build up your immunity before cold and flu season starts. The manager of your local drugstore will wonder why his cold remedies aren't moving as well as they used to.

Go salt-free when gargling. Remember your grandmother forcing you to gargle every winter morning with salt water, swearing it would keep away colds and flu? Well, she was right. But if, like us, the idea of gargling with warm salt water makes you gag, skip the salt. Studies find gargling plain water works just as well, says Susan Montauk, M.D., professor of clinical family medicine at the University of Cincinnati's College of Medicine, who recommends it for her patients. In fact, she says, statistically you'll do better with plain water than with salt water.

Get a CRP for sinusitis. Instead of just swallowing the antibiotics your doctor hands you—and the line that all sinus infections are bacterial in nature—ask for a CRP test, an inexpensive blood test that measures levels of an inflammatory marker and is given primarily to test for heart problems (see page 18). If levels are high, you have a bacterial infection and will need antibiotics, thank you very much. But if levels are low, your infection is viral and only time will clear it up. One Danish study found doctors using the CRP test for sinusitis wrote 20 percent fewer prescriptions for antibiotics than those who didn't—great news as we try to stem the growth of antibiotic-resistant bacteria.

Get a CT scan for that chronic cough. Doctors are pretty bad at diagnosing the reason behind a chronic cough. Instead, they'll probably just write you a prescription for a nasal medication to dry up secretions. But a study from Mayo Clinic doctors who performed CT scans on the sinuses of those with chronic cough found more than a third of them had chronic sinusitis, an infection, or inflammation that could cause coughing and sneezing. The treatment? Antibiotics, nasal steroids, or decongestants. ◄

Staying Heart-Healthy
10 Little-Known Ways to Help Prevent Heart-Related Disorders

Take your niacin. LDL, LDL, LDL. If that's all you're hearing when you ask for your cholesterol results, then you're only getting half the story. High levels of HDL—the so-called good cholesterol—are just as important, if not *more* important, in predicting heart attack risk as LDL levels and other blood fat markers. But if all your doctor does is prescribe a statin, you're missing the boat. Talk to your doctor about high-dose niacin—a B vitamin shown to increase HDL levels. Don't be thrown by negative talk about flushing as a side effect of niacin. Today, new formulations, including an over-the-counter form called SLO-niacin and a prescription form called Niaspan, provide all the benefits of niacin without the red face. Problem is, there aren't any drug companies pushing vitamins, so your doctor may not be up on the latest about this important treatment.

Get heart-healthy with chocolate. It seems to go against all of the nutritional advice Mom ever gave, but dark chocolate truly is a healthful food—proven in studies to lower your blood pressure. With its heart-healthy monounsaturated fat, antioxidants, and other beneficial plant chemicals, dark chocolate is actually more akin to nuts than it is to candy. It also provides fiber and magnesium. Scientists who fed people 100 grams of dark chocolate every day for two weeks found that their blood pressure dropped a significant amount—on average, 5 points on the systolic reading (the top number) and 2 points on the diastolic (the bottom number). The one hitch: The test subjects had to forgo other sweets or junk food in their diets to compensate for the added calories. So eat 100 grams of Hershey's Special Dark Chocolate every day, and pass up 531 calories' worth of pies, cakes, ice cream, and chips that you would have eaten otherwise.

Replace butter with avocados in your food. We have nothing personal against dairy farmers, but avocados are a tasty, heart-protecting substitute for butter and cream. When you mash them, they take on the same creamy texture as butter. Use them to thicken your soup or make your mashed potatoes creamier. Avocados are one of the only two fruits (along with olives) that are high in fat—but it's the heart-healthy variety called monounsaturated fat.

SECRET WEAPON

Milk

Mom always told you to drink your milk to build strong bones. We're telling you to drink it to reduce blood pressure. A study published in the journal *Hypertension* that evaluated nearly 5,000 men and women found those getting three or more servings of low-fat dairy a day were 36 percent less likely to have high blood pressure than those eating half a serving a day.

Ask about diuretics for high blood pressure. Pity the poor doctor. With dozens of medications available to treat high blood pressure, patients coming and going at all times, and that stack of medical journals piling up on her desk, who can blame her for prescribing what she knows best—rather than what the research shows works best. And that would be simple diuretics, one of the oldest—and cheapest—classes of drugs to treat high blood pressure. Yet the most-prescribed drugs for high blood pressure are beta blockers. Now an analysis of more than 13 studies involving 105,000 patients finds that people on beta blockers have a 16 percent higher risk of stroke than those on diuretics. The difference was so striking that the Swedish researchers conducting the study recommended beta blockers *not* be the first choice to treat hypertension. Talk to your doctor about switching.

Get tested beyond HDL/LDL. Bad news, your doctor says with a grim look. Your cholesterol is a bit high. Before he can whip out his prescription pad and start you on a statin, ask for more details. Specifically, a lipoprotein phenotyping, which, in addition to measuring HDL (good) and LDL (bad) cholesterol, measures amounts of two other types of blood fats: chylomicrons and very low-density lipoproteins (VLDL). High levels of either can be far more risky in terms of developing heart disease than a high LDL. Plus, statins may have no effect on VLDL or chylomicron levels. The results of the tests will let you know how serious your cholesterol levels are and whether you should start immediately on a statin or give lifestyle changes a try first.

Ask your doctor to check your CRP. Chances are your doctor hasn't. Yet this simple, $15 blood test can tell you more about your risk of a heart attack than ten cholesterol tests. The high-sensitivity C-reactive protein (hs-CRP) test measures a marker for inflammation—a risk factor for stroke or heart attack. In fact, a study published in the *New England Journal of Medicine* found the test is twice as effective as a standard cholesterol test in predicting heart attacks and strokes. The good news? Statins, the most commonly prescribed drug for high cholesterol, also reduce CRP levels.

Take horse chestnut extract to prevent clots when flying. Although you'd rather have your fingernails pulled out with pincers than fly in a cramped coach seat these days, sometimes there's no way to avoid it. If you simply must suffer through a long flight, take double the recommended dose of horse chestnut extract before heading for the airport, says Mary Hardy, M.D., director of Integrative Medicine at the Ted Mann Family Resource Center at the University of California, Los Angeles. The herb helps reduce leg swelling, minimizing your risk of blood clots.

Measure your waist to determine heart risk. That beer belly you're toting around does more than force your pants down around your knees; it's also a big, fat sign that you're at risk for a heart attack (and/or diabetes). Abdominal fat is more inflammatory than fat on your rear or hips, and those inflammatory chemicals it puts out are devastating to your coronary arteries. A simple tape measure can tell you if you're carrying around this risk factor, but the Shape of the Nations Report from the World Health Federation in Switzerland found 62 percent of doctors surveyed said they don't measure their patients' waistlines to check for overweight and obesity. The survey quizzed doctors and patients in the United States, Canada, and 25 other countries. Ninety-five percent of women at risk for heart disease said their doctors never measured their waist circumference, and 71 percent said that their doctors never told them that excess weight, including high-risk abdominal fat, boosted their risk for heart disease. So bring a tape measure with you to your next doctor visit and teach your physician how to do a waist measurement:

- Raise your shirt above your stomach.
- Place the measuring tape around your waist halfway between the top of your hip bone and the bottom of your rib cage.
- Relax and breathe out while measuring. If your waist is no more than 35 inches (89 cm) for women or 40 inches (101 cm) for men, you're okay. Any more and you better hit the gym.

Get a roommate to cut heart disease. And no, your cat doesn't count. Given the latest research out of Denmark, we think it's worth giving up a bit of privacy and learning to share the refrigerator shelves. The Danish study found that people living alone have twice the risk of serious heart disease compared to those who live with someone. We hear craigslist (the online bulletin board at www.craigslist.org, where you can find everything from roommates to a used dining room table) is a good place to advertise that spare room!

Keep working to reduce heart risk. Yeah, yeah, you're two years away from retirement and your boss makes the Meryl Streep character in the movie *The Devil Wears Prada* look good. You're dying to quit or even get yourself fired so you can take early retirement and get out of the rat race. Hold on. A study of more than 12,000 Americans finds that losing your job late in your career dou-bles your risk of heart attack or stroke. So suck it up, keep your head down, and document everything. In fact, continuing to work through your golden years, volunteering, and even just taking the stairs instead of the elevator are the kind of daily activities researchers at the National Institute on Aging found could help you live longer. Even better? The researchers found these non-exercise activities packed as much longevity punch as actually working out! ◄

EBCT: The Test Your Doctor Probably Won't Recommend

If you've been relying on cholesterol readings or treadmill tests to judge your risk of a heart attack, you're missing the boat. William Davis, M.D., medical director of Milwaukee Heart Scan and author of the book *Track Your Plaque*, notes: "Using cholesterol testing to identify people with heart disease is like trying to predict who is going to die on a high-speed freeway." That's because half of all heart attacks occur in people with levels of the "bad" LDL cholesterol below 134 (anything over 129 is borderline high).

Instead, he recommends a ten-minute, $200 test called an electron beam computed tomograph, or EBCT. The scans take fast pictures of the heart for 20 seconds inside an open machine that uses about the same amount of radiation contained in dental x-rays. The scans show the amount of calcium in your coronary arteries (20 percent of artery-clogging plaque is calcium) and provides a far more accurate picture of your heart disease risk.

Why hasn't your doctor recommended this simple test? "Everyone focuses on LDL cholesterol because high cholesterol is a profitable disease," says Dr. Davis. Doctors are also waiting for the results of a long-term trial of the screening test due in 2008. We say, don't wait. Three studies published in major medical journals in 2006 found the test worked great at predicting heart attack risk. It's recommended for all American men over age 45 and most women over 55.

Secrets of Good Sleep
7 Easy but Rarely Disclosed Ways to Make the Most of Your Slumber Time

Get your ZZZ's for better memory. If you go to your doctor complaining that you no longer remember the cat's name and you forgot your dentist appointment twice, he might give you a short quiz, pat you on the back, and tell you that you're fine—we're all getting older. But will he ask you the critical question: How much sleep are you getting? Probably not. And that's a shame, because a major study from Harvard Medical School sleep researchers found that the amount and quality of sleep you get significantly affects your memory, particularly the type of memory that helps you remember facts and events in time.

Skip the sleeping pill. Ever wonder why docs are so quick to whip out the prescription pad when you complain about insomnia? Because it's easy, quick, and it works—temporarily. They also have only five minutes before they need to see their next patient, and it would take longer than that to explain the most effective therapy for insomnia—cognitive behavior therapy, or CBT. This therapy teaches you to realistically evaluate your insomnia and find ways to address it. For instance, you might learn that missing a night's sleep isn't so terrible. That, in turn, helps you feel less anxious about not falling asleep so you can, well, fall asleep! One study followed 63 adults with insomnia for eight weeks and found CBT worked better than the prescription medication Ambien (zolpidem).

Check your meds if you can't sleep. Doctors are always supposed to ask you what medications you're taking (or know by looking at your chart), but we've found they rarely do. So when you complain of insomnia, they may not think to connect your sleeplessness with some drug you're taking. Yet many medications can interfere with sleep, says Dr. Mary Hardy of UCLA. These include beta blockers, thyroid medication, certain antidepressants like the selective serotonin reuptake inhibitors (SSRIs), decongestants, corticosteroids, and medications with caffeine (like Excedrin). If you're seeing your doctor about insomnia, make a list of all drugs you're taking—including over-the-counter medications and herbal and nutritional supplements. List the dosages you're taking, too, and take them to the doctor with you.

Boil some lettuce for a good night's sleep. It sounds yucky (and might make a bit of a mess) but lettuce contains a compound called lectucarium, which works similarly to opium in your brain. Since opium is a bit difficult to get these days (not to mention illegal), try this: Simmer three to four large lettuce leaves in a cup of water for 15 minutes. Remove from heat, add two sprigs of mint, strain, and sip just before bed. Any kind of lettuce works, so go for the cheapest—plain ol' iceberg.

Calm those restless legs with a bar of soap. It's a common cause of insomnia: You go to bed, tired and ready to get a solid eight hours. Just as you're drifting off, however, your legs jerk. And they continue to do this throughout the night, either keeping you from falling

☐ The most frequently prescribed medications for chronic insomnia have never been tested or approved for that purpose. In fact, while the antidepressant Desyrel (trazodone) is the most prescribed drug for insomnia, just one quality study has been published on its use for insomnia. That study found that after a week, Desyrel worked no better at relieving insomnia than a placebo.

☐ All over-the-counter sleeping aids, from Tylenol PM to Sominex and everything in between, contain the same active ingredient—diphenhydramine or some other antihistamine. So for the occasional sleepless night, Dr. Mary Hardy says, skip the expensive store brands and pick up any generic antihistamine. Just make sure it doesn't say "non-drowsy" on the label!

asleep or waking you up. While there is now an approved prescription medication for restless legs syndrome (there seems to be a drug for everything these days) side effects include confusion, dizziness, nausea and hallucinations. We have a better solution: Slip a bar of Ivory soap under your legs and the restlessness should disappear in about 3 to 5 minutes, says Dr. Lou Schlachter. It must be plain soap, she says, not a deodorant bar like Dial or Zest. The high magnesium content of the soap helps, she says. And, indeed, research links low levels of magnesium to restless legs. In one study of ten patients with restless legs syndrome, those taking 150 to 300 milligrams of elemental magnesium and 300 to 600 milligrams of calcium a half hour before bed woke less often and experienced fewer jerks after supplementing for four to six weeks.

Take a vitamin for better sleep.
If your restless legs are keeping you awake, by all means try the bar of soap recommended above. But also pop a B vitamin. In one small study, researchers found that women with restless legs syndrome were deficient in folic acid, which is required for proper brain and nerve function. Supplementing with this vitamin, however, improved symptoms. Take 400 to 800 micrograms of folic acid a day, along with a 50-milligram B complex supplement to maintain a balance of B vitamins.

Exercise at the right time. It has been shown time and again that even mild exercise, like a half-hour of walking, can help you sleep better. But *when* you exercise is also important. Exercise is stimulating; it's not something to do just before bedtime. Instead, plan your exercise for early evening—about four to six hours before bedtime. This is the time it takes for your body's metabolism and temperature to drop after exercise, which primes your body for sleep. ◁

Alleviating Depression
6 Secrets for Handling Distressing Down-in-the-Dumps Moods

Find a new friend to prevent depression. Research finds that fewer of us have close friends today than people did 30 years ago. Research also finds much higher rates of depression today than 30 years ago. While there's no evidence (yet!) that the two are linked, we think they might be. That's because there's so much evidence showing that supportive relationships—whether friend or family—can protect you against major depression, particularly if you're a woman. Since family members are all too often the *cause* of depression, we think finding new friends is important. How to make friends when you're no longer in school? Join a group, sign up for a committee, invite a coworker out to lunch or for an after-work drink.

Get a dog to lift your spirits. With more than 147 million prescriptions for antidepressants like Prozac written each year in the United States and Canada, it might seem like everyone and their mother is popping happy pills. Shoot, veterinarians are even prescribing Prozac and its cousins for puppies. But instead of medicating your dog, you should play with it, especially if you're sad or depressed. That's what researchers from the University of Missouri found when they studied levels of mood-related chemicals in people after they'd played with a dog for just a few minutes. Playing with Fido increased levels of feel-good hormones. Rufff!

Find happiness in eating fish. Why are so many of us depressed? Could it be that we're not getting enough fish? That's what a growing body of evidence shows. The link, researchers say, is related to omega-3 fatty acids, "good" fats that help nerve cells, like those in the brain, communicate with one another. Among the many studies looking at fish consumption and depression, one found that people eating a healthy diet with fatty fish like salmon two or three times a week for five years had significantly fewer feelings of depression and hostility than a similar group of people who weren't getting as much fish. If you can't stand fish, you have a couple of other options: 3 grams a day of fish oil or 2 tablespoons a day of ground flaxseed, another great source of omega-3s. ◄

WHAT THE DRUG COMPANIES DON'T WANT YOU TO KNOW ABOUT Therapy

Cognitive therapy, a form of therapy that helps patients view the world differently as a way of addressing their depression, is at least as effective as drugs when it comes to treating severe depression. And the therapy has no side effects and costs less. Those findings come from researchers at the University of Pennsylvania and Vanderbilt University who followed 240 patients for 16 months—an unusually large and long study for depression. They even found that the therapy's effects lasted longer after patients stopped the therapy than when they stopped the medication.

Alleviating Anxiety

12 Little-Known Ways to Deal with Anxiety and Life's Stresses

Plan an outdoor vacation for winter. Unless you live in Florida or California, you know that February is actually 35 days long—at least, that's how it feels. By this point in the winter, you're likely dragging from the lack of sunshine, the lousy weather, the lack of a significant break, and the general crappiness of the world. So cruising the islands or even skiing in Utah can give you a powerful dose of mood-lightening natural light, says UCLA's Dr. Mary Hardy. You don't have to be super-wealthy for such a trip. Even a cut-rate hotel in Florida will work—as long as it has a balcony for sunbathing. Once you return home, you'll not only be refreshed and revitalized but you'll only have a few weeks left until spring arrives.

Skip a night of sleep to end depression. If you struggle with depression, here's a surprising finding that might give your spirits a lift: Researchers find that skipping an entire night of sleep can quell depression for as long as a month. No one's sure why this works, but speculation is that depriving yourself of sleep "resets" your internal clock and enables people who are depressed to actually sleep better.

Indulge yourself to avoid regrets later. You only order a single scoop of vanilla, shop at Wal-Mart, and fly coach—and then only to visit your aunt Ruth in Topeka. Someday, you say, you'll upgrade to first class, buy cashmere, indulge in a banana split every week. Don't wait too long … a study from researchers at Columbia University found that denying yourself life's little pleasures leads to more than a dull life. It leads to serious regret as you age. Over time, the regret gets worse, while the guilt over indulging fades.

Ask your doctor for this blood test for anxiety. We've always said how great it would be if there were a simple blood test to diagnose mental health conditions like depression and anxiety. Now there is, at least for anxiety. A blood test to measure levels of the protein acetylcholinesterase, a chemical you release when you're under stress, and the enzymes butyrylcholinesterase (BChE) and paraoxonase (PON), accurately predicted the presence of an anxiety disorder 90 percent of the time in Israeli trials. Although the researchers hope to have a commercial test for these chemicals on the market soon, your doctor can order the test through a hospital or specialty laboratory.

SECRET WEAPON

Basil Tea

If you're feeling rattled, rankled, and wound up, relief is as close as your herb garden or your supermarket. Basil tea is a calming concoction for many people. Just put three fresh basil leaves in a cup of hot water and steep for ten minutes before drinking. Fresh basil is easy to find in the produce section of your supermarket too.

Avoid the stress of telling lies. Pinocchio learned well: No good can come from lying. Not to mention it increases levels of stress hormones that, over time, can cause lasting harm. Don't believe us? How do you think polygraph tests work? By picking up on your body's response to stress, such as increased blood pressure, heart rate, and breathing rate. The stress response is so strong that researchers are developing a "sniffer test" to measure stress hormone levels on your breath.

Quit the caffeine to reduce jitters. We have one question for you: If you have a tendency to get anxious, and you know that coffee and other highly caffeinated beverages and foods make people jittery, then what are you doing with a Starbucks card? Seriously, quit the caffeine. It blocks the calming effects of the brain chemical adenosine, which usually helps promote calmness and sleepiness. And you don't have to chug it all at once to get these effects; one study found drinking the equivalent of two cups of coffee over five hours could make you as jittery and anxious as if you'd chugged two cups of coffee all at once.

Learn the calming effect of breath control. You know how when you're anxious, your heart beats like a locomotive coming full speed up the tracks, and try as you might, you can't seem to get enough oxygen in your lungs? Forget the old breathe-in-a-paper-bag trick. Instead, try this the next time you feel the beginnings of that anxious feeling, says Michael Crabtree, Ph.D., a professor of psychology at Washington & Jefferson College in Washington, Pennsylvania, and a licensed clinical psychologist.

- Lie on the floor, place your hand on your chest, and try to reduce the amount of movement, while continuing to breathe normally. You need to breathe for five minutes and allow your hand to feel the breathing. But you don't want your chest to move, you want the other parts of your body to take over the breathing—using your diaphragm, instead of the big chest inhalation and exhalation.

- Make yourself aware of your breathing in non-stress situations, such as reading or watching television.

- Try to employ the breathing you experience in non-stress situations in more stressful situations—such as traffic jams or conflicts with the kids. "Use the power of getting yourself more focused and relaxed," says Crabtree.

- Develop this non-stress type of breathing as your sustained way of life. "Make it your normal way of breathing," he says.

- Be aware that chest breathing still has a purpose, but only as a point of context. It should only be used in periods of extreme emotional arousal—like running away or fighting.

Try an antibiotic to cut fear of public speaking. Given the growing problem of antibiotic resistance, getting your doctor to prescribe one is getting as difficult as convincing an accountant to take a week off in April. But here's one reason to prescribe the drug: to help you get over socially related anxiety quicker. This type of anxiety hits when you have to do something in public, like give a speech. When researchers from Emory University gave 13 patients undergoing therapy for their anxiety the antibiotic D-cycloserine (DCS) and compared them to a similar group undergoing therapy but not getting the drug, they found those getting the antibiotic learned to overcome their social fears quicker. D-cycloserine is typically used to treat tuberculosis, but studies find it can also enhance learning, which may be why it helped, the researchers speculate.

How I Do It A Spirituality Expert Counters Anger

The secret is selective silence. "As soon as you realize that you are about to express anger over a situation, hush up," says Mick Quinn, the author of *Power and Grace: The Wisdom of Awakening*. "This was the position Gandhi took, and note the fantastic results."

As you interact in your relationships ...

☐ Pay attention to the arising of thoughts (or feelings) of anger or anxiety.

☐ Ask yourself this question: "Do I care more about this other person than I do about myself?" A positive response reveals a truly selfless person and a friend anyone would want to have, keep, and cherish.

☐ Be prepared for the sometimes overwhelming need to express negative thoughts or emotions without regard for the consequences on your relationship(s).

☐ Choose to not express those thoughts and feelings by being *selectively silent*.

☐ "Discern, decide, and disregard." Discern that a thought is not beneficial to your current objective, decide not to express it in conversation or action, and through introspection and selective silence, disregard it.

Pop some sunflower seeds to lower anxiety. You've got a big speech to deliver tomorrow and already you can feel your palms sweating and heart racing. Here's what you do, says Dr. Mary Hardy: Munch on sunflower seeds for a few hours before the presentation. Why? Because low levels of magnesium contribute to anxiety. Anxiety, in turn, depletes your body of magnesium as a result of the fight-or-flight response. But magnesium-rich sunflower seeds can break this vicious cycle. One more thing: Before you go to bed tonight and first thing in the morning, take 200 milligrams of this valuable mineral.

Watch some funny movies to bust stress. Yes, line up an Adam Sandler marathon, the complete works of The Three Stooges, and the last three seasons of *Seinfeld*. Then every day you'll have something funny to look forward to. That in itself is enough to boost stress-busting hormones like endorphins and growth hormones, and drop stress-inducing hormones like cortisol and epinephrine, according to a University of California-Irvine College of Medicine study. Researchers there tested 16 men, half of whom knew they were going to watch a funny video three days before they did. The ones who knew the yucks were coming had huge decreases in stress-inducing hormones and increases in relaxation-enhancing hormones even before watching the film. Those who didn't get to see the movie had no changes.

Bang on a drum to relieve stress. It might sound a little New Age, but drumming—yeah, beating on a drum with a group of people—is a great way to relieve stress (especially if you picture your boss's head as the drum). Researchers at Meadville Medical Center in Pennsylvania compared 50 people who either participated in a drumming circle or just listened to drumming and found the drummers had much lower levels of the stress hormone cortisol and much higher levels of immune-enhancing chemicals called natural killer cells. You can find a drumming circle in your area by looking in the newspaper or checking with an alternative health center or practitioner.

Create a space where you can cool out. Paint the room a calming light blue or green. Add a scented candle designed to help relax you, such as lavender, lights on a dimmer switch, and a comfortable chair with a soft throw. This is your relaxing room, a place you can go when you need to calm down—after work, for instance. The colors are important because they've been shown to help people feel calm and relax, says Larina Kase,

Psy.D., a psychologist at the Center for Treatment and Study of Anxiety at the University of Pennsylvania and president of Performance and Success Coaching, LLC.

Become an art lover to cut stress. You could start attending art auctions, visit a museum, or simply frame and hang your kids' pictures on your walls. Regardless, studies find that viewing works of art, no matter how much they're worth monetarily, can reduce stress hormones! Another option: Make your own art. Any kind of creative activity like painting or drawing also reduces stress hormones. Oh, and talk to your doctor about those blank white walls in her office.

Ask for a prescription before a stressful situation. We're not one to advocate medication for all woes, but this one from Susan Montauk, M.D., professor of clinical family medicine at the University of Cincinnati College of Medicine, really made sense. She prescribes a 24-hour beta blocker called atenolol (Tenormin) for patients who have test anxiety or become anxious in other situations. "It's wonderful for those who get a little bit of heart palpitation," she says. You know, that feeling you get just before giving a presentation like you've had six cups of coffee and run two miles? Dr. Montauk has her patients take the medication on a day when they're not going to have any anxiety, just to make sure it works and doesn't have any side effects. Of course, you need to talk to your health care provider about this. Beta blockers are only available with a prescription.

Just say no to stressful demands. Repeat after me: "No, I cannot serve on the bake sale committee." "No, I do not want to spend every night and weekend driving vast distances to take my child to elite soccer games." "No, I cannot loan you the money for a new car ... allow you to move back home ... take on the fired employee's job." Yeah, it sounds simple, but most of us have no clue how to say the "n" word without feeling guilty; and if you're feeling guilty, what's the point? So Susan Newman, Ph.D., a social psychologist and author of *The Book of No: 250 Ways to Say It—and Mean It*, provides this handy five-step plan:

- Count the number of yeses you've given out during the past week. Make a list of them. The number will shock you.

- For one week, track how you spend your time every hour and who you're with. You may discover one friend is monopolizing you or one family member is very demanding. If you're managing your time well, however, you'll keep some in reserve for yourself.

- Decide who is first on your list: your spouse, child, boss. What about yourself?

- Know your limits. How long can you listen to a friend's sad story again without choking her? How many more PTA meetings can you sit through without screaming?

- Pick one thing a week to cede control of. Maybe it's paying the bills, cutting the grass (does it *have* to be perfect, or can your 12-year-old do it?), fixing dinner every night (there's some great, healthy takeout available these days). ◀

Dental Secrets
9 Simple Tricks You Can Use to Keep Tooth Problems at Bay

Use an extract on that sore tooth. The pain from your sore tooth is so bad you're ready to tie one end of a string around it and the other around a doorknob and slam the door shut. Hang on. Before you destroy that beautiful grin, put a couple of drops of oil of clove on a cotton ball, put the cotton ball over your sore tooth, and bite down. Hold for several minutes. This elixir made from the dried, unopened flower buds of the tropical clove tree is a great multitasker when it comes to tooth pain—numbing the pain and killing bacteria and other germs that could make whatever's causing the pain worse. You can do the same thing with vanilla extract. After three or four minutes of biting down, spit out the cotton ball and swish 6 ounces water mixed with 1/4 teaspoon salt and several drops of the extract in your mouth for 30 seconds. This will kill more bacteria. Spit—don't swallow. This solution is only temporary, however; make an appointment with your dentist to see what's causing the pain.

Chew gum to prevent cavities. Chewing gum used to *cause* cavities, but these days it can actually prevent them. Just make sure your gum contains xylitol, says Dr. Mary Hardy. Not only does the gum chewing help maintain saliva flow to flush away bacteria, but studies find that it makes bacteria less likely to adhere to your teeth. You may want to avoid gum altogether, however, if you have bridges, crowns, veneers, or other reconstructive dental work; the constant chewing may help loosen the materials.

You don't really need to have your teeth checked every six months unless you have gum disease, smoke, or have other high-risk factors for dental problems (such as diabetes). Studies comparing dental problems to the number of dentist visits find that visiting the dentist at least once a year (along with regular flossing and brushing) provides good dental health.

Another tooth-friendly chewing gum. Next time you're in the checkout line at the grocery store, toss a few packs of Big Red chewing gum onto the counter. The spicy cinnamon gum contains the ingredient cinnamic aldehyde, a plant oil that keeps nasty bacteria from growing, helping reduce cavities and gum infections. Don't like cinnamon? You can get similar results with Arm & Hammer Baking Soda Gum and gum made from the tree bark pycnogenol (available in health food stores).

Brew a pot of tea for oral health. It's the second most commonly drunk beverage on the planet (second only to water), yet tea gets a bad rap when it comes to your teeth because the tannins in tea can stain. We say, fuggedaboutit. With all the great tooth bleaching tools out there, today you can have your tea and drink it too. That's a good thing, since studies find that tea drinkers have fewer dental cavities, while rinsing with green tea after brushing can reduce overall plaque and the risk of gum disease.

Floss, floss, and then floss again. Sure, it's something you *tell* your dentist you do, but deep inside you know it's been at least three years since you bought that unopened container of dental floss gathering dust at the bottom of your bathroom drawer. Well, it's time to pull it out. Study after study confirms that having gum disease significantly increases your risk of not only tooth loss but also heart disease, and flossing can prevent gum disease. Diseased gums apparently release high levels of compounds that increase inflammation—everywhere in your body. So pull out the floss, toss it into your purse or pocket, and use it after every meal and before bed.

Try this new way to floss. Admit it—you'd rather clean under your fingernails with a scalpel than floss your teeth. What if we told you about a tool that's easier to use and works better than regular dental floss at reducing plaque and gum inflammation? It's true—researchers at the University of Pennsylvania School of Dental Medicine compared flossing with BrushPicks (which have a narrow, three-sided blade at one end, and a probe with six bristles at the other end) with regular dental floss and found the "cleaning aid" was significantly better than the old-fashioned floss.

Avoid hidden sugar sources. You choose apples over apple pie, carrots over caramels and water over soda, but what about those hidden sources of sugar? Like a spy, cavity-contributing sugar lurks everywhere, including antacid tablets, cough drops, liquid medications, and chewable tablets, including vitamins. The sugar content of these over-the-counter preparations is particularly high in children's versions, and research shows they contribute to dental cavities. What to do? Your dentist won't tell you, but we will: Brush your teeth after chewing a couple of antacids or sucking a throat lozenge, just as you'd do after that piece of apple pie.

Swallow, don't chew, your vitamin C. Yes, they're as big as horse pills, but swallowing vitamin C supplements could save your teeth. Chewing them significantly increases the acidity of your saliva, which, combined with the high sugar content in the tablets, can really do a number on your tooth enamel.

Use an electric toothbrush. Put a little spin in your morning routine with an electric toothbrush instead of a manual one. A review of 21 studies over the past 37 years found less dental plaque and gum disease in people who used the battery-powered tools. ◁

Eye Care
4 Secret Ways to Prevent Difficulties with Your Vision

Eat fish for dry eyes. How much fish have you been eating lately? And no, the fried shrimp at Captain D's doesn't count. If you find yourself rubbing your eyes a lot and practically mainlining Visine, then the two—lack of fish and dry eyes—could be related. Fish contains valuable omega-3 fatty acids, which make your tears oilier so they coat the surface of your eyes better. They also reduce inflammation, another cause of reduced tear production. Either eat a fatty fish like salmon or mackerel two or three times a week, or take 3 grams of fish oil daily.

SECRET WEAPON

Sunglasses

You wear sunscreen for your skin, don't you? Well, you need the equivalent for your eyes too. In fact, sun exposure is one of the leading contributors to potentially blinding diseases such as age-related macular degeneration and cataracts. Not just any pair of sunglasses will do, however, so listen up. You want glasses that transmit no more than 1 percent UVB and 1 percent UVA rays, wraparound to prevent sunlight from leaking in the sides of the glasses, and gray lenses because they provide the best protection. If you wear contact lenses, get yours with ultraviolet light protection. "Class 1" contact lenses, a designation from the U.S. Food and Drug Administration, provide the best sun protection. But since contacts don't cover the entire eye, it's best to wear proper sunglasses.

Eat spinach for eye nutrients. You know why Popeye is always affiliated with spinach? Because when he was invented back in the early 1930s, a misprint in a medical study gave spinach ten times the amount of iron it actually had. We don't really care where the idea linking spinach to strength came from. What's most important is that Popeye never went blind. Today we know that spinach is rich in eye-protecting carotenoids like lutein and zeaxanthin. Numerous studies find that diets rich in these nutrients can prevent or slow the progress of age-related macular degeneration. But raw spinach won't cut it; you need to cook spinach a bit to release the full amount of carotenoids. So sauté a bag of prewashed spinach in 2 tablespoons extra-virgin olive oil and a garlic clove just until the spinach wilts. Toss a pinch of dried red peppers over the greens, place over pasta, and sprinkle the whole thing with grated Parmesan cheese.

Get your bilberries for night vision. Here's a fact we're pretty sure neither you nor your doctor knows: Pilots in the Royal Air Force in Britain used to eat tons of bilberry jam to improve their night vision before flying sorties. They knew then what science is only now learning: Bilberries, also called English blueberries, can preserve the health and integrity of your retina and improve night vision. Take a 160-milligram supplement twice a day.

Try acupuncture for dry eyes. No, not *in* your eyes, but in other parts of your body. Numerous studies find that this ancient Chinese treatment significantly increases eye moisture, although, as with many alternative approaches, we're not sure why. But you know what? We also don't know why or how a lot of drugs work! And don't worry: If you're afraid of needles, most acupuncturists today can use acupressure or other non-needle approaches. ◁

Caring for Your Ears
6 Little-Known Tricks for Staving Off Problems with Hearing

Get exercise to hear better. Now, this is something we know your doctor doesn't know—but the more physically active you are, the better your hearing is likely to be! Why? Because aerobic activity such as biking and walking brings more oxygen into your lungs, which increases blood flow throughout your body (including your ears). That, in turn, improves your hearing! At least, that's what we hear from researchers.

Eat avocado to help your hearing. Mmm, like eating solid butter—but oh, so much better for you! The green fruit is rich in magnesium, a mineral that helps protect your hearing from noise-related hearing loss. Just make sure the fruit is uniformly dark when you buy it and yields slightly—but not too much—when you press on it. You can store a ripe avocado in the fridge for two or three days.

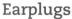

SECRET WEAPON

Earplugs

You don't have to have spent your youth following the Grateful Dead around to damage your hearing with loud noises. The noises of everyday life—lawn mower, leaf blowers, cars backfiring, even the ubiquitous iPods attached to everyone's ears these days—are more than enough. So get a few pairs of earplugs, scatter them around the house, in your car and purse, and use them to turn down the volume of your world.

Drink wine to prevent hearing loss. Okay, when's the last time your doctor told you to drink? Probably never, even though everyone, particularly Morley Safer of *60 Minutes*, knows that wine is good for your heart. But even Morley probably doesn't know it's also good for your ears. That's what researchers evaluating 3,000 people in Beaver Dam, Wisconsin, found. Just one to three glasses of wine or beer a day could actually protect against age-related hearing loss. Stop right there, though. Once you hit four or more servings of booze, not only do you have a drinking problem, but you may be contributing to hearing loss.

Take care of your teeth to protect hearing. Trust us, you want to keep your original teeth. The more teeth you have, it seems, the better your hearing as you age. That's what researchers found when they compared dental health and hearing loss in more than 1,000 veterans (why they thought to link the two, no one knows). Every tooth you lose more than doubles your risk of hearing loss. Scientists aren't sure why, but suspect it has something to do with the position of the jaw or maybe lack of muscle activity that affects the auditory tube. Regardless, brush and floss twice a day!

Be aware of your partner's snoring. While your doctor may warn you about obvious loud noises like gunshots and lawn mowers, you may never hear about the dangerous effects of snoring on your hearing. Yes, snoring. Research shows that the sound of snoring can be louder decibel-wise than the sound of city traffic. And any loud noise damages your ears over time. After proving to your partner that yes, he or she *does* indeed snore—a tape recorder may help—suggest a visit to a sleep center. Snoring can be a sign of sleep apnea, a breathing disorder that could lead to heart disease.

Take ginkgo biloba to open up your ears. If you have a doctor who recommends herbal supplements as part of a healthy life, good for you. The rest of us buy books like this. Because it's a rare doctor who's going to recommend ginkgo biloba for your hearing. Yet several European studies find that the herb improves hearing, even restoring hearing suddenly lost. One study compared it to the drug pentoxifylline, used to increase blood flow in cases of sudden hearing loss, and found the herb worked better than the drug! Take between 12 and 120 milligrams twice a day, depending on the extent of your hearing loss. ◄

EXPERT INSTANT ADVICE

Clean Out Your Own Ears (Thanks Anyway, Doc)

Ever notice your general practitioner is a little too, ahem, *eager* to get at the wax in your ears? No, it's not some strange fetish. But when they clean out your ears, they get to bill your insurance company (or you) for a separate service, since cleaning out earwax is actually considered a surgical procedure. Maybe that's why U.S. physicians clear impacted wax, or cerumen, from an estimated 150,000 ears each week! Save the money and do it yourself. Mix 1 tablespoon hydrogen peroxide with 1/2 cup warm water. Fill an ear bulb syringe (the blue things you use to clear an infant's nose) with the mixture, tilt your head sideways, and release the solution at the opening to your ear (don't stick the dropper tip into the ear). You'll hear and feel bubbling, but don't worry. Those bubbles help loosen the earwax so it can make its way to the surface for removal. Then, after a few seconds or when the bubbling stops, turn your head the other way to drain the ear.

For extensive earwax, get the over-the-counter wax softener Cerumenex (it's prescription-only in Canada). Fill the canal of the ear with several drops and plug with a cotton ball before going to sleep. In the morning, remove the cotton, shower, and wash your hair. This usually rinses out all but the most severe plugs.

Coping with M.D.'s
11 Tricks for Getting the Most Out of Medical Exams and Visits to Doctors

Get the first appointment of the day. What is it with doctors that they think *their* time is more valuable than yours, leaving you to cool your heels in the waiting room for an hour or more past your scheduled appointment? One way to get around this is to make sure you get the first appointment of the day or the first appointment after lunch, says UCLA's Mary Hardy, M.D. No one will have tied up the doctor or staff before you, and everyone will be more refreshed and less rushed than if they're running between you, the "chronic cough," and the "foot fungus."

Do your homework on your condition. The days of trusting implicitly in your doctor are over. These days, you have to be an active participant in your health care. And that means learning about your condition and the best way to treat it. No, you don't need to go to medical school. Thanks to the Internet, national guidelines for treating many health conditions are just a few mouse clicks away. Start with guidelines based on the latest scientific evidence at the National Guidelines Clearinghouse at www.guideline.gov. Then make sure you ask your doctor if *your* treatment is based on the latest evidence.

Find out what your doctor isn't telling you. There are procedures, tests, and treatments that could help you, but since your health insurance doesn't cover them, your doctor isn't telling you about them. That's the finding from a survey of 1,124 U.S. physicians, which showed that one in three docs withhold information from their patients about useful medical services that aren't covered by the patient's insurance. The remedy: Be an informed patient, do your own research, and look your doctor in the eye as you ask: "Is there anything else I could do? Even if it's not covered by my health insurance?"

Ask to sample a drug first. When your doctor prescribes a brand-name medication, ask if you can have samples. Drug company representatives often give doctors free samples, and it will cost your doctor nothing to pass them along to you. You'll get a "free ride" for several days, and if you have a bad reaction to the medicine, you'll find out without having paid a cent. You may actually end up giving that pharmaceutical company *less* of your cash for a change. One caveat: Check the expiration date on the drugs first.

Ask for three months of meds. The next time your doctor writes you a prescription, ask for enough to last you three months rather than a shorter duration. That way, you only have to pay one co-pay for a three-month supply, instead of three monthly co-pays for the same amount of medication. Check the prescription before leaving the doctor's office, however, to make sure it's written correctly.

Tell your doctor what you can afford. Studies find that doctors won't ask you if you can afford your medication, but if you tell them you can't, they'll come up with strategies so you can get your drugs and still have money to pay the rent and eat. Some options:

Many so-called objective patient websites and consumer health organizations are heavily funded by drug companies. Even some national campaigns highlighting a particular disease—like one that popped up in mid-2006 explaining that a virus causes cervical cancer—come from drug companies. That cervical cancer campaign? Funded by Wyeth-Ayerst in the months before it received FDA approval for the first HPV vaccine. The message: Be an informed consumer. Check websites for information on board members and funders and be aware of messages designed to steer you toward a particular drug or diagnosis.

writing prescriptions for generics instead of brand names, reducing dosages, stopping some medications, teaching you how to split pills, and referring you to pharmaceutical assistance programs. So forget the "don't ask, don't tell" policy on income when it comes to your health.

Schedule your skin checkup for winter. If you call your dermatologist in June and ask for an appointment for your annual skin check in August, is the receptionist going to say, "Why don't you wait until December when you don't have a tan and it's easier to see any irregularities?" No, most likely she will go right ahead and make your appointment without passing along this vital information. But now *you* know, so hold off on that exam until winter.

Time your Pap test. Okay, guys, you can tune out here. This is just for the ladies. Before you schedule that annual Pap test, check your calendar. The best time for the test is the week before or after you ovulate, usually the first or third week of your menstrual cycle, says Dr. Mary Hardy. This is when the cervical opening is widest, so it's easier to get a sample, and the cervical mucus is thinnest, increasing the accuracy of the test.

Time your mammogram. Another one for the ladies, so guys, consider this the book's version of a commercial you can tune out. Ladies, whether anyone talks about it or not, having your breasts squeezed between two glass plates in a futile attempt to make them as flat as a pancake *hurts*. But it must be done (every year or two from age 40 onward). To reduce the pain, time your mammogram for the week after your period, suggests the American Cancer Society. Your breasts are less tender and, an added bonus, a major study found mammograms taken during this time are more accurate. They're less likely to result in false positives, while mammograms taken during the second half of your menstrual cycle are twice as likely to miss a cancer.

Eat only liquids before a colonoscopy. Just the thought of it gives us the shivers, but once you turn 50, a colonoscopy should be as much a part of that passage as a midlife crisis.

You can make the whole thing easier on yourself by following a liquid diet for two days before the procedure so during the pre-procedure "clean-out" you don't have the, ahem, "matter" to clean out.

Ask for a warm blanket for that PET scan. No one likes lying on the cold metal bed of a PET scanner waiting to learn if he has cancer. But if you're covered with a warm blanket, the test will not only be more comfortable, but more accurate. That's because special tissue called "brown fat," the kind that keeps you warm, also tends to absorb the radioactive tracer used in a PET scan to identify cancers, misleading doctors into thinking the fat cells are cancer cells or even hiding actual cancer cells. The warm blanket, however, can reduce the amount of tracer the fat takes in by 62 percent. Other ways to ensure an accurate PET scan include abstaining from strenuous activity and caffeinated beverages before the scan. ◁

Hospital Savvy

5 Surprising Tips for Making Hospital Stays as Brief and Safe as Possible

Avoid hospitals and emergency rooms in July and August. In the U.S., new medical students, interns, and residents start work July 1 and medical errors spike. There's even a name for it: The "July phenomenon." One study found that the odds of interns nearly missing important information in a blood test were more than twice that in their first month on rotation as during the following 11 months of their intern years. A primary reason for the near misses? "Inexperience and unfamiliarity with hospital systems," say researchers. Another study found the average length of stay in hospitals increased 2 percent in July, August, and September, while the average death rate increased 4 percent. You can wait until Christmas for that hernia repair, can't you?

Never check into a hospital on a weekend. Unless it's an emergency—if you're just having tests or elective surgery—don't check into the hospital on a weekend (or a holiday). Chances are good that you will do nothing but lie in bed for the weekend at a cost of more than $1,200 a day. Doctors try to discharge patients by Friday, so hospitals want to fill the empty beds on weekends. For both your monetary and physical health, insist on checking in as close to the test or surgery time as possible.

Check out a hospital, especially if you're a woman. Hospitals today are spending millions to lure women as patients, splurging on such features as fancy atriums with three-story fountains, maternity wards with wood floors, down comforters, and flat-screen televisions. But we know that you can't judge a book by its cover. And, in fact, many of those hospitals wouldn't appear quite so inviting if they revealed that you're 40 percent more likely to die of a heart attack or stroke there than if you chose the hospital down the road for your cardiac bypass operation or to treat your heart attack. That's what a three-year study of more than 2.1 million hospitalizations at more than 2,100 hospitals found when it analyzed six heart-related procedures and diagnoses for the hospital's female patients. Overall, there was a 40 percent difference in death rates between the nation's best-performing hospitals and the nation's worst, and a 23 percent difference in death rates between the best-performing hospitals and those that were only average. If all the hospitals performed as well as the best hospitals, 30,548 additional women might have survived their hospitalization for heart disease and stroke. To find out where your hospital ranks, visit www.healthgrades.com.

Ask: Have you washed your hands?
How gross is this: The nurse changes the sheets of your roommate who just had his appendix out, then comes right over to work on yours. Did she wash her hands? Nooooo. In fact, although the primary way to reduce the spread of hospital-borne infections is hand washing, studies find most hospital workers comply with basic hand-washing requirements less than half the time. One way to make sure the nurses or doctors do wash their hands before examining you? Ask. One study found when patients checked whether health-care workers washed their hands, the workers washed their hands more often and used more soap.

Ask for a less unpleasant catheter.
It's one of the most humiliating and painful parts of hospitalization (if you're a man). Having a nurse stick a catheter up your private part. It's also probably the reason you got that nasty urinary tract infection during your hospital stay. Next time you have to go to the hospital, ask for an external, or "condom," catheter. This form of catheter, also called a "Texas catheter" (don't ask), is a rubber latex sheath with a tube at the end that fits tightly on the penis, rather than having to be inserted *in* the penis. The first-ever study comparing the two types of catheters found the condom catheter, which is much more pleasant and less painful, reduced the risk of urinary tract infections by 80 percent. That could mean a shorter hospital stay, not to mention a quicker overall recovery. Of course, this type of catheter doesn't work if the reason for using a catheter is a constricted urinary tract because of prostate problems or bladder surgery. ◁

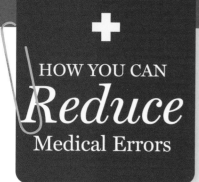

HOW YOU CAN
Reduce
Medical Errors

A groundbreaking Institute of Medicine report issued in 1999 found that 44,000 to 98,000 Americans die in hospitals each year, not from the medical conditions they checked in with but from preventable medical errors. While the health-care system as a whole is working on ways to reduce those dreadful figures, there are also things you, as a patient, can do. Here are the top ten recommendations from the U.S. Agency for Healthcare Research and Quality.

☐ Be an active member of your health-care team. Don't just blindly nod when your doctor hands you a prescription or says you need surgery. Question everything, ask for studies, find out about your doctor's experience in a particular procedure. Research shows that patients who are more involved with their care tend to get better results.

☐ Make sure *all* your doctors know *everything* you're taking. That includes prescription and over-the-counter medicines, and dietary supplements such as vitamins and herbs. But it also includes illegal drugs. Don't worry—your doctor is bound by confidentiality rules not to disclose the information to anyone. So once a year, toss all your meds into a paper bag and take them to your annual checkup.

☐ When your doctor writes you a prescription, make sure you can read it. If you can read it, chances are good the pharmacist can too. And that will help reduce medication errors.

☐ Ask for information about your medicines in terms you can understand—both when your medicines are prescribed

and when you receive them. Studies find that doctors are terrible at explaining to patients how to take medications, what their side effects are, and how long they should be taken. Ask the following questions:

What is the medicine for?

How am I supposed to take it, and for how long?

What side effects are likely? What do I do if they occur?

Is this medicine safe to take with other medicines or dietary supplements I am taking?

What food, drink, or activities should I avoid while taking this medicine?

☐ Make sure you understand the medication label. For instance, does "four doses daily" mean a dose every six hours or just during regular waking hours?

☐ If you have a test, don't assume that no news is good news. Ask about the results.

☐ When you're discharged from the hospital, ask your doctor to explain the treatment plan you will use at home. This includes learning about your medicines and finding out when you can get back to your

regular activities. Research shows that at discharge time, doctors think their patients understand more than they really do about what they should or shouldn't do when they return home.

☐ If you're having surgery, make sure you, your doctor, and your surgeon all agree and are clear on exactly what will be done. In fact, ask your doctor to sign his/her initials on the site of the surgery—for instance, the left knee—then double-check that it's the correct site. That's what the American Academy of Orthopaedic Surgeons urges its members to do.

☐ Make sure that someone, such as your personal doctor, is in charge of your care. This is especially important if you have many health problems or are in a hospital.

☐ Ask a family member or friend to be there with you and to be your advocate (someone who can help get things done and speak up for you if you can't). Even if you think you don't need help now, you might need it later.

Using Meds Effectively
7 Secrets You Should Know About Taking Prescription and OTC Drugs

Buy drugs late in the month. Filling your prescription on the first of the month significantly increases the likelihood you'll get the wrong dose or drug. A study from researchers at the San Diego Center for Patient Safety found that since government checks such as Social Security go out at the beginning of the month, that's when many people get their prescriptions filled. That, in turn, overwhelms many already-overwhelmed pharmacists. And those overwhelmed pharmacists may be part of the reason that University of San Diego researchers found deaths related to pharmacy medication errors spiked 25 percent at the beginning of the month. So get yourself on a mid- or late-month refill schedule.

Check your meds at the drugstore. Before you hand over the charge card, check the medicine in the bag and ask, "Is this what my doctor prescribed?" A study from the Massachusetts College of Pharmacy and Allied Health Sciences found that 88 percent of medicine errors involved the wrong drug or the wrong dose.

Check the ingredients of cold remedies. If your child has the sniffles, you may be tempted to provide him with all manner of over-the-counter treatments to provide comfort. But you could be putting your child's health at risk unless you read the fine print carefully. The corner drugstore will happily sell you cold treatments by the basketload, but make sure that you aren't inadvertently harming your child by giving him too much of particular ingredients. You might give him the proper dosage of acetaminophen tablets, for instance, but not notice that the cough medicine you're also providing contains the same drug. Too much acetaminophen can cause liver damage. So check the fine print on the packaging of all medications.

Swallow your penicillin with live-culture yogurt. Your doctor isn't going to tell you this as he writes the prescription, but antibiotics can have some annoying side effects, including diarrhea and yeast infections (in women). The easy way to prevent these problems is by eating at least two cups of live-culture yogurt (you can find it in the dairy case) a day while taking antibiotics. The "good" bacteria in the yogurt restores the "good" bacteria that the antibiotic wipes out.

SECRET WEAPON

Water

Sure, it's the elixir of life. But did you know that studies find that getting at least five 8-ounce glasses of water a day, particularly if you're over 65, can reduce your risk of falls, constipation, coronary heart disease, and even bladder cancer (in men)? In fact, one study found that nearly half of older adults admitted to the hospital from the emergency room were dehydrated—and didn't even know it. A good way to get enough water is to fill one-third of a gallon-size pitcher with water and keep it in your refrigerator. When the pitcher is empty, you've consumed your 40-ounce minimum for the day.

Measure medicine properly.
Studies find that many people don't understand how to measure liquid meds. Too often, they use a regular teaspoon, which doesn't deliver the right amount. Save the teaspoon for cereal and pick up a medicine spoon or syringe for the drugs.

Get off the Pill to quit smoking.
You've tried the patch, the gum, even the inhaler, but nothing seems to work and you're still smoking half a pack a day. Now try switching your birth control pill for a nonestrogen form of contraception, such as an IUD or a diaphragm. Women apparently not only metabolize nicotine faster than men, but the effects are even more pronounced in women who are taking oral contraceptives. Researchers from the University of California, San Francisco, who conducted the study that found this effect, say this sex difference may be one reason women have a harder time quitting smoking than men.

Take your meds—or else. Or else you could die. No kidding. A report analyzing 21 studies found that people who take their medicine regularly—*even if their medicine is a sugar pill*—have a lower risk of dying during a certain time period than those who don't follow the instructions. Don't count on your doctor to remind you how important it is to take your meds, however; numerous studies find docs are notoriously bad when it comes to counseling patients regarding the most important thing about a prescribed drug: If you don't take it, it won't work! ◄

Alleviating Pain
8 Little-Known Facts You Should Know About Coping with Aches and Pains

Don't take Tylenol for arthritis.
If your doctor is still recommending Tylenol for arthritis pain, then she's not reading the medical journals. A major study published in the respected *Archives of Internal Medicine* found that Tylenol, or acetaminophen, worked no better than a sugar pill at relieving arthritis pain. Plus, in large doses it could cause kidney damage and liver damage. Instead, work with your doctor to find alternative means of managing your pain, ranging from exercise to non-steroidal medications like ibuprofen, which studies find works much better than acetaminophen for this type of inflammatory pain.

Don't mix pain relievers for different pains. You're taking ibuprofen for your arthritis and acetaminophen for your headache and an over-the-counter flu remedy that, unbeknownst to you, also contains acetaminophen. Whoa! You've just overwhelmed your liver. So read the labels of your pain relievers and cold and flu remedies before popping another pill.

Go for the lowest dose of painkillers. First you pop an all-day naproxen for your sore back. But a few hours later, your back still sore, you unthinkingly shake out a couple of Motrin from the bottle in your purse. That night before you go to bed, you take a couple of Tylenol PM to help you sleep. Keep on this way and you're putting yourself at risk for high blood pressure. Seems that women who consume high doses of non-aspirin pain

Many surgeries have little or no clinical evidence proving their effectiveness, and some show no more benefit than a placebo, or sham, surgery. That's because no government agency has to "approve" new surgical techniques in the way that the FDA approves new drugs.

Back surgery is a prime area to be cautious. Many doctors recommend spinal fusion surgery for chronic back pain. But a study comparing the surgery to exercise found that each was just as effective in reducing pain.

Disk bulges and protrusions found on MRI are just as common in people without back pain as in people with back pain, according to a study published in the *New England Journal of Medicine*. That means if your surgeon tells you that you need surgery to correct a bulging disk, get a second opinion. The disk may not have anything to do with your pain.

Another major study found that a common surgery performed on patients with arthritis of the knee was no better at relieving pain or improving knee function than a sham, or fake, operation in which incisions were made but no surgery was performed.

Bottom line: If your doctor recommends surgery for chronic pain or other chronic conditions, get a second and even a third opinion, and don't go under the knife until you exhaust all your other options.

---

relievers like acetaminophen and ibuprofen are much more likely to develop high blood pressure than women who don't. Start keeping a medication diary in which you note the time, dose, and type of over-the-counter drugs you're taking; the total amount just might surprise you.

Pick pain medication on price, not symptom. Even though it's become a major marketing ploy for over-the-counter pain relievers to tout their "specialty" on the label (for instance, Excedrin Migraine), such products all contain the same basic ingredient regardless of the type of pain they're purported to address. So check the label of the product you're interested in, note the amount of active ingredient in each dose, then pick up the cheapest generic brand containing the same thing and save yourself a few bucks (and another headache!)

Burn out arthritis pain with chile-pepper salve. There are no fancy, 30-second television spots or national campaigns, and since no one is marketing it to your doctor, you may never hear about it, but chile peppers (to be more precise, the active ingredient in chile peppers—capsaicin) are one of the most effective pain relievers around for arthritis pain. You don't swallow capsaicin, however; you apply a cream containing it to the painful area. Experts think it works by depleting something called substance P, a chemical that transmits pain messages to your brain. Give it time: You have to apply capsaicin four times a day for several days before it kicks in, but the relief will be worth it. If you can find the cream combined with glyceryl-trinitrate (GTN), a compound that stimulates the release of nitric oxide, grab it. Not only does GTN reduce the stinging that occurs when you first apply the capsaicin cream, but the two together seem to work better than either alone at reducing pain. Keep your hands away from your face and eyes when applying, and wash your hands immediately after each application.

Take fish oil for neck and back pain. More than 70 million people in the U.S. alone take prescription non-steroidal anti-inflammatory drugs (NSAIDs) to reduce inflammation and pain. Yet these drugs are now the leading cause of health problems and death related to prescription medications, says the U.S. Food and Drug Administration. Imagine if there was a completely natural compound that would not only relieve your pain, but provide additional health benefits as well? No ifs, ands, or buts about it: fish oil supplements can. When researchers from the neurosurgery department at the University of Pittsburgh asked 125 people with back and neck pain who were already taking NSAIDs to add 2,400 milligrams a day of omega-3 fatty acids for two weeks, followed by 1,200 milligrams per day thereafter, 59 percent said they completely stopped their NSAID medication after two weeks and were pain-free, while 60 percent of the rest of the partici-pants who were still taking NSAIDs said their overall level of pain had improved when they added the fish oil. Look for pharmaceutical-grade fish oil, which is guaranteed toxin-free.

Wrap your pain with warmth. The drug companies aren't going to tout this study, but you can get more pain relief from a muscle-warming wrap like ThermaCare Heat Wrap than you can from ibuprofen or acetaminophen. At least, that's what a well-designed study of 371 people with low back pain found. Plus, if you wear the wrap overnight, you'll have less pain for least two days—even without the wrap! However, in the interest of full disclosure, we should tell you that the wrap's manufacturer—Procter & Gamble—sponsored the study. We say, go ahead and try it any-way. It certainly isn't going to increase your risk of liver, kidney, and heart dam-age the way over-the-counter pain relievers can!

Try this nondrug tactic to relieve a headache. Got a headache? Before you make the cash registers ring at the local pharmacy, try this drug-free remedy: From a standing position, bend forward from the hips and settle your forehead onto the padding of a chair. Relax in this position for 30 seconds, feeling the gentle pressure against your head. Then sit down in the chair, spread your fin-gers, slide them into your hair, and make a fist. Pull your hair gently away from your scalp, hold for three seconds, and release. This relieves tension in the connective tissues underlying your scalp. Continue this process of grabbing handfuls of hair and pulling gently. Work your way from the top of your head to the sides and finally to the back. With the tension relieved in your entire scalp, you should feel refreshed and ready to resume your day. ◁

How to Navigate a **Health Food Store**

Finding your way safely around a health food store is much like navigating a minefield. There are a lot of traps—hidden behind a lot of hype, misinformation, and outright ignorance—to be on the lookout for while trying to find useful products. The following advice comes from UCLA's Dr. Mary Hardy.

Ask about employee training

The clerk behind the counter should know the difference between various forms of calcium, why liquid echinacea is preferred over tablets, and why you shouldn't take kava kava if you have liver disease. But he usually doesn't. In one published report, a researcher from the University of Hawaii posed as the daughter of a breast cancer patient and visited 40 health food stores. She was frequently told to take shark cartilage, a remedy linked to liver toxicity, nausea, fever, and other ill effects in cancer patients. A Canadian study in which employees of 34 retail health food stores were asked what they'd recommend for a patient with breast cancer found 33 different products recommended, none of which had any significant research behind them. Only eight employees discussed the potential for drug interactions, and one actually suggested the patient stop taking tamoxifen (a proven cancer treatment). So ask about the clerk's training (large chains say they invest in training) and don't follow any recommendations if the clerk doesn't at least ask about your health and other medications you're taking.

Stay away from memberships

If you're being pitched a membership in a health food club, get out of there. Health food stores should be dedicated to helping you find the best remedy for your needs, not plying you with stuff you don't need.

Do your research before you hit the store

Don't walk in looking for "something to help the pain in my knee." At least know to ask for glucosamine.

Read the labels

Compare the amounts of active ingredients and the types of ingredients in the supplement, dosages, and number of doses in the bottle. Such comparisons will lead you to the best value for your money.

Ask to see third-party literature

If all you're handed regarding the benefits of a supplement is literature from the manufacturers, you're in the wrong store. First of all, manufacturers can't make disease claims about their products (for instance, "improves fertility"). Second, you need some unbiased information. If the supplements don't mention the brand name and come from experts not connected with the manufacturer, ask to see additional information.

Supplement Secrets
8 Tricks for Getting the Most Out of Vitamins and Other Supplements

Take vitamins with food. Popping your multivitamin any old time is about as effective as trying to put out a fire with a watering can. If your body can't absorb the vitamins and minerals in that horse-size pill, it's not doing you any good. To maximize absorption, take all vitamins and minerals with food.

Don't take supplements with coffee. If you're used to popping a handful of vitamins and minerals with your morning coffee, you could be missing out on important benefits, says Viviana Simon, Ph.D., director of scientific programs at the Society for Women's Health Research. Seems caffeine interferes with your body's ability to absorb calcium, manganese, zinc and copper, as well as vitamins C, A and B. Wait an hour before consuming anything with caffeine after taking your supplements.

Take children's vitamins if you have a swallowing problem. Gummi vitamins for children are a godsend for older adults and anyone else who has problems swallowing vitamins, or who gets stomach irritation from a single large dose of several supplements. Instead, take two children's vitamins in the morning and two at night. Try the gummi vitamins—they're delish!

Be sure to take vitamin D. Vitamin D is beginning to look like the miracle vitamin. Also called the sunshine vitamin, it can protect against colon cancer, help maintain strong bone, reduce the risk of developing type 2 diabetes and multiple sclerosis, and improve immunity and brain function, among other benefits, according to research. Yet studies also find many North Americans, particularly those in northern climates, don't get enough of this vital vitamin because the sun is our primary source. In fact, findings showing significant vitamin D deficiencies in certain populations led the Institute of Medicine in 2005 to recommend higher daily intakes of this supplement. Dark-skinned individuals, elderly people, and those who don't get enough sunlight (most of us in the winter months) should get an extra 1,000 IU per day from food or supplements. You can get that with three cups of vitamin-D fortified milk, one cup of vitamin D-fortified orange juice, and 600 IU of vitamin D supplements. The rest of us should aim for at least 600 IU a day.

Check your calcium source. Drug company marketers don't exactly ballyhoo this on the packaging of their supplements, but the human body is better at absorbing one common form of calcium than another. Favor sources of calcium citrate (such as Citracal) instead of the other variety, calcium carbonate, which is often found in antacids such as Tums. Calcium citrate is absorbed two and a half times more easily. If you choose this form, however, says Dr. Mary Hardy, double your dose. Calcium citrate contains less elemental calcium (the stuff that matters) than calcium carbonate.

Stifle the gas with enzymes. First, the facts on flatulence: Everyone does it, on average about a pint a day or about 14 discharges a day (it doesn't take much to make the odor). Now, how to stop doing it so much: Take a dose of digestive enzymes, either fruit-based papain and bromelain, which come from papaya and pineapple, or animal-based trypsin and pepsin, with each meal. That's the recommendation of Dr. Hardy. Many over-the-counter digestive enzymes contain both types. The enzymes will help you better digest your food, leaving less to ferment in your colon and produce the stinky gas that gets you those weird looks in the elevator.

Check out a supplement before taking it. Supplements often don't contain the amount of active ingredient—or even *any* active ingredient—listed on their labels. If you want to check out the quality of your supplement before you plunk down $25, go to www.consumer lab.com. This independent laboratory tests supplements and provides reports on their ingredients. You'll need a membership for the full report, but even the partial reports provide good information. If the supplement isn't listed, it either wasn't tested or was tested and found wanting. The site only posts products that passed testing. Another way to ensure quality is to buy store brands from leading retailers such as Wal-Mart, CVS, and Eckerd Drugs. They have a reputation to protect and are more likely to use reputable manufacturers and manufacturing processes.

Stay away from sex-enhancement supplements. If you head online to buy herbs and other supplements to make you more powerful in bed, hold on. The U.S. Food and Drug Administration warns that numerous online sexual enhancement products contain drugs, herbs, and other products that aren't listed on the labels. These could be dangerous, potentially interacting with other drugs you're taking or triggering a life-threatening allergy. Specific ones to watch out for are Zimaxx, Libidus, Neophase, Nasutra, Vigor-25, Actra-Rx, or 4EVERON. If you need to get your blood moving, good old magazines and videos are a better choice. ◄|

WHAT SUPPLEMENT MAKERS DON'T WANT YOU TO KNOW ABOUT Contaminants

We're so accustomed to assuming that anything sold in a drug or health food store is safe, that it probably never occurred to you that your Ayurvedic health remedies could contain dangerous levels of lead and other heavy metals. But when Boston doctors bought dozens of the remedies at stores throughout the region and tested them, they found 20 percent had significant amounts of lead, mercury, or arsenic, sometimes at very high levels. What to do? Buy your herbs from a trusted herbalist and ask where the remedy originated. Those grown in India, China, and other third-world countries are more likely to contain the contaminants.

10 MUST-HAVE
healing herbs
and Supplements

There's a whole new arsenal of supplements that natural medicine experts "prescribe" for themselves and their patients—because they're backed by compelling research that proves they really work. Your doctor isn't likely to tell you about them. You'll have to discover them for yourself. Here are the top ten natural remedies that live up to their promise. All are widely available at health food stores.

1 Andrographis

Although it isn't as well known as echinacea, andrographis has been used for centuries to treat colds and fevers, and it seems to work better, reducing inflammation and stimulating the immune system. TriMune (which also includes vitamin C, zinc, and echinacea) and Kold Kare are two common brands.

2 Arnica

Ointments and creams made from this herb can be used to ease swelling and promote healing of injuries that cause inflammation. Use it to treat bruises and burns; strains, sprains, and sore muscles; bursitis and tendinitis; and even carpal tunnel syndrome. Just take care not to use it on broken or bleeding skin.

3 Bromelain

Derived from pineapple stems, bromelain is an enzyme that encourages good digestion. Bromelain supplements help break down food and complete digestion, making them helpful for conditions such as flatulence or inflammatory bowel disease. Bromelain also eases swelling and bruising by blocking body chemicals that cause inflammation, helpful for treating bruises, muscle soreness, and bee stings.

4 Capsaicin

Capsaicin is the chemical that gives hot peppers their heat. It helps relieve pain by short-circuiting pain signals from skin nerves to the brain. It's available as a cream in strengths ranging from 0.025 to 0.075 percent. Apply it to the skin for osteoarthritis, shingles, neck ache, or carpal tunnel syndrome, or as a patch for back pain. An initial burning feeling fades quickly. Start with the mildest form and wash your hands after applying. Never use capsaicin on broken skin or blisters. Leaving a patch on too long may cause skin irritation.

5 Devil's Claw

This bitter-tasting African herb contains compounds called harpagosides that reduce inflammation, making it helpful for conditions such as chronic back pain, neck aches, and osteoarthritis. It's commonly available in a liquid and as a powder.

6 Elderberry and Elderflower

During flu season, keep Sambucol, a concentrated extract of elderberries, on hand. When you feel flu symptoms coming on, take a tablespoon four times a day for three to five days to boost your immune system and shorten the duration of the attack. Also keep a jar of elderflowers; a tea made from them will help you sweat and help break a fever.

7 Evening Primrose Oil

Made by pressing tiny seeds of the evening primrose flower, this remedy is rich in an essential fatty acid that eases inflammation and can be used to treat asthma, rheumatoid arthritis, PMS bloating and menstrual cramps, and impotence. It also helps moisturize skin, hair, and nails and can be taken orally to help brittle nails and dry hair from the inside out. It comes as an oil or in gel-filled capsules.

8 Lemon Balm

Lemon balm is an old-time remedy and as a tea is used for treating insomnia, shingles, and—mixed with dandelion and crushed fennel seeds—inflammatory bowel disease. It has been found to contain compounds that are potent virus fighters and is also available as a concentrated ointment that is used to speed recovery from a cold sore outbreak.

9 Lysine

Lysine is an amino acid that has been shown to help fight viruses, especially herpes, by blocking the activity of arginine, another amino acid that viruses need to replicate. Taking the supplement can help control outbreaks of oral and genital herpes, when combined with restrictions on arginine-rich foods, such as nuts, chocolate, and raisins. It also helps to eat lysine-rich foods, such as cheese, eggs, chicken, milk, and lima beans.

10 Quercetin

Quercetin is an antioxidant derived from plants that acts much like an antihistamine. Take it to relieve or help prevent allergy symptoms, such as watery eyes, stuffy nose, and sneezing, or to help ease airway inflammation in asthma.

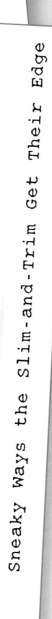

Healthy Food Choices

11 Secrets for Selecting Foods That Will Make Your Meals More Nutritious

Start meals with vegetables. If you find it hard to get excited about the veggies on your plate, try starting your meal with veggies *only*. Before you even bring out the chicken or lasagna, eat a double portion of salad, green beans, or broccoli—whatever vegetable you're serving that night. Or a hearty vegetable soup. Then sit and chat with your dinner companion for 15 minutes before getting the next course. You'll eat less of the rest of the meal!

Choose cleaned, bagged veggies. While it may cost a bit more, cleaned, bagged vegetables are the best thing to hit grocery stores since Starbucks counters. Numerous consumer studies find that we're more likely to buy bagged salads and other produce. These days, you get much more than just lettuce. How about green beans, peeled and diced butternut squash, washed and chopped kale—we're all for it. In fact, the introduction of bagged, prewashed spinach in the late 1990s is touted as the main reason spinach consumption increased 16.3 percent in North America between 1999 and 2001.

Stock up on frozen vegetables. Probably not something your supermarket manager is going to like (fresh usually costs more), but frozen veggies may actually be more nutritious (since they're often flash frozen just hours after picking) and they're a heck of a lot more appealing than the mushy rotting mess that often fills our refrigerator vegetable drawer. Try microwaving an entire bag's worth of frozen broccoli or green beans (in a microwaveable container), drizzling a couple of tablespoons of low-fat dressing over them, and sprinkling with low-fat Parmesan cheese for a quick lunch or dinner.

Pop some soybeans. Soy is a high-protein, low-fat vegetable that tastes so good you might expect the nutrition police to come after you. But forget tofu. We're talking edamame, or soybeans. Buy them frozen or fresh, steam for 5 minutes, and sprinkle with some coarse salt. Now pop the beans out of the pod. Make a lot—you can't eat just one!

Make fries from sweet potatoes. Instead of plain potatoes, make sweet potato "fries." Slice a scrubbed, large sweet potato into one-inch (2.5-cm) strips, coat with a tablespoon of canola oil, and bake in a preheated oven (450°F or 230°C) for about ten minutes. Shake the pan to turn the fries and continue baking until crispy, about another 15 minutes.

Buy whole-grain bread. Bread manufacturers aren't going to tell you this, but all too often the "wheat" bread they're marketing is nothing but regular white bread browned with molasses. To make sure you're getting the real thing, the first ingredient in any whole-grain product should have the word "whole" in it, as in "whole wheat," or "whole grain." If it says multi-grain, seven-grain, nutria-grain, cracked wheat, stone-ground wheat, unbromated wheat, or enriched wheat, it's not whole wheat, and thus is lacking some of the vitamins and minerals, not to mention fiber, of whole grains.

Serve whipped butter at the table. Julia Child always said to use real butter when you wanted butter, and we agree. But she never told you what *type* of butter! We recommend whipped. It's still the real thing, but at 60 calories a serving compared to stick butter's 100, and with 5 grams of saturated fat compared to regular butter's 7, you'll use less, saving calories. Let it soften before using; it spreads easier, ensuring you'll use even less!

Eat mushrooms for antioxidants. If you're as sick of hearing about the health benefits of "brightly colored vegetables" as we are, here's some good news: Researchers at Pennsylvania

---

EXPERT INSTANT ADVICE

5 Great Uses for Beans

Beans are packed with fiber (15 grams in just a cup of black beans) and, since they come canned, they're so easy to use. Just rinse them first to remove excess sodium (or look for the no-salt-added variety). Not sure what to do with them?

1. Puree a can of cannellini beans with 2 garlic cloves, 1 tablespoon lemon juice, and 1 tablespoon olive oil. Use as a dip for veggies and whole-grain crackers.

2. Spread nonfat refried beans on a whole-wheat burrito and sprinkle with chopped chicken and shredded cheese.

3. Use 1/4 cup black beans and salsa as a filling for your morning omelet.

4. Make a bean salad with canned black beans, fresh or frozen corn kernels, chopped cilantro, chopped onion, and chopped tomato. Drizzle with olive oil and a dash of vinegar, salt, and pepper.

5. Make your own chili pizza. Top a prepared (whole-wheat) pizza crust with kidney beans, shredded cheese, and ground turkey cooked with chili flavorings.

State University found you can get the same levels of disease-fighting antioxidants in portobello and cremini mushrooms as in the ubiquitous carrots and green peppers. We prefer ours grilled, please, with just dash of balsamic vinegar.

An apple a day to keep fractures away. You already know about the benefits of calcium and vitamin D for strong bones. But what about fruit and vegetables? Yup, chalk up another health advantage to these amazing foods—the more fruits and veggies you eat, the higher your bone mineral content, a fancy way of saying you have stronger bones and are less likely to develop osteoporosis or fractures.

Eat chocolate—the right kind. In case you missed it on page 17, dark chocolate is packed with healthy antioxidants. But what you may not know is that it's also packed with magnesium, says Kevin Gianni, a personal trainer in Danbury, Connecticut, and creator of "The 50-Second Fitness Quick Fix" health and fitness tip video-zine. That magnesium can help moderate your appetite!

Buy condiments that add flavor. If you select the right condiments, you'll have the underpinnings for wonderful sauces, low-fat marinades, and even low-salt flavorings that will greatly improve the taste of your meals. Some of these condiments have a high salt or sugar content, so the secret is to use them judiciously to add flavor or to look for low-sodium or sugar-free versions. One great benefit of these tasty meal flavor-adders is that they'll help you stay away from less healthy fatty condiments, such as mayonnaise, butter, stick margarine, and creamy salad dressings. These delightful flavorings include:

- Flavored ketchups and barbecue sauces, chili sauce, and salsas (look for sugar-free varieties)
- Horseradish and various types of mustards
- Jarred spaghetti, bruschetta, and pesto sauces (the latter is luscious spooned atop salmon and baked)
- Jarred olives, capers, sun-dried tomatoes, anchovies, and roasted red peppers
- Worcestershire, hot pepper, soy, and teriyaki sauces (look for low-sodium varieties)
- Extra-virgin olive, sesame, and walnut oils (the healthy oils)
- Flavored vinegars and various kinds of marmalades. ◂

Better Breakfasts

6 Simple Strategies for Starting the Day Without All the Usual Grease and Sugar

Drink tomato juice for breakfast.
Instead of high-sugar orange juice in the morning, substitute a cup of low-sodium tomato juice. It's more filling, is less likely to spike your blood sugar, and provides more nutrients and fiber.

Drink a fruit smoothie. What about drinking your fruit instead of eating it? No, not in fruit juice—which is often high in sugar and stripped of the fruit's fiber—but in a smoothie. Just toss a cup of berries—strawberries, blueberries, raspberries—and a sliced (but not peeled) apple, peach, or pear into your blender. Add 1/2 cup skim milk and a frozen banana, maybe a cup of ice if you like it thicker, and blend. Mmmmm good!

Mix your cereals half and half.
We agree that eating some of those high-fiber cereals is tantamount to munching on cardboard. So try this: Mix 1/3 cup of the hearty stuff with your favorite cereal. Choose a high-fiber cereal such as All-Bran, with 8.5 grams of fiber, and you're more than one-third of the way toward the recommended 25 grams of fiber a day.

Eat an Israeli-style breakfast.
Instead of the sugary cereals, starchy breads, and greasy meat and eggs that make up the typical North American breakfast, do what Robyn Frankel of St. Louis, Missouri, did after visiting Israel. She switched to Israeli breakfasts: hummus, cottage cheese, tomatoes or fruit, plus sometimes a slice of raisin bread. For the first time in her life she's eating breakfast regularly, which studies find is critical if you're going to lose weight and keep it off. The 57-year-old public rela-tions consultant carries just 128 pounds on her 5-foot, 2-inch frame.

Eat half a grapefruit twice a week.
Grapefruits are loaded with folate, which has been found to significantly reduce the risk of stroke. But be cautious if you're taking regular medications. Grapefruit and its juice can interact with medications that have to be processed through the liver. Check with your doctor about any possible interactions between grapefruits and any medications you are taking.

Sprinkle half a cup of blueberries on your cereal. Studies find that these tiny purple berries are loaded with valuable antioxidants that can slow brain aging and protect your memory. Not into cereal? Try baking blueberries into oatmeal to create your own oatmeal-blueberry granola bar or mixing them into whole-wheat pancake or waffle batter. ◄

Cooking Techniques
6 Tricks the Home Chef Can Use to Make Dishes More Healthy

Don't pour oil, mist it. Those supersized jugs of olive oil you buy at warehouse stores may be a good deal financially, but they can get you in trouble calorically. To avoid pouring too much, get a nonaerosol sprayer (like a Misto) and fill with your favorite oil. Use for flavoring foods, coating pans and grills, or spraying directly on bread or salad. You'll use less—much less!

Fake the cream in sauces. You want to make your mother's famous cream of tomato sauce and creamy beef stroganoff, but you don't want the extra fat and calories of heavy cream. No problem! Just open a can of nonfat condensed milk. You'll get the creaminess without the fat and calories—promise!

Sneak vegetables into your entrées. Here are two simple ways to increase your intake of vegetables by adding them to main dishes as you cook:

- Always start with *mire poix* (pronounced MEER-pwah). This blend of onions, celery, and carrots (ratio of 2:1:1 or 3:2:1) with parsley and bay leaves is worth learning a bit of French for. It's a great way to sneak veggies into nearly every entrée you prepare. Sauté a cup (or more) of the mixture (which you can buy already cut up and prepared in some groceries) in a tablespoon of canola oil, then use as a starter for sauces, stews, and soups.

- Whether you're making homemade or jarred spaghetti sauce, adding 1/2 cup or more of pureed veggies (red peppers, cauliflower, carrots, or broccoli) provides just the right touch of antioxidants, vitamins, and—don't forget!—flavor. Or add 1 cup grated or mashed carrots, zucchini, squash, sweet potatoes, or pumpkin to muffins and other quick breads.

Try a different take on potatoes. If you are like most of us, you always make potatoes the same way—peeled, boiled, and mashed with lots of butter. It's a lot of carbs and a lot of calories. Here are two alternatives to try:

- Add boiled and pureed cauliflower to your mashed potatoes. You won't be able to taste the difference, but you'll get less starch and more fiber. Also, to cut back on the amount of butter you add, blend in a little low-fat milk.

- Instead of mashed, serve potatoes boiled with the skin on and cut into cubes. Even better, select new potatoes, which have fewer simple carbs than other types of potatoes.

Stretch the meat. This is a closely related trick—one your parents or grandparents probably used during the Depression, when a pound (500 grams) of hamburger had to feed 12. They stretched it with mashed potatoes, grated carrots, beans, and other vegetables. Well, even though you can afford sirloin these days, we recommend the same approach. Add grated vegetables (try carrots or onions) to ground turkey or beef to stretch the meat, reduce the fat, and punch up the fiber content of meat loaf, hamburgers, chili, and soups. You can buy veggies already cut up and prepared in many supermarkets. Even better: Learn to use soy, beans, and lentils as delicious protein sources instead of meat in dishes like stews, spaghetti sauce, and lasagna.

Add some fat to that salad. Your nutritionist may not tell you this, but the key to getting the most out of all those fruits and vegetables is … wait for it … *fat!* That's because many of those vitamins and other nutrients are fat soluble, meaning they need some fat present if your body is going to absorb them. For instance, researchers from Ohio State in Columbus compared salads and salsas made with and without avocado (high in monounsaturated fat). When it came to the salsa, participants absorbed up to 4.4 times more lycopene and 2.6 times more beta

5 Ways to Have Your Cheese and Eat It Too

EXPERT INSTANT ADVICE

1. **Choose hard cheeses.** Parmesan and Romano (the real stuff, not the stuff in the green can) pack a wallop of flavor in a small amount. Two grated tablespoons contain less than 4 grams of fat, about 2 of them saturated. Even better: Look for low-fat versions.

2. **Shred your cheese.** Then just sprinkle over your burrito or salad instead of laying on slices or tossing in chunks. You'll use less, saving calories and fat.

3. **Go for soft cheeses.** Skim or nonfat ricotta or farmer's cheese, goat cheese, and feta are often lower in fat than other cheeses. And like hard cheeses, a little goes a long way.

4. **Go for the flavor.** Just a tiny bit of strongly flavored cheese such as blue cheese can transform a salad without transforming your waistline.

5. **Have a slice.** An ounce (28 grams) of processed cheese has just 4 grams of fat per slice and 60 calories, compared to cheddar, with 9 grams of fat and 114 calories.

carotene (valuable antioxidants) than when they ate plain salsa.

The researchers saw similar results with the salad—adding avocado upped the absorption of lutein up to 7 times and of beta carotene by nearly 18 times! Without the added fat from the avocado, the salad had a mere 2 percent of its calories from fat, and participants absorbed barely any of the carotenoids. That doesn't mean you have to douse all your healthy veggies and fruits in fat. If you're eating a steak, for instance, you've got plenty of fat to carry the nutrients in the salad throughout your body, so stick to nonfat dressing and skip the cheese (and avocado) in that instance. ◁

9
WAYS TO GET
nine servings
without even trying

You know you're supposed to get nine servings of fruits and vegetables, but the thought of all that healthy stuff makes you, well, nauseated. What if we told you that when it comes to fruits and veggies, a serving is really a relatively tiny amount? Here are easy ways to get your nine in one day (without throwing up):

1 Make a super salad

One 7-ounce (198-gram) bag of washed lettuce equals a bit more than one serving. Add a sliced tomato, a cut-up apple, and 1/4 cup raisins and you've just eaten four servings. Top your super salad with cooked chicken or diced, hard-boiled egg whites for protein and you've got lunch.

2 Munch 'em as a snack

Freeze 1/4 cup blueberries and 1/4 cup grapes and munch on them during your favorite TV program. That gets you up to six servings.

3 Dip 'em

For a before-dinner snack, dip 1/2 cup carrots into low-fat ranch dressing. Now you're up to seven.

4 Add some nuts

Sprinkle chopped, toasted pecans or walnuts over green beans.

5 Drink 'em

Eight ounces (225 ml) of low-sodium V8 juice provides two vegetable servings. Voilà! You've hit the magic nine and it's not even dinnertime.

6 Add some sweetness

Drizzle honey, maple syrup, or fruit juice on steamed carrots or sweet potatoes.

7 Roast 'em

Nothing brings out the natural sweetness of veggies like roasting. You can roast nearly anything, but our favorites are carrots, onions, beets, turnips, rutabagas, and Brussels sprouts. Just cut into chunks, mix with enough canola oil to coat, sprinkle with kosher salt, and spread in a single layer on a greased pan. Roast in a preheated 450°F (230°C) oven until browned on the outside and fork tender on the inside.

8 Make popcorn

Cut the florets off a cauliflower and cut them up into bite-size pieces. Mix the cauliflower pieces with 2 tablespoons canola oil and sprinkle with kosher salt. Preheat the oven to 450°F. Spread the pieces on a cookie sheet and bake them until they are brown, turning them once. Now pop a movie in the DVD player; then settle back and pop this healthy version of popcorn in your mouth.

9 Sauce 'em

There's a reason spaghetti squash got its moniker—the strands of golden squash really do look like spaghetti, only they pack a much more powerful punch. Take the pretend pasta one step further by topping the strands with tomato sauce and a curl of fresh Parmesan cheese.

Tracking Diet Progress

3 Simple Tricks for Creating a Revealing Record of Your Food Intake

Write down everything you eat. This is where the restaurant industry could be in trouble. If you start writing down everything you eat during the day, especially meals eaten out, the shock of how much is actually going in should be enough to get you to toss those neighborhood restaurant takeout menus. While you're at it, check your weight every day. Studies find that careful monitoring of what you eat and what you weigh helps you lose more weight than those who aren't tracking their progress. One study of 40 obese people found that those who followed the tracking advice lost nearly twice as much as those who didn't. Another study found that those who weighed themselves every day lost more weight (or gained less weight) than those who didn't.

Use your cell phone to track your food. Here's a new take on the traditional food diary—which numerous studies find can help with weight loss. Instead of writing down everything you eat, snap a picture with your cell phone or digital camera, then upload onto your computer. *Seeing* what you've eaten in a day can be far more effective in showing you where you're making nutritional, high-calorie mistakes than just reading about it. If you want a formal way to do this, you can sign up online for www.nutrax.com, a service that allows you to build an online food picture log. For $8 a week, a dietitian offers meal-by-meal feedback.

Give yourself a shiny star. It might sound elementary, but do it anyway: Buy a package of those little shiny metallic star stickers. Every day you meet your fitness or nutritional goal (for instance, a 30-minute walk and fixing a healthy meal instead of ordering pizza), give yourself a sticker. "As silly as it sounds, sometimes seeing a whole month of shiny stickers can make you really proud," says Lindsay Wombold, Healthy Horizons program assistant at Butler University in Indianapolis, Indiana. "It's tangible proof of how well you're doing." ◁

WHAT **WEIGHT WATCHERS** AND **ATKINS** DON'T WANT YOU TO KNOW ABOUT Diets

What's most important when it comes to losing weight is *following* the diet, no matter which weight-loss program you choose. That's what a study published in the *Journal of the American Medical Association* found. Researchers compared the effectiveness of Weight Watchers, which limits calories and portions; Atkins, which limits carbohydrate intake; the Zone, which moderates foods based on glycemic value; and the very-low-fat Ornish diets.

The scientists found that sticking with the plan is more important than the plan itself.

However, researchers also found that regardless of the diet, none of the participants stuck with it long-term, with 21 percent quitting before two months, and 42 percent quitting before six months.

Trimming Sugar and Salt
5 Simple Tricks for Cutting Your and Your Family's Intake of These Ingredients

Cut out high-fructose corn syrup. What if we told you that there's one ingredient in food today that, more than anything else nutritionally related, is making us fat? No, it's not fat. And it's not even sugar—at least, not all forms of sugar. It's high-fructose corn syrup (HFCS), which didn't even exist 40 years ago. Today, however, this sweetener is found in nearly every processed food you buy—from fast-food hamburger buns to ketchup, juice, cereal, and even mayonnaise. It's much more dangerous than plain sugar, because your body doesn't metabolize it in the same way, leading to higher levels of blood fats such as triglycerides and VLDL (very low density lipoprotein) cholesterol, which is even worse for you than regular cholesterol.

Even more frightening: It doesn't affect the hormones that suppress hunger. So even if you're getting an extra 500 calories a day from HFCS, your body still thinks it needs more, explains Linda Bacon, Ph.D., associate professor of nutrition at the University of California, Davis. The easiest way to avoid HFCS is to eschew processed foods and, when it comes to condiments and cereals, buy organic (and read the ingredients list carefully). You can make a big dent in your HFCS consumption just by giving up regular soda and fruit juices and other sweetened beverages such as tea, which has become very popular.

Crack the sugar code. Manufacturers are deathly afraid that you'll quit using their products if they aren't dripping with sugary taste. After all, North Americans slurp down about 34 teaspoons of sugar a day—more than three times the limit recommended by the USDA. So sugar gets hidden in products everywhere you turn, including cough medicine, chewing gum, tomato sauce, baked beans, and lunch meats. You'll even find sugar in some prescription medications. Identifying sugary foods can be tricky, however, because manufacturers often substitute code words on their labels. So look for these terms: corn syrup, dextrin, dextrose, fructose, fruit juice concentrate, high-fructose corn syrup, galactose, glucose, honey, hydrogenated starch, invert

---

WHAT CANDY MANUFACTURERS DON'T WANT YOU TO KNOW ABOUT Fruit

If you have a sweet tooth, you can assuage that need for sweets with fruit just as well as with candy, cakes, and cookies. It's a scientific fact. Researchers from Ohio State found that sweet-snack lovers eat more fruits than salty-snack lovers, and fruit lovers eat more sweet snacks than vegetable lovers. The moral of the research? Reach for a juicy peach next time you're craving a Mars bar and see if it doesn't fill that craving just as well.

sugar maltose, lactose, mannitol, maple syrup, molasses, polyols, raw sugar, sorghum, sucrose, sorbitol, turbinado sugar, and xylitol.

Substitute kelp powder for salt.

Sea vegetables have some of the highest mineral content of any plant on earth, says personal trainer Kevin Gianni. Plus, since they're from the sea, they're salty! You can find kelp powder at health food stores. Sprinkle it over vegetables, mix a tablespoon into sauces—use anywhere you'd normally use salt.

Look out for non-salt sources of sodium.

Although salt is the prime culprit that adds sodium to our diets, it is not the only one. Check food labels for sodium, Na, monosodium glutamate or MSG, sodium citrate, baking soda, baking powder, and sodium bicarbonate. They are all forms of sodium.

Break the salt habit gradually.

Don't expect to be able to dramatically cut the amount of sodium you consume overnight—or even over a week. It takes time for your taste buds to adjust and begin to recognize the subtle favors masked by salt. Until then, everything that doesn't have salt will be bland tasting. When cooking, slowly cut back on the amount of salt you add to dishes. Another way to get on the path of less sodium intake is to mix low-sodium foods with regular salted foods. Mix no-salt peanuts with regular salted peanuts, unsalted peanut butter with regular peanut butter, or lite salt with regular salt, suggests Lila Ojeda, R.D., a bionutritionist at Oregon Health Services University. Slowly increase the amount of the salt-free product as you decrease the amount of the salted version until you're only eating the salt-free food. ◄

Your Eating Mind-Set
5 Ways Your Mind Can Triumph over Matter in Fighting the Battle of the Bulge

Learn to eat intuitively. It's the last thing the weight-loss and exercise industries want you to do, but if you simply stop trying to remake your body and accept it for the way it is, you're more likely to eat better and may even lose weight unintentionally. That's what researchers at Ohio State in Marion found through a series of studies on "intuitive" eating, which teaches people to eat based on feelings of hunger or fullness, not for emotional or situational reasons. The studies evaluated 597 college women, finding that those who were intuitive eaters appreciated their bodies more, and were more likely to agree with statements like, "Despite its flaws, I accept my body for what it is." An earlier study by the same researchers found that women who ate intuitively were also more likely to have a lower body mass index than women who didn't.

Hypnotize yourself. We do it all the time when we daydream or become so engrossed in a book, movie, or task that we lose track of time, says Susan Neri-Friedwald, a certified hypnosis therapist from New York and author of the CDs *Take Control of Your Eating* and *Eat What You Like and Lose Weight*. Every night, just before falling asleep, repeat four to five times out loud (whispering is fine, and any added emotional intensity strengthens it), "I am in the process of becoming thinner and thinner." Repeat every night for 30 consecutive nights, and it will become your automatic subconscious thought. The last thing you tell yourself before falling asleep will be repeated all night long by your subconscious, she says, and you should begin to see results almost immediately. The evidence supports her: Several studies find that adding hypnosis to weight-loss programs not only improves the amount of weight lost, but participants tend to lose more weight over the long term compared to those who aren't hypnotized.

Go interactive on the Internet.

Weight-loss programs like eDiets proliferate online, but they're probably not going to share this with you: You'd do better getting weekly advice from a behavioral therapist online than simply reading about diet and exercise and filling out tracking forms. That's the result of a study from Brown University. Researchers found that dieters who received such advice lost three times as much weight over six months as those who took a more passive approach to online weight-loss info. One reason is that those getting online advice logged on twice as often those who didn't. Another is that the structured program with continued contact simply works better than just providing information. A later study by the same researchers found that it doesn't matter if the feedback is real, via e-mail from a human, or automated.

Pray your way to weight loss.

Several studies find that women enrolled in church-based weight-loss programs lose more weight than those who try to lose on their own. One of the best designed and most recent studies involved 15 Baltimore churches and 529 overweight women. During the yearlong study, one-third of the participants attended weekly nutrition and physical activity sessions at the church, one-third added spiritual content and prayer to the regimen, and one-third received education materials on healthy living. Those getting the on-site help—with or without the spiritual content and prayer—lost significantly more weight than those just handed educational materials, with women who weighed the most at the beginning of the study losing an average of 20 pounds.

Get ready for bed right after dinner.

No, you don't have to put your PJs on, but go ahead and brush your teeth and wash and moisturize your hands, says Marina Kamen, a 47-year-old mother of three who lost 100 pounds in her late 30s and has kept it off for more than ten years. "Now that you are fresh and clean, you might think twice before dipping your hand into a greasy bag of chips or messing up your minty mouth with a sugary cookie," she says. ◁

Subversive Habits

4 Surprising Changes in Everyday Non-Eating Behaviors That Can Help You Lose Weight

Turn off the television. There's probably no simpler way to lose weight than to stop watching television. A study involving 486 low-income-housing residents in Boston, two-thirds of whom were overweight or obese, found every hour of television viewing was associated with 144 fewer steps walked—or an average of 520 fewer steps a day for those who spent 3.6 hours in front of the television. Additionally, for each hour of television that participants watched, they were 16 percent less likely to achieve the 10,000-steps-per-day goal. For those who watched the 3.6 hours a day of TV on average, their odds of walking 10,000 steps a day were 47 percent less than non-television-watchers. Researchers estimate that 10,000 steps a day measured with a pedometer roughly approximates the recommended level of daily activity.

If you can limit yourself to just two hours a day of TV or less, you're likely to consume fewer calories and fewer nutritionally bereft snacks than those who watch more. And when you *do* watch TV, leave the snacks in the kitchen. Another study found that if you snack while watching TV, you're much more likely to be obese.

Don't overdo your hours at work. This isn't something your boss is going to encourage, but who cares what she thinks? The fact is, if you work more than nine hours a day (and lunch is included in here as part of your nine hours, whether you work through it or not) you're more likely to be overweight.

And while you're at it, find a less stressful job—the more stressful your job, the more likely you are to be overweight.

Get a solid eight hours of sleep. No, we're not recommending the "sleep diet" described on page 69, but there is compelling evidence that hitting the sack before midnight and getting a solid seven or eight hours can prevent obesity. Researchers from the University of Warwick in Coventry, England, reviewed the cases of more than 15,000 adults and found that sleep deprivation is associated with almost twice the risk of being obese. They also found that the less you sleep, the more your body mass index and waist size increase over time.

What would cause this? Probably hormonal changes produced by sleep deprivation. Other studies find that lack of sleep stimulates production of ghrelin, a hormone that stimulates appetite, and reduces production of leptin, a hormone that suppresses appetite.

Take a walk before dinner. Going for a short walk does more than burn calories. Like most exercise, it also cuts your appetite. And if you do it just before dinnertime, you won't want to eat as much as usual. In a study of 10 excessively overweight women conducted at the University of Glasgow in Scotland, 20 minutes of walking reduced appetite and increased the sensations of fullness as effectively as a light meal. ◁

10
FRUITS & VEGGIES TO
enhance
your meals

When you see them in grocery stores, you may turn up your nose at them, and even wonder, Who the heck buys this stuff? Well, starting today, *you* do. Here are ten to try, along with recipe ideas.

Garlic

We don't recommend doing this alone. Find someone you love, and share. Remove the loose paper covering from a head of garlic, cut off the tops, drizzle olive oil over it, wrap in foil, and bake in a 350°F (175°C) oven until soft, about an hour. Then squeeze the soft heads of garlic onto toasted bread and spread. You'll be getting fabulous amounts of plant nutrients called thioallyls that dramatically lower blood cholesterol levels, as well as prevent blood from becoming sticky and clumping into heart-damaging clots. Scientists believe you can lower your total cholesterol about 9 percent with just 1.5 to 3 cloves of fresh garlic daily for 2 to 6 months.

Avocados

Yeah, yeah, yeah, they're high in fat. But it's "good" fat—the monounsaturated kind that helps lower cholesterol. Try mashing a ripe avocado with a bit of lemon juice, onion, and chopped tomato as a topping for baked potatoes.

Fennel

Also known as sweet anise, fennel has a sweet, mild licorice flavor. The feathery fronds can be used as an herb, like dillweed, to flavor soups and stews. The broad, bulbous base is treated like a vegetable and can be eaten raw or sliced and diced for stews, soups, and stuffing. Try it roasted for a sweet treat.

Bok Choy

An Oriental cabbage, bok choy is like the Chinese version of spinach, only better. It doesn't get mushy, it retains its crunch, and it is the perfect vehicle for soy sauce. Serve it chopped and stir-fried in a bit of peanut oil and soy sauce. Or toss a chopped bunch into a hearty vegetable soup just before serving.

Jicama

Known as the Mexican potato, jicama (pronounced HE-kuh-muh) is a root tuber (like potatoes). Buy it smooth and firm with unblemished roots. Serve it cold and raw, or in soups, stews, or salads. Great as a substitute for water chestnuts.

Chayote Squash

A summer squash native to Latin America, chayote (pronounced chy-O-tay) squash is also known as the vegetable pear because of its shape and color. It has a mild taste, like zucchini, with a slightly citrus tang. You don't have to peel it, and the seeds inside are edible. Just cut into cubes, add 1/4 cup water, cover, and microwave for about 8 minutes.

Kohlrabi

A member of the turnip family, it is often called a cabbage turnip, but it's sweeter, juicier, crisper, and more delicate in flavor than a turnip. The cooked leaves have a kale or collard flavor. Trim and pare the bulb to remove all traces of the fibrous layer just beneath the skin, then eat it raw, boil it, steam it, microwave or sauté it, or add it to potato casseroles.

Belgian Endive

This type of lettuce has a mild, slightly bitter flavor and is packed with fiber, iron, and potassium. Use it in salads and instead of crackers with vegetable dips.

Guava

Yes, we never thought of actually *buying* it either, let alone eating it. But this fruit is awesome—and not just plain. Add the flesh to smoothies, dice it into fruit salads and salsas, and puree it for a fabulous sauce for fish or chicken. An added benefit? Researchers had 50 people with high blood pressure and high cholesterol eat four to seven guavas a day for 12 weeks. They found that the guava eaters had much lower blood pressure and LDL cholesterol (the bad stuff), and they had higher HDL cholesterol (the good kind) than 50 people who didn't add the fruit to their diets.

Prunes

These days the politically correct term is "dried plums," but we'll never stop thinking of them as prunes. Blend prunes with water into a puree and use this to replace oils and fats in baking, add prunes to stews for a delicious sweetness, or chop them and sprinkle over salads, yogurt, cottage cheese, or cereal. Prunes have a special kind of soluble fiber called pectin, which forms a gel in your intestines that absorbs excess cholesterol, sweeping it from your body. When 41 men with mildly high cholesterol levels added 12 prunes a day to their diets for four weeks, their LDL levels dropped more than when they drank grape juice for four weeks.

Cutting Calories

8 Secrets for Reducing the Temptations That Compel You to Eat More Than You Need

Clear out all tempting foods. You know the saying: "You don't miss what you don't have." Add another iteration on this: "You can't eat what you don't have." Go through every cabinet, the refrigerator, freezer, and pantry, and toss (or donate) every food product you don't trust yourself with. It's better to waste it by putting it in the trash than putting it in your mouth, says Lindsay Wombold, Healthy Horizons program assistant at Butler University in Indianapolis, Indiana.

Pay a few extra cents for smaller packs. Your accountant won't like it, since the small packs actually cost *more* per ounce (gram) than the large packs, but your doctor will. It turns out that people tend to eat less when they get several small packages than when they get one large package containing the same amount, says Raphael Calzadilla, exercise guru from eDiets.com. Part of the reason is that the smaller packages provide obvious stopping points at which to consider whether you want to keep eating. We have another reason: The added cost might persuade you to be more frugal with your snacks—for instance, sticking to one bag at a time instead of several in a day.

Shop at the supermarket, not the warehouse club. This carries the same idea one step further. Costco, Sam's, and BJ's may take a contract out on you, but you'll probably wind up eating less. Yup, it turns out that having large stockpiles of food products at home like those huge boxes and bottles of food you get at wholesale club stores

makes the products more visible and appetite-provoking than less plentiful ones. So those mega-containers contribute to overconsumption and, possibly, to overweight.

Find lower-calorie alternatives to the foods you crave. You will shave off pounds without feeling deprived if you find reasonable substitutes for the high-calorie foods you crave. We're talking baked veggie chips in place of fried Lay's; nonfat, sugar-free ice cream or fruit pops in place of Häagan-Dazs; baked "fried" chicken instead of the real thing. You get the idea!

Hide the candy dish. If your major munching occurs at work, here's some advice that will not only cut back on the calories but also save you bucks in the candy aisle at Costco: Hide the candy dish, use an opaque dish, or better yet, get it off your desk. A four-week study looking at how much chocolate candy 40 secretaries ate found that people ate an average of 2.2 more candies each day when they could see them (for instance, in a clear dish), and 1.8 more candies when they were on their desks, as opposed to just a couple of feet away. (Hey, it's rough, but someone has to do the tough studies!)

Crack your own nuts. Don't buy shelled nuts, says Susan Burke, R.D., vice president of nutrition at eDiets.com. Shelled nuts make it too easy to eat too much. Besides, their nutrient value drops with processing. A little elbow grease with the nutcracker not only helps to limit portions but burns calories, provides the freshest nut, and gives the most nutritional bang for your buck.

Every meal, eat a pear, apple, or some strawberries. The snack-food industry will gasp in horror, but what they don't know won't hurt 'em. And what they don't know is that each of these fruits contains 4 grams of fiber. Getting just that much extra fiber a day (although more is better) is enough to reduce your risk of being overweight fivefold, according to a study from Tufts University. Not only does fiber fill you up without filling you out (because its calories are not absorbed), but it boosts hormones that send the "I'm full" message to your brain.

Try frozen dinners for portion control. Sometimes frozen is best, particularly when it comes to weight loss. That's what researchers from the University of Illinois at Urbana-Champaign found when they compared weight loss between two groups of overweight and obese men. One group ate two frozen meals a day (they could choose among 24 varieties of Uncle Ben's Bowls) plus other foods. The other group fixed their own meals. Both followed government nutritional guidelines and contained about 1,700 calories. While all participants lost weight, those who got their grub from the freezer lost an average of five more pounds (2.5 kg) than those fixing their own meals, and their average body mass index dropped more. A similar study showed similar results for overweight women. The reason for the difference? The automatic portion control. ◁

The 5 Most Nutrition-Packed Foods

EXPERT INSTANT ADVICE

The following comes from Susan Burke, R.D., vice president of nutrition for eDiets.com, and Jeff Novick, director of nutrition for the Pritikin Longevity Center & Spa in Aventura, Florida.

1. **Fish.** Choose any fish for high-quality, lean protein that is low in saturated fat and cholesterol. (One caveat: Avoid large deepwater varieties such as tilefish, kingfish, and swordfish, which are chock-full of mercury.) Vary your fish choices: Fatty fish (salmon, sardines, mackerel, and tuna) are full of healthy omega-3 fatty acids, but you shouldn't eat them every day. And don't ignore shellfish: Although it contains dietary cholesterol, this type of cholesterol is not linked to heart disease.

2. **Beans.** Beans are the richest source of vegetable protein to be found. They're dense in nutrients, low in calories, and are loaded with fiber—especially soluble fiber, the type that lowers blood cholesterol.

3. **Fruit.** All fruits are fantastic as long as you eat them whole, as opposed to drinking processed juices. But super fruits like blueberries, kiwis, and strawberries pack the most nutritional punch in terms of antioxidants and fiber.

4. **Sweet potatoes.** When you see orange, think nutrition. Orange means beta carotene, which produces the antioxidant vitamin A. Sweet potatoes are also rich in vitamin C and B_6, and they're full of fiber.

5. **Oatmeal.** Studies find that people who eat oatmeal on a regular basis maintain a stable weight and a healthy cholesterol level. That's because oatmeal provides a high-fiber, high-protein source of magnesium and selenium. Just mix 1/2 cup whole oats and 1 cup water and microwave for 1 minute. Add blueberries or raisins for an additional treat.

Snack Control
3 Strategies for Limiting the Damage Caused by the Urge to Nibble

Don't be duped by "energy" bars.
In food-industry lingo, energy doesn't mean vim and vigor; it means calories. And that's what "energy bars" have plenty of. They use the imagery of hard-driving athletes who need a quick dose of calories to supply their muscles enough energy to finish the marathon. However, there aren't enough marathoners or long-distance cyclists or cross-country skiers to provide the demand to keep all the high-profit energy bars on the shelves. So most of them wind up being bought by armchair athletes who eat them instead of lunch or just for snacks. Researchers say that most of the bars do contain some ingredients that are good for you (nuts, fruit, and oats, for example), held together with goo that makes them taste good. As a lunch, energy bars are better than corn chips and soda, but not as good as an apple and a salad. If you think you need them during your workout, just be sure you're burning more calories during the workout than you're eating in the bar. And if by chance you are eating these bars because you really *do* need a shot of calories, then eat the bars slowly, advise experts. Like one bite every ten minutes.

Choose the plain chips. Snack chip manufacturers fall all over themselves to entice you with new flavorings, backed up with glitzy advertising campaigns and fancy packaging. Mesquite this, sour-cream-and-onion that. What they don't tell you is that such chip flavorings typically come with hefty additional doses of salt—often twice the normal amount. And excessive salt can lead to high blood pressure, heart and kidney problems, and bone disorders. So save your exotic cravings for fresh foods and keep your chip choices simple.

Don't want to eat it? Don't buy it.
Are you or your kids engaged in a constant struggle to resist those tantalizing chips, dips, and frozen desserts beckoning from the refrigerator and pantry? Here's a simple secret that the junk food manufacturers hope you don't catch on to: Once these foods have crossed the threshold of your house, they have already won the battle. Most likely, if you've bought it, you'll eat it. So the place to start just saying no is at the store. Research shows that among the factors contributing to our unfortunate tendency to stuff ourselves and get fat is proximity. If food is easy to get, you're more likely to eat too much of it. If you're trying to avoid specific foods or certain kinds of food, keep them out of the house. And it's not just for you. The person who does the shopping and fixes most of the meals has the most influence over what others in the household eat, according to Dr. Brian Wansink, director of the Food and Brand Lab at Cornell University. He calls that person the "nutritional gatekeeper" (no longer always the mother). Dr. Wansink has found that Americans make about 248 food decisions every day, many of them without much thought, and that the "gatekeeper" controls 72 percent of those decisions. ◁

Burning Calories

4 Tricks for Losing Fat by Increasing Your Metabolism and Your Daily Activities

Drink plain ice water. The Gatorade people aren't going to feature you in any commercials this way, but here's the truth: Not only does water have zero calories, but when it's very cold, you actually *burn* calories warming and absorbing it. Once you finish burning those calories, your metabolic rate remains 30 percent higher than before you quaffed the liquid—for another 90 minutes!

Keep a glass of ice water next to you all day and continually sip from it, refilling it with fresh water when it gets warm or you finish the glass. That way you'll never get dehydrated. Why should you care? When you're dehydrated, your metabolism slows so it can wring every drop out of whatever liquid it is getting, says Mary Hardy, M.D., director of Integrative Medicine at the Ted Mann Family Resource Center at the University of California, Los Angeles. In fact, it can actually lead to 45 fewer calories burned a day. That might not sound like much, but it adds up to 4.5 pounds (2 kg) a year!

Eat hot peppers to rev your metabolism. Don't you pity the vendors of "miracle" weight-loss products? While they're begging you to shell out big bucks for secret (and dubious) formulas, scientists have identified a simple and inexpensive food that may turbocharge your weight loss. It's right there in the produce section. Hot peppers not only liven up a meal, but some studies show that very spicy foods can temporarily increase your metabolism, or the rate at which you burn calories. Some enticing uses for hot peppers: Spice up your morning omelet with minced jalapeño, or fire up some beef stew with half a diced banana pepper.

Walk the stairs. Just four minutes of stair climbing a day can lead to a four-pound (1.8 kg) weight loss in just a year, says Michelle Cederberg, a Canadian fitness and wellness consultant. Here's the math: An average 160-pound (73-kg) person will burn about 50 calories climbing up stairs for four minutes (and down for one minute). If that same person takes the stairs for the same length of time five days a week, by the end of the year he'll burn about 12,700 calories (or about four pounds of fat). You can track your efforts at Health Canada's Stairway to Health online calculator at http://stairway.hc-sc.gc.ca/calcalc.aro.

Keep moving after dieting. You've heard the statistics: Most people who diet regain the weight they lost—and then some—when they end their diets. Well, you're not a statistic and you can avoid becoming one if you spend 30 minutes, four days a week, cycling, walking, or water jogging during and after your diet. That's because the low-intensity exercise can prevent the decrease in metabolism and fat burning that often occurs during and after a diet. ◁

Eating Out

6 Tricks for Avoiding Overconsumption When You Go Out to Eat at a Restaurant

Skip the romantic restaurants. It's not something any restaurateur is going to admit, but the reason they keep the lights low and play soft music is that they know this atmosphere encourages you to eat slower for a longer amount of time. It also makes you more likely to order dessert and another drink. How do they know? Research proves it.

Double up on appetizers. Your waiter will roll his eyes, because he wants you to order one of those oversized entrées. However, you can often trim back on calories—and cost too—if you order two appetizers for dinner and skip the entrée altogether—particularly if the restaurant has a nice selection of seafood- and vegetable-based starters. Just say *nada* to anything fried.

Keep your salad simple. Restaurant managers can't help themselves. They take a pleasantly simple offering like veggie salad and have to pile on the calorie-laden (and more expensive) extras—such as cheese, salami, spicy ham, croutons, and mayo-based dressing. By all means order a salad, but insist on vegetables only.

Skip the cocktail. What's the first thing the waiter wants to bring you in a sit-down restaurant? A cocktail, wine or beer, of course. Waiters know instinctively what was confirmed in a study in England—people who have an alcoholic drink before dinner tend to eat more. The study found that men who drank a glass of beer 30 minutes before a meal ate more during the meal than men who consumed a nonalcoholic beverage.

Those who drank alcohol also ate more fatty and salty foods and felt hungrier after the meal than men who didn't have alcohol. So if you're trying to control your weight, have your alcohol after your meal rather than before.

Check fast-food calories on the Web. Many of the highly hyped meals at fast-food restaurants are little more than a heaping helping of fat and calories. You won't be able to tell this by reading that menu over the service counter, of course. If you like the convenience of fast food but also want to keep your arteries free and clear, here's the best way to find the most healthful foods: Go to the Internet site of each chain store you frequent and click your way to the nutritional breakdowns for each offering. You'll quickly discover that the French fries, other fried foods, hamburgers, and mayo-based sauces are a shocking nutritional minefield. You'll see the wisdom of ordering smaller portions and heart-healthy sandwiches.

Keep your coffee order simple. That pricey coffeehouse wants you to order your brew in as fancy a form as possible. Not only does this drive up the tab for each visit, but it also stacks on hundreds of calories—from the whole milk, whipped cream, sugar and syrups. A regular cuppa joe made from good beans and with a dash of skim milk is heaven in itself, so protect your wallet and your arteries by keeping things simple. ◁

At the Table

7 Secrets for Reducing Your Food Intake When You Sit Down to Eat

Limit your food choices. This is something the owner of that Mongolian buffet down the road really doesn't want you to know, but the more variety you are offered in a meal, the more you'll eat. University of Pennsylvania researchers found this out when they offered people either three or one flavor of yogurt. Those with the choice ate an average of 23 percent more. So keep down the number of different things to eat on your home table.

Eat alone or with one other person. Pull a Greta Garbo and tell your partner you "vant to be alone." It might just save you unwanted weight. Researchers find that meals eaten with one other person are one-third larger than those eaten alone, and the amount increases as the number of people you're eating with increases. By the time you sit down to dine with six people, you're eating 72 percent more than if you'd just eaten alone.

Don't read or watch TV while eating. It's not on the Weight Watchers list of weight-loss tips, but distractions such as television, reading, movies, and even sporting events take your attention away from your eating to the point that you eat more. So no more meals on automatic pilot. Declare a media blackout and focus on what you are putting into your mouth.

Keep the physical sizes of dishes smaller. Researchers at Cornell University threw an ice-cream social to test whether oversized bowls (34 ounces [960 grams] versus 17 ounces [480 grams]) and extra-large ice-cream scoops (3 ounces [85 grams] versus 2 ounces [55 grams]) led to overeating. They found that doubling the size of someone's bowl increased how much participants took by 31 percent. The larger scoop increased the amount of ice cream by 14.5 percent. Yet all but 3 of the 85 participants finished all of the ice cream in their bowls. The moral of the story: Serve it up in smaller dishes!

Keep serving bowls smaller too. Rather than pile all of the mashed potatoes into one oversized bowl and bring it to the table, split it into two bowls. You'll wind up eating less. That's what Cornell University researchers found when they invited college students to a

Medicine That Cuts Weight

EXPERT INSTANT ADVICE

If you have a serious weight problem, you may want to talk to your doctor about prescribing a drug that is most commonly used to treat depression and smoking habituation but that has been shown to be effective in helping people lose weight. Researchers studied women who were taking bupropion, marketed as Wellbutrin for depression and Zyban for smoking cessation, for 24 weeks. The women followed a 1,600-calorie-a-day diet and lost significantly more weight and fatty tissue than women who only cut calories. Even better: The women taking bupropion kept the weight off for at least two years. The drug acts on the neurotransmitters norepinephrine and dopamine, which play a role in reward and pleasure in the brain.

Super Bowl party (get it, Super *Bowl?*) and offered them snacks from one of two tables. One table had a large bowl of snacks, and the other had two smaller bowls of snacks that, together, equaled the same amount as the large bowl. Students taking from the large bowls ate 56 percent more (142 calories) than those who served themselves from the smaller bowls.

Use chopsticks for all your food.

Using chopsticks might be messier, but you'll also eat less. When researchers compared patrons dining in Chinese restaurants, they found that those who were overweight were more likely to be using silverware than chopsticks, while normal-weight patrons chose the more labor-intensive chopsticks.

Add the color blue to your table.

The designers of fast-food restaurants avoid the color blue like the plague. For good reason: That particular color suppresses the appetite. So give yourself one more weapon in the war against bulging waistlines. Use blue dinner plates, cover the dinner table with a blue tablecloth, and dress in blue as well. Avoid using red, yellow, and orange in your dining areas. These colors encourage eating. ◁

Exercise Motivation
7 Surprising Ways to Set Your Mind on Getting Active and Getting Fit

Make your fitness goals known. Tell your family, friends, and coworkers about your fitness goals and encourage them to ask you how you're doing with meeting them. Knowing that everyone is watching you provides great motivation to stick to your goals, says Lindsay Wombold, Healthy Horizons program assistant at Butler University in Indianapolis, Indiana.

Make an appointment with your doctor. This isn't something docs are very good at, so it's up to you to start the conversation. Ask about your health and how becoming more physically fit can help you become healthier. Then ask for some advice. A government study found just three hours of advice and counseling by doctors and other health-care professionals over two years boosted couch potatoes' physical fitness.

Hire a personal trainer for one hour. In addition to the workout you'll get, ask the trainer to set your fitness goals for the year. A study from researchers at McMaster University in Hamilton, Ontario, found that if you're new to exercising, you'll do better if you have a fitness professional determine your goals rather than going it alone. That means setting the weights on machines for you, determining how long you should walk or run, giving you a time limit for the treadmill, StairMaster, or elliptical trainer. The reason for the improved results? The self-confidence you get when an expert believes in you and thinks you can reach a certain goal. You only need to hire the trainer for an hour to get your goals set. Of course, if you want to continue working with him or her, that's a good thing too!

Think *fit living*, not just *workouts*. The exercise industry makes more money when everyone thinks of fitness only in terms of formal workouts. But even if you spend three hours a week in the gym, what of the other 100-plus waking hours we have each week? Truth is, fit people go about their entire day living in a high-energy way. Not only is it fun and motivating; these ongoing spurts of everyday activity add up to a whole lot of fitness. So how do you live fit? Here are easy examples:

- Stand up and walk around whenever you get on the phone.
- Always take the steps, not the escalator or elevator.
- And when you take the steps, try for two at a time!
- Stand up and move around during every TV commercial break.
- Routinely stretch your arms, legs, and back.
- Carry stuff more often—garden supplies, groceries, laundry.

Do it for charity. Some of us get greater satisfaction helping others than helping ourselves. If you fall in that category, then find a way to use your charitable nature to motivate you to exercise. For example, donate $1 to a favorite charity for every mile you walk. Donate $10 for every pound you lose. Or commit to several fund-raising events per year that involve walking, biking, dancing, or a sports match.

Be creative with your measurements. There are so many ways to measure fitness that you can quickly become paralyzed by them all. Is it my weight? Body mass index? Pulse? Is it mileage covered, pounds lifted, calories burned, minutes of activity? For maximum motivation, focus on what matters most to you: Do you feel better than you used to? Do you look better than you used to? Are your clothes less tight? Can you see a difference in the mirror? Are your improvements getting noticed by others?

Fly to your next race. Sign up for a walkathon or race that requires an airline flight to get there. Book your flight at the same time that you sign up for the race, even if it's six months away. The motivation to train for the race (which will cost you in terms of a lost reservation if you chicken out) will keep you more motivated than any personal coach. ◁

SECRET WEAPON

A Personal Trainer's Tool Kit

If these work for personal trainers and nutritionists, they can work for you, says Raphael Calzadilla, fitness expert for eDiets.com:

- Body composition calipers, for checking body fat vs. lean tissue
- A digital, easy-to-read scale, to help monitor the above
- A tape measure, to gauge inches lost or gained
- A camera, to take a "before" photo
- A workout chart, for monitoring strength increases
- A heart rate monitor, for gauging target heart rate during aerobic exercise
- Plastic replicas of five pounds (2.25 kg) of human fat and five pounds of human muscle, to show the value of gaining muscle and losing fat.

Working Out

6 Tricks for Making the Most of the Time You Spend Exercising

Increase your intensity, not your time. Forget hour-long spinning classes and five-mile (8-km) runs. A study from the exercise gurus at McMaster University in Hamilton, Ontario, found that just six minutes of intense exercise a week could provide the same physical benefits as hours of moderate exercise. Now, by "intense exercise," we're not talking about a stroll in the park, and the six minutes were spread over three exercise sessions that also included some recovery time. The researchers had their subjects do between four and seven 30-second "bursts" of all-out cycling on stationary bikes, each followed by four minutes of regular cycling three times a week for two weeks. (Another alternative would be full-out running for 30 seconds in the midst of a leisurely jog or walk.) All told, the time the "sprinters" spent exercising each week was 20 percent of the time spent by the moderate exercisers (1 1/4 hours versus 5 1/4 hours).

Exercise first thing in the morning. Don't think about it. Just roll out of bed, put on your shoes (oh, and please brush your teeth), and go. You're more likely to get your workout in if you do it in the morning, research shows. An added benefit: You'll sleep better at night.

Weigh the benefits of free weights. The salespeople hawking enormous—and expensive—multi-exercise workout machines hope you don't catch on to this: Inexpensive free weights actually offer a number of advantages in terms of fitness and convenience. When you use free weights, you can exercise both sides of your body separately, eliminating muscle imbalances. Only some exercise machines allow that. If you have a slight body, the typical exercise machine—designed for men—may not fit you no matter how much you fiddle with the settings. If you like working out at home, you may have trouble working a gargantuan machine into the décor of your family room. Dumbbells, on the other hand, are compact, inexpensive, and easy to use.

Drink a glass of cherry juice before working out. Who woulda thunk a glass of red juice could make a difference in muscle strength? But that's just what researchers at the University of Vermont in Burlington found when they had 14 volunteers drink either fresh cherry juice blended with commercial apple juice twice a day for three days before exercise and for four days afterward, or a dummy mixture containing no cherry juice. The cherry juice drinkers lost far less muscle strength in the days after their workouts than those drinking the fake mixture (4 percent vs. 22 percent). The cherry juice drinkers also had much less pain after working out than the other juice drinkers. Plus, the cherry juice drinkers said their pain peaked at about 24 hours, while it lasted twice that long for those getting the placebo juice. The researchers suspect the high levels of antioxidant and anti-inflammatory compounds in cherry juice are behind its benefits.

Stick to drinking water when exercising. The television ads show elite athletes slurping down sports drinks to

How I Do It **This Skinny PR Pro Hated to Exercise**

When Dan Collins graduated from college in 1984, he was 21, just a hair under 5 feet, 11 inches (180 cm), weighed 239 pounds (108 kg), and had high blood pressure.

"You're coming to see me once a month, every month," his doctor told him. And the fear of the white coat kicked in. "I'd tried other ways of losing weight, such as the 'sleep diet' during summer vacation when I slept as long as I could—the logic being if you're asleep, you're not eating," explains Collins, a senior director of media relations at Mercy Medical Center in Baltimore.

He lost the weight—but promptly gained it back, plus 20 pounds.

But the "power of the white lab coat," as he calls it, worked. Hearing he was in trouble from a doctor finally gave him the motivation he needed to lose weight permanently. He stopped night eating—the bane of many with a food addiction. As the weight came off, however, it became important for him to find some way to keep it off. The problem: He had never found a way of exercising that agreed with him. Until the day he stopped at the local YMCA. He had intended to

sign up for a class on automotive maintenance, but he became intrigued instead by a class called Fencing for Beginners.

"I felt good enough about myself at that time to dare to don the very unforgiving whites and met a man named Ray Gordon, the instructor." Twenty years later, Collins weighs a healthy 190 pounds. Gordon remains his closest male friend, and they continue to fence. At last word, the two swashbucklers were in training to set the first Guinness World Record in fencing.

replenish their body chemistry and thus enhance their performance. Well, this has little relevance to us normal folk. Research does show that top-performing endurance athletes need higher levels of sodium and far more to drink than everyday people. Sports drinks like Gatorade fill that need—they're rich in salt, which not only provides the needed sodium but also keeps the athlete thirsty for more fluids. Here's the reality check, however: The extra salt provides no benefit at all to everyday people. Even if you exercise regularly, unless you are testing your body's physical limits for extended periods, water will quench your thirst nicely.

Use music to help increase your pace. Program your iPod or other portable music player to start out with

slow music (think classical and easy listening) and gradually build to rapid-fire dance music (any club music should do nicely). That arrangement, studies find, will result in your working harder and longer than those who start with fast or slow music and stick with it, or move from fast music to slow music.

And here's another use for your favorite toy: Use it when you're walking. A study published in the journal *Chest* found that people who listened to music while walking covered four more miles (6.4 km) during the eight-week study than a similar group that didn't listen to music. The participants had serious respiratory disease, and researchers think that listening distracted them from the negative symptoms of exercise (such as boredom and fatigue) and reduced shortness of breath. ◄

10

SECRETS FOR
choosing
a health club

Here's how to choose a gym—advice from Lindsay Wombold, who works for a health and wellness program at Butler University in Indianapolis, Indiana, and Raphael Calzadilla, a fitness expert for eDiets.com.

1 Health clubs can *always* waive the "enrollment fee." That fee is just a way for them to get more money out of you. If you don't want to pay it, just tell the sales rep you're going to join somewhere else. You're pretty much guaranteed to have the fee waived.

2 Make sure you can cancel at any time. You may even need to write on your contract that "per [salesperson's name], I can cancel this membership anytime with no fees." Have the salesperson sign and date it. Even better, have the manager sign and date it in case there's turnover and your salesperson no longer works there.

3 Find out when the gym is busiest, and make sure that works with your preferences. For instance, if you prefer to work out during a quiet time but the only time you can get to the gym is after work when the machines are mobbed, this might not be the best gym for you.

4 Ask for a one-week trial and bring a friend. Your friend might be able to spot problems you didn't see.

5 Insist on a free personal training session if you join. If they already provide one, ask for two.

6 Ask how often the equipment is serviced and cleaned. Cleaning should be done daily; servicing at least once a month.

7 When you get a tour of the facility, check for torn benches and antiquated-looking cardio equipment, and inspect the cleanliness of the locker area.

8 If the sales rep is wooing you with visions of Pilates and yoga classes, ask about additional fees. Many make you pay more for such classes.

9 Fitness clubs oversell memberships in the hope that people won't go. If just 20 percent of the members showed up at one time, most clubs would not have enough space or equipment to support them. Ask when the busiest times are, and show up then to see if the place is too crowded for your taste.

10 Personal trainers at gyms are on commission plus a small hourly rate. So beware of trainers who hound you to sign up for sessions—they're most likely under pressure to make a sales goal. Instead, get a sense of the trainer's genuine passion for fitness. If he or she doesn't pressure you, that's a good sign.

Women's Exercise Concerns
5 Things Every Woman Should Know to Get More Out of Her Workouts

Time your exercise to your menstrual cycle. Don't tell your health club manager, but the next time he sees you climbing like mad on the StairMaster, it's because you're in the latter part of your menstrual cycle. A study from the University of Adelaide in Australia found that women who exercise during this time of the month, when levels of estrogen and progesterone are highest, burn more fat for energy, leading to less exercise-related fatigue.

Check your iron levels. No, not the kind of iron you pump, the kind that enables your blood cells to carry much-needed oxygen to your body tissues. A study from Cornell University found that women with low levels of iron—but not low enough to be classified as anemic—find it more difficult to maintain exercise and training than women with normal levels. An estimated 16 percent of North American women have this level of iron deficiency and don't know it. Women who are physically active, dieting, or vegetarians are particularly at risk.

Don't despair! Supplementing with 100 milligrams a day of iron can double your exercise endurance compared to iron-deficient women who don't supplement. Don't try this on your own, however—this is prescription-strength iron that should only be taken under your doctor's supervision. Good sources of dietary iron include red meat, seafood, and citrus fruit or juice taken with meals to improve absorption from iron-rich foods such as legumes, whole grains, and green vegetables.

Ignore the mirrors at gyms. The designers of fitness clubs can't resist throwing up a wall of mirrors anytime they install an exercise room. The assumption is that you want to watch yourself work out. But observing your own stepping, lunging, and arm swinging might actually work against you. One study found that women who exercised in front of a mirror felt less calm and more fatigued after 30 minutes of working out than those who exercised without mirrors. Some exercise gyms are now catching on and offering "reflection-free" zones. If yours doesn't, talk to the gym manager.

Pass on star-centered videos. You could pack the Hollywood Bowl with all of the svelte models and skinny celebrities who are hoping you'll buy their exercise videos. But experts say such videos may actually undermine your motivation to work out. A study at McMaster University in Hamilton, Ontario, Canada, found that people felt less confident about their fitness and less inclined to exercise in the future when they used videos featuring super-slim models with amazing muscles and revealing thongs. Oddly enough, the effect was even worse with videos featuring an ultra-slender host leading a group of plumper, normal-looking women. Apparently that scenario further emphasizes the divide between exercise divas and everyday folks.

If you want a motivating exercise video or class, researchers say you should look for a teacher you can trust. Find a teacher with a fitness background who, like the rest of us, needs to exercise in order to look great. Videos created by personal trainers and exercise physiologists, or classes taught by them, are a good bet.

You can be both healthy and heavy. Many women think they are too heavy to benefit from exercising; others get discouraged when they don't see significant weight loss after weeks of exercise. But the most important benefit of exercise is keeping your heart healthy. And research shows that the amount of activity you get, not your weight, is the chief predictor of heart disease. One study in particular, published in 2004 in the *Journal of the American Medical Association*, evaluated more than 900 women, three-quarters of whom were overweight or obese. Researchers assessed them for weight, body mass index, and level of physical activity, then gave them angiograms to detect heart disease. The results were clear-cut: Weight didn't matter, but exercise did: It wasn't the heaviest women who showed the most evidence of heart problems, but the least active women. So get moving, whatever your size.◁

Walking

7 Secret Ways to Make the Most of the Ultimate Healthy No-Cost, Low-Impact Activity

Walk to control your body weight. Don't think this mild activity can help? In one significant study, a group of sedentary people were given a daily goal of 10,000 steps of brisk activity, as measured by their pedometers. They improved their fitness levels, blood pressure, and body fat just as much as a group that followed a traditional gym-based aerobic program. Overall, studies find that getting 8,000 to 10,000 steps a day (about five miles or 8 km) helps you lose weight, while adding to that another 2,000 steps (an extra one mile or 1.6 km a day), helps you maintain your current weight and stop gaining weight.

Walk for entertainment one day a week. Instead of walking around your neighborhood, walk through the zoo, an art museum, or an upscale shopping mall. First, circle the perimeter of your location at your usual brisk pace. Then wander through again more slowly to take in the sights.

Walk in the prettiest neighborhood. Okay, we admit it. Just circling the same streets can get plenty boring. Heck, even our dog got bored after two years of walking the same neighborhood. So do what we did: Get in the car and drive to a new neighborhood. And make it a nice one. When researchers from the University of Wollongong in New South Wales, Australia, surveyed walkers about their walking habits, they found that men who perceived their neighborhoods to be "aesthetic" were more consistent about walking around them. Other research finds that neighborhoods with well-maintained sidewalks and safe and well-lit walking areas encourage walking more than neighborhoods that don't have those features. Also, people who live in so-called walkable neighborhoods walk an average of 70 more minutes each week than people who live in neighborhoods lacking such characteristics.

Walk faster earlier in your walk. If you want to increase the amount of fat you burn during your walk, add some bursts of faster walking toward the *beginning* of your walk. Many walkers wait until the end of the walk to speed up, treating their faster walking as a finishing kick. Yet a study published in the *European Journal of Applied Physiology* found that exercisers burned more fat and felt less fatigued when they inserted their faster segments toward the beginning of a workout rather than closer to the end. It works because you speed up your heart rate early and keep it elevated for the rest of your walk.

Walk when you shop. Online shopping is great in terms of convenience and selection, but it stinks when it comes to burning calories. Walking around the mall, however, can burn about 200 calories an hour, much more than what you'll burn sitting on your butt as you surf the Net. You can increase the effectiveness of your walk and shop time by doing a lap around the mall between store visits.

Walk to fund-raise for a cause. You, you, you. That's all you think about! Instead, start thinking about the Susan G. Komen Breast Cancer Foundation, the National Multiple Sclerosis Society, The Terry Fox Run, or the Red Cross. All are charities that sponsor walk- and

runathons to raise funds. You don't even have to formally join the event. Just pledge to contribute. You'll take pride in the fact that you're walking for something beyond yourself, which will motivate you to go longer and faster. After every walk, mark the amount you owe on a chart, and when you reach $100, send a check. Whoever thought exercise could be tax deductible?

SECRET WEAPON

Pedometer

The manager at your local gym will hate you, because once you figure out the benefits of this palm-size gadget, your days on the treadmill are history. You wear pedometers on your waist. The device senses your body motion and counts your footsteps, then converts the count into distance based on the length of your stride.

Don't skimp on quality when you buy a pedometer. A study published in the online edition of the *British Journal of Sports Medicine* found that cheap pedometers are not only less likely to accurately measure steps taken, but most overestimated participants' steps, which could lead to a false sense of accomplishment.

Walk around the office or house. Are you stuck at your desk working all day, practically chained to your PC? Get up and walk around for five minutes at least every two hours. A brisk five-minute walk every two hours will parlay into an extra 20-minute walk by the end of the workday. And getting a break will make you less likely to reach for snacks out of antsiness. It's good idea to get up and walk around for a few minutes every hour or so if you are sitting for long periods of time at home reading, watching television, Web surfing, or pursuing a hobby. ◁

Secret Workouts
8 Easy Ways to Sneak Some Beneficial Exercises into Your Daily Routine

Squeeze for a tight rear. Your gluteus maximus, also affectionately known as your butt, is the largest muscle group in your body. Fire it up and you'll burn calories, says Michelle Cederberg, a fitness and wellness consultant from Calgary, Alberta. Whether you're standing or sitting, an invisible butt squeeze (tighten, hold for two seconds, release) repeated 10 to 15 times, one to three times a day, will tighten your tush and burn calories.

Practice proper posture. By making an effort to stand "tall and proud," you contract dozens of muscles from your legs up to your neck, says Cederberg. This burns calories and builds muscle. Whether you're ironing, doing dishes, or standing in a line at the bank, concentrate on keeping a solid foot stance, a slight bend in your knees, an open chest (that is, standing tall, not slouched), with shoulders depressed and head up. Another secret workout: Imagine you're squeezing a pencil between your shoulder blades and you have to hold the muscles tight so the pencil doesn't fall. It doesn't take long before the muscles in your back start to fatigue. Anytime you realign your posture, sit or stand a bit taller, and get away from a slumped posture, you're exercising your back and core muscles.

Do leg exercises while doing laundry. Whether you're folding clothes, ironing (yes, some of us still iron!), or waiting for the rinse cycle, "captive time" is ideal for adding in some lovely leg work, Cederberg says. Perform 10 to 15 plié squats (think ballerina). Position your heels just beyond shoulder width

with your toes rotated out to 45 degrees. As you drop into your squat, keep your knees in line with your toes and make sure your head, shoulders, and hips align, or "stack up," as you drop down. Return to the starting position, and squeeze the muscles in your butt as you stand tall.

Play games with the kids. Instead of sitting around watching your kids play sports, dive in. That's the advice from Beth Brody of Stockton, New Jersey, who lost 20 pounds (9 kg) and kept them off for a year by inventing active games with her five- and seven-year-old sons. Together they invented the game Mommy Monster, "an exhausting game of chasing them until I catch one for tickling," she explains. They also play dodgeball and soccer. "If I don't move fast enough, I get hit with the ball or kicked in the shin." These days, she's down to a size 6 dress from a size 10, and she doesn't get winded during her three-mile (4.8-km) jogs. Best of all: "Dodging the shin kicks has certainly made me more agile."

Do isometric exercises. Remember the term? It dates back to the Charles Atlas days. Isometric exercises, put simply, are exercises in which muscles are tensed without movement. For example, pushing as hard as you can against a brick wall is an isometric exercise, because neither you nor the wall moves. Research has shown that isometric exercises provide lots of value, particularly for those people with a limited range of motion. And you can do them anytime, anyplace. The basic rule: Hold the tension for 5 to 10 seconds, then relax for a few seconds. Repeat the cycle five to eight times. Here are some simple isometric exercises to try:

- Tense your abdominal muscles and hold.
- Put your hands together in front of you, as if praying, and press your hands together as hard as you can.
- Stand with your legs apart about a foot from a wall. Push against the wall with your hands as if you were trying to move it.
- Stand inside a doorway and, with your arms straight down and by your sides, put the backs of your hands against each door frame. Push your hands against the doorway as hard as you can, as if you were trying to widen the door space.
- While still inside the doorway, push your palms against the frame above you, as if you were trying to lift the building.
- Sit down in a chair, feet flat on the ground. Push your legs into the ground as hard as you can.

Get outdoors at least three hours every weekend. Ever notice how so much of the equipment at a health club—treadmills, stationary bikes, climbing walls, rowing machines— merely replicates what you would be doing if you were outside? Truth is, one of the best indications of a fit lifestyle is how much time you are outdoors. Why? Even if you are just strolling, gardening, washing the car, or taking a child to a playground, you are being far more active than you would be sitting indoors. Plus, it's terrific for your attitude—and a whole lot cheaper than paying for a health club membership. Best of all, once you get in the habit of being outside on your free days, you'll soon be hankering for more active pursuits: bike riding, nature hiking, even taking up a sport again—anyone can shoot baskets in the driveway for fun and exercise!

Lengthen and speed up your stride while walking. Not just occasionally— all the time! Become a high-energy walker—fast, confident, with good posture and healthy arm swinging. Just this little everyday adjustment will deliver lots of extra calories burned, stronger legs, and a shapelier behind over time.

Make cooking an easy, everyday workout. By adjusting your gear, your food supplies, and your storage, you can make every meal healthier to create! Here are a few ways:

- Switch your primary cooking knife to a cleaver. It's heavier, giving your hands, wrists, and forearms a better workout while chopping.
- Switch to cast-iron skillets and soup pots. Again, they are much heavier to lift (plus, they cook terrifically well).
- Buy milk and other drinks in larger containers. This turns pouring into an exercise.
- Defy wisdom and put the pantry and cooking items you use most either very high or very low. Stretch slowly and deliberately as you reach up or squat down for items.
- Learn the master-chef trick of tossing your food while it cooks, rather than stirring. This means picking up your sauté pan by the handle and literally tossing the ingredients up in the air to turn them. It takes a lot more strength than mixing the food around with a spoon, and it looks impressive to those watching you cook! ◀

Food Labels

10 Tricks for Deciphering the Real Truth from the Information on Packaged Foods

Look for short ingredient lists.
When you find a packaged food in the supermarket with a long list of ingredients on the label, just set it back on the shelf and look for a simpler version of the food. (We're talking here about the "Ingredients" part of the label. "Nutrition Facts" is another part, and more about that later.) The alarming truth is, many of those ingredients are various kinds of sugars and chemical additives, and they're not put there for you—they're there to benefit the company that processes the food. They "enhance" the looks, taste, or shelf life—which is all about marketing and shipping and not at all about your health. Most additives aren't known to be harmful (although the health effects of some are still open to question), but they aren't about nutrition or taste as nature intended taste to be. In fact, one of their main purposes is to make up for a lack of those things. So check the list of ingredients every time. Marion Nestle, a professor of nutrition at New York University, says that almost always, the shorter the better.

Think twice about "no cholesterol" claims. Cholesterol is a fat that occurs only in animal products (meat, fish, eggs, milk, and butter, for instance). So why do some plant-derived products claim in large letters that they contain no cholesterol? Because the food companies know that people care about their cholesterol levels, and they know that most people probably have forgotten or never knew that plants don't contain any. Some of the offenders are cereal, bread, cookies, salad dressings, and, especially, oils and margarine. Oils are obviously fats, so the makers think you'll be reassured to see that there's no cholesterol in the corn oil, safflower oil, or olive oil. Next time you see the claim, just say to yourself, "Duh! It's a plant product! Of course it doesn't contain cholesterol."

Learn what "organic" really means. There's considerable confusion about the use of the word "organic" on food labels, just as there is about almost everything having to do with labeling. For starters, the organic label is earned through a certification process, and it means the producer adhered to a strict set of rules and procedures.

- *For organic fruits and vegetables,* U.S. Department of Agriculture rules—and virtually identical regulations in Canada—say that they must be grown without any of these things: genetically modified seeds, fertilizers made from chemicals or

sewage sludge, chemical pesticides or herbicides, and irradiation. Growers are also required to keep records and present them upon demand by accredited inspectors. Foods may also be labeled "100 percent organic," "organic" (95 to 99 percent organic), "made with organic ingredients" (74 to 94 percent organic), or, for organic content of lesser amount, the specific organic ingredients may be listed.

- *On meat,* the organic seal means the animals may be fed only certified organic feed and no by-products of other animals. The animals can't be given hormones or antibiotics. They must be allowed access to the outdoors and treated humanely.

All organic farms must keep records and be inspected by accredited inspectors. There isn't enough organic food being produced to meet the demand for it, but its availability is increasing all the time. Many supermarkets now carry some organic food, and there is at least one chain (Whole Foods Market) that

---

WHAT THE FOOD INDUSTRY DOESN'T WANT YOU TO KNOW ABOUT Food Politics

The food industry would have you believe that buying food is all about price and convenience. To some degree, it is. But more importantly, buying food is about the health of you and your family. It's also about agriculture, the environment, and your local economy, to name just some issues that are involved every time you buy food. Think of your purchases as votes. You can vote for or against the use of pesticides, herbicides, antibiotics, chemical fertilizers, and preservatives. You can vote for food that is locally produced or food that has been trucked hundreds or even thousands of miles. You can vote for or against humane treatment of animals.

sells mostly organic. In addition, farmers' markets, health food stores, and individual farms are good sources of organic food.

Be suspicious of "natural" labels. The food labels "natural" and "organic" are pretty much interchangeable, right? That's exactly what food companies want you to think. But here's the truth: Use of "natural" on labels is a much more loosey-goosey affair than use of the term "organic." There's no single set of requirements for products claiming to be natural, but such labels are supposed to be accurate. If, for example, meat is claimed to be natural because the animal was not fed antibiotics or hormones, the label should say that and it should be true. Farmers or food companies that use the "natural" label are not subject to inspections as a condition of using the label. You just have to take their word for it.

Be wary of the serving size. Many "Nutrition Facts" labels are designed to make you think you're getting fewer calories than you really are. For example, labels list the nutrients on a per-serving basis. But be sure to check the "serving size" and "servings per container" lines. The candy bar that most people would eat all by themselves in a single sitting may say that it contains two servings. If you saw "100 calories" on the label, you must make a mental adjustment—you're actually eating two servings, so you're getting 200 calories.

Use a pocket calculator to compare items. A calculator is the best tool for helping you figure out what the food industry doesn't want you to know: the actual value of the nutrients in the food you're buying. For example,

say you're trying to find out which breakfast cereal is more nutritious, General Mills' Multi Grain Cheerios or Kellogg's Frosted Mini-Wheats (the whole-grain version). The Cheerios serving size is listed as one cup, but the Mini-Wheats serving is "about 24 biscuits." You can't really open the box in the store to see how that stacks up against the one cup, so the only way to compare unit to unit is to use grams, which are listed on both packages. The 59-gram Mini-Wheats serving is almost twice the size of the 29-gram Cheerios, so you have to cut in half the nutrients listed on the Mini-Wheats label. Gram for gram, their nutrients are very similar: roughly the same calories, fiber, carbs, protein, and fat. Even the amount of sugars is about the same, despite the fact that the Cheerios box proclaims the contents to be "lightly sweetened" and the Mini-Wheats have frosting! This might come as a surprise to a lot of nutritional gatekeepers.

Get the "whole" story. Marketers know that nutrition-conscious shoppers are interested in whole grains these days. Don't be deceived into buying a product that's labeled "wheat bread," however. What you really want is "whole wheat" or "whole grain" bread (for more, see page 47).

Don't confuse cereal hype with facts. If you want a healthy breakfast cereal, not one that just claims to be, ignore the large-type claims on the package and go right to the labels. Look for a short list of ingredients. Look for a whole grain as the first ingredient. Look for one that has no sugar. (You can always add sugar yourself if necessary.) Then look at the per-serving nutrients on the nutrition label. Look for a cereal with a lot of

No wonder North Americans are getting fat. If all the food production in North America were measured as calories and distributed evenly among the entire population, it would average about 3,900 calories per day for every person. Yet adults need only about 2,000 to 3,000 calories per day, except for those who get a lot of exercise. (And those who are overweight, as well as young children, should usually be eating fewer than 2,000.) What happens to all the calories you eat but don't burn? They get stored as fat, of course. So you can easily see part of the problem: One reason food companies go to such lengths to get you to buy more and eat more, without regard to the consequences, is that there's too much food being produced.

fiber in each serving. Highly sweetened cereals, when fed regularly to young children, condition their taste for sugar at an early age, forming habits that are hard to break. Nutrition professor Marion Nestle says that most breakfast cereals are now processed and sugared to such a degree that "they might as well be cookies—low-fat cookies."

Don't get soaked for watery foods. Water is the magic ingredient in prepared foods, and if it's first on the list of ingredients, that's a clue that there's a long list of additives to follow to give that water some taste and texture. You might not be surprised to see water at the top of the list of ingredients in soups. After all, soup does take a lot of water. It's more surprising to find it so prominent in SpaghettiOs. Many, many salad dressings contain more water than anything else, and since oil and water don't mix, it takes a bunch of additives to hold everything together. Water is cheap, so the food industry likes it.

Scan the can for MSG. Check out the ingredient list on the labels of prepared foods—on soups, for example. Keep reading, because it's pretty far down on a long list (although if there is no MSG, that's usually prominently mentioned at the top). MSG (monosodium glutamate) is sometimes listed under its own name but often under other names, among them hydrolyzed soy protein, autolyzed yeast, and sodium caseinate. MSG is a synthetic version of the substance *umami*, as it is known in Japan, which occurs naturally in some foods, including Parmesan cheese, soy sauce, and mushrooms. MSG, widely used in Asian cooking, went out of favor when it became associated with headaches and other unpleasant symptoms. Now many Asian restaurants proudly advertise "No MSG" on their menus, but the food industry still sneaks it in as a flavor enhancer. So if you're concerned about MSG, look for it under all of its names. ◁

Buying Produce
8 Strategies for Getting the Best-Tasting and Most Nutritious Fruits and Vegetables

Study "fresh" produce with a skeptic's eye. Unless the produce you're buying in your supermarket was locally grown, it has probably spent at least a week and possibly as much as 10 days being picked, trucked, packed, hauled, transferred, unpacked, displayed, arranged, misted, and rearranged. Furthermore, some fruits and vegetables are picked before they are really ripe so they won't spoil during the time lag. Some produce has been treated with gases, washed, cut, and bagged. Even then, it may sit in your refrigerator for a day or more before you use it. All the while, the produce is losing taste and nutritional value, which are affected by light, heat, and oxygen. If produce had to be labeled with its country of origin, that would offer a clue as to how long the produce had been on the road. But the food industry has resisted any such requirement for years. Some stores (Whole Foods Market, for example) voluntarily say where their produce comes from so customers can draw their own conclusions about just how fresh it might be. Otherwise, you're on your own.

Let common sense be your guide. If you live in Minnesota and your supermarket has strawberries in February, you can be pretty sure they've come a long way. Also, go by looks. If the lettuce is limp, it's been around too long. But paradoxically, fruits and veggies that are too shiny and waxy also may be stale. The spit and polish may be cloaking flaccid cukes or peppers, for instance. Stores do often label produce as "local," when they have it, because for many customers something locally raised is a real treat. Early in the season the locally grown may be a little more expensive, but as the season goes on, it gets cheaper.

For freshness, buy frozen. If you have any doubts about the freshness of the produce in your supermarket, here's an insider tip: Sometimes the frozen fruits and vegetables are fresher than what you'll find in the "fresh" produce section. How could that be? Frozen fruits and vegetables are picked when they're fully ripe, and they're frozen on the same day. Freezing does change the texture somewhat, but very little nutritional value is lost in the processing. The vitamin content may be somewhat reduced, but the protein, fat, minerals, fiber, and calories are the same. However, that only goes for the single-item packages of fruit and vegetables, which don't take up most of the real estate in the frozen-food aisles of your supermarket. Most of the space is given over to highly processed, prepared dishes or meals, which are more profitable for the food companies.

When it comes to limes, any (real) lime will do. Do you really need Key limes for Key lime pie or Key lime bars? Key lime growers want you to think you do, but tasters in a blind taste test split over which was better, the bars made with Key limes or those made with regular lime juice. Key limes are a trifle sweeter than the others, but the difference isn't great—except in the amount of work it takes to get at that juice. It takes about six Keys to get the same amount of juice you can get from one regular lime. Easiest of all is bottled lime juice, but testers found it bitter and an unacceptable substitute for any kind of lime, Key or otherwise.

Pick your own fruits and veggies. If you can't grow your own produce, then do the next best thing: Pick your own. PYO farms are one alternative to agribusiness food. Strawberries, raspberries, blueberries, apples, and pumpkins all lend themselves to the PYO treatment, and you get to trade your labor for part of the price of the produce. You'll get the freshest food possible, for less money than you'd have to pay in the grocery store, and you and the family will get some good exercise to boot. Some places also provide entertainment such as hayrides and petting zoos. You won't read about them in glossy magazine ads, but you might find out about one from a small ad in your local newspaper, a poster nailed to a telephone pole, or a roadside sign. Many do their best advertising by word of mouth.

Subscribe to a farm. Here's another non-agribusiness option: community-supported agriculture, or CSA. You get good, fresh food, and you also contribute to the survival of a small farm—the kind that big farms are always driving out. In a CSA, subscribers pay a farmer (usually at least partly up front) for a certain amount of food every week for the season. You get whatever's available, and the farmer gets cash to help keep the farm going. Your bag or box of food may be cheaper than what you'd pay for the same items at the grocery store, but that isn't always the case and isn't the only reason, or even the main reason, to try this arrangement. There's no requirement that CSAs be organic, but many are. One of the hardest parts is finding one, because they don't usually have marketing budgets. You won't find a flyer in your mailbox advertising the weekly specials. Ask at your local health food store for suggestions or contact a local or regional organic farming organization.

Eat for free in fields of greens. Some of the most nutritious vegetables in existence await you just outside your door. Plants with dark green leaves, such as dandelion greens, have more nutrients per ounce than any other food. Even the dandelion blossoms are good— in pancakes, fritters, salad and, with a little time and practice, as the basis for an interesting wine. And dandelions are just the beginning. Another good green

---

EXPERT INSTANT ADVICE

Use Imagery to Picture a Healthy Meal

Food companies make more money from their highly processed foods than from the simple ones, and that's why we're barraged with their advertising and images of snack food, cookies, complicated frozen dishes, chips, dips, and other salty, sugary food. Despite the best efforts of the U.S. Department of Agriculture and Health Canada to get us to eat more fruits and vegetables, we aren't. And the veggies eaten most often aren't the most nutritious ones. Dr. Douglas Husbands, a certified clinical nutritionist in San Carlos, California, has devised a way to help his patients visualize what they should be eating. He tells them to picture a plate of food divided like this: Half is filled with brightly colored or dark green, leafy vegetables. (Notice that French fries and iceberg lettuce don't qualify.) A quarter of the plate holds a serving of food with lean protein, such as fish, free-range chicken, or grass-fed beef. Finally, the last quarter has a healthy starch such as brown rice, a sweet potato, or a slice of whole-grain bread.

is *Chenopodium album*, commonly called pigweed or lamb's-quarters. (The Latin name is important because plants sometimes have different common names in different locales.) It's a common garden weed and grows just about anywhere in disturbed soil. Ramps, or wild leeks, are so prized that some communities in the South build whole festivals around them.

Two important warnings: Beware of gathering wild plants in any area where herbicides or other poisons have been applied, and avoid anything that can be mistaken for a poisonous plant. Buy a good field guide, such as *A Field Guide to Edible Wild Plants* by Lee Allen Peterson. If you're interested in mushrooms—and there are many wonderful wild ones—they're in a category all by themselves, and your best bet is to take a class from an expert. Wild food is about as anti-agribusiness as you can get. If you start learning about it and using it, you'll not only eat better, you'll have found an interesting new hobby.

Ripen fruit in a paper bag. Unless you're buying locally grown fruit, you rarely get it fully ripe from the supermarket. If it was picked at its peak, it would spoil during the time it takes to move the fruit from the grower to you. You may have heard that putting fruit in a paper bag concentrates the ethylene gas and speeds ripening. To make it ripen even faster, put some fully ripe fruit (bananas, for example) into the bag with it. The ripe fruit is giving off more ethylene, which the unripe fruit can use. Don't use plastic bags; the fruit will just spoil. The paper bag trick only works with fruits that will continue to ripen after they've been picked. Among them

are apples, avocados, bananas, blueberries, cantaloupe, kiwis, mangoes, peaches, pears, plums, and tomatoes. It pays to know which fruits don't ripen after picking, so you can avoid buying unripe ones in the first place. They include citrus fruits, pineapples, cherries, grapes, raspberries, strawberries, and honeydew melons.

Eat the fruit, skip the juice. The fruit juice industry has done a great job of persuading people that juice is a wonderful food, and the earlier you get your kids started on it, the better. Well, there's *some* truth in that. Fresh orange juice, with plenty of pulp, has vitamins, fiber, some minerals, just about no fat, and it tastes good. But there's little need to chug down OJ like it's water—a mere four ounces (125 ml), or half a cup, would supply about 60 mg vitamin C, well above the recommendations of 40 mg per day for men and 30 mg for women. What you don't hear so much about is all the calories in juice. Eight ounces (250 ml) of orange juice has 112 calories, a bit more than the 106 in the same amount of Coke. (Of course the diet version has no calories, but it does have artificial sweeteners—another story altogether.) These days, some young children nurse bottles of juice more or less all day. So the first problem is that juice drinkers usually drink way too much of it. Go for whole fruit instead. It's not as easy to chow down on a couple of oranges as it is to drink two cups of juice. A second problem is that the food companies have created tons of juice-like products, such as "juice drink," that are mostly sugar and water, with varying amounts of juice thrown in. Because these cost less, many people choose them over 100 percent juice. ◂

START YOUR OWN
community
Agribusiness

Who says growing, marketing, and distributing food has to be done on a global scale? A community-supported agriculture organization does it all on the local level. The marketing is rudimentary, and the distribution system usually extends less than 100 miles (160 km) from the farm—not the thousands of miles that big agribusiness covers.

Most CSAs are started by the farmer, who must go out and sell the idea to subscribers. But Sprout CSA in Richmond, Virginia, provides another model: a CSA started by the subscribers, who went out and found a farmer. Noah Scalin, a graphic artist, was the seed behind Sprout. When he returned to his native Richmond in 2001 after ten years in New York City, he soon began to miss the farmers' markets and other sources of organic food he had enjoyed in New York. So he organized a group of like-minded people, and they found a farmer to provide the food. Scalin did most of the marketing and he and other subscribers also helped with harvesting and distribution.

In 2002, Sprout's first year, there were nine subscribers, and the number grew every year until it reached 130. That turned out to be too big a workload, so it scaled back to 75 subscribers. At this writing, the subscribers were paying $575 for the season, May through October. Each week they received a box of whatever the farm had in its gardens. In one week in mid-July, for example,

subscribers got cucumbers, cabbage, kale, onions, and potatoes.

A CSA doesn't supply all of the vegetables one might want, and the output can be hurt by bad weather. But Scalin said he not only loves the food but also loves the idea that he's contributing to healthy farming practices (Sprout's farm is organic, although not all are) and helping a small farm to sustain itself.

If you want to know more about community-supported agriculture, organic farming, and other alternatives to supermarket produce, these organizations will put you on the fast track:

Alternative Farming Systems Information Center, National Agricultural Library, ARS, USDA, 10301 Baltimore Avenue, Room 132, Beltsville, MD 20705-2351; 301-504-6559; afsic.nal.usda.gov

National Sustainable Agriculture Information Service, P.O. Box 3657, Fayetteville AR 72702; 800-346-9140; attra.ncat.org

Canadian Organic Growers, 323 Chapel Street, Ottawa, Ontario K1N 7Z2; 888-375-7383; www.cog.ca

Robyn Van En Center for CSA Resources, Wilson College, Fulton

Center for Sustainable Living, 1015 Philadelphia Avenue, Chambersburg PA 17201; 717-264-4141, ext. 3352; www.csacenter.org

Biodynamic Farming and Gardening Association, 25844 Butler Road, Junction City, OR 97448; 888-516-7797; www.biodynamics.com

Organic Consumers Association, 6771 South Silver Hill Drive, Finland MN 55603; 218-226-4164; organic consumers.org

Ecological Agriculture Projects, McGill University (Macdonald Campus), Ste.-Anne-de-Bellevue, Quebec H9X 3V9; 514-398-7771; eap.mcgill.ca

Organic Trade Association, P.O. Box 547, Greenfield MA 01302; 413-774-7511; info@ota.com; www.ota.com

Tomato Tricks

5 Surprising Ways to Make the Most of This Popular Vegetable That's Technically a Fruit

Store tomatoes at room temperature. Ripe, juicy, just-picked tomatoes have a rich, vibrant taste. But it isn't improved by refrigeration. Keep good tomatoes in the pantry in a basket so air can circulate around them.

Capture the flavor of tomatoes at their peak. Even if you don't grow your own, it's worth it to get good tomatoes in season from a farmers' market or farm stand and preserve them for future use. Older cookbooks told you how to can tomatoes, but canning takes a long time and makes a mess. To freeze tomatoes, just cut out the tough part of the core, put the whole tomatoes on a baking sheet and into the freezer, says Jyl Steinback, author of *The Busy Mom's Slow Cooker Cookbook*. After they've frozen, transfer them to a plastic zipper bag and put them back into the freezer. When you want to use them, you can

easily peel them if you allow them to thaw until they're just barely soft on the outside. Then just rub off the skins. Or you can run warm tap water over them and peel them immediately. Use them in recipes for any cooked dish.

Avoid crushed and ground canned tomatoes. They're convenient, yes, because you don't have to cut up the tomatoes. But they're often packed in poor-quality tomato paste that has a metallic aftertaste. Use whole canned tomatoes instead. If you're making sauce in a hurry and don't have time to cook down all that juice, just pour it off and save it. And instead of cutting up the tomatoes, just break them up with your hands as you add them to the sauce. Canned tomatoes are often very good and always better than poor-quality fresh ones. While you're at it, avoid most plum tomatoes too. They are often used in cooking because they have more pulp and less juice and seeds, so they cook down faster than some of their juicier relatives. But plum tomatoes in general are quite tasteless, and Roma (the most common in North America) is one of the least flavorful.

Make tomato sauce without simmering all day. *Mamma mia!* The tomato sauce that simmers for hours does taste great. But a fresh tomato sauce that takes just minutes to cook has a charm all of its own—especially when it's made with local tomatoes at the height of their flavor. There are many excellent versions of this sauce. This one comes from *The Sopranos Family Cookbook: As Compiled by Artie Bucco*. Cook 2 large, smashed garlic cloves in 1/4 cup olive oil over medium heat for about 4 minutes or until the garlic is golden. Add 2 pounds (1 kg) very ripe tomatoes, peeled, drained, and chopped. (If fresh ones are not in season, use one 28-ounce [540-ml] can Italian tomatoes, drained and chopped.) Add salt to taste and simmer for 15 to 20 minutes, until the sauce is thick. Stir in 8 to 10 fresh basil leaves, torn into pieces. Serve over hot, cooked pasta. This sauce doesn't have the complexity of its long-simmered cousin, but that isn't the only kind of sauce, as the ads for the canned supermarket sauces would have you believe.

Keep the tomato seeds and skin.
A sauce with peels and seeds in it—horrors! That's some people's opinion, and they're entitled to it. But it's all a matter of taste. The skin and seeds both contribute a great deal to the flavor of a tomato sauce, but if you want to remove the evidence, put the sauce through a food mill. Or make a somewhat coarser sauce with a blender or food processor. Or let it be, with skins and seeds intact. Another sauce tip: When you've seen one tomato, you haven't seen them all. Different varieties have different tastes, and even a single tomato has several aspects to its character. It can be sweet, sour, and salty, all at the same time. You can choose different flavorings to bring out the different facets. Basil, chives, sweet peppers, and even mint will bring out sweetness. Wine, citrus, capers, and vinegars will bring out the sour. The salty aspect will respond to anchovies, olives, capers, and cured meats. ◁

Make Your Own Salad Dressings

EXPERT INSTANT ADVICE

The food companies don't want you to know this, but making salad dressings is not a big deal. You can make any oil-and-vinegar-based dressing from a basic vinaigrette and the additions of your choice. The vinaigrette is simple as can be.

> Mix 3 parts good olive oil to one part good vinegar, then add salt and pepper to taste.

Keep that on hand in the refrigerator all the time. If you want blue cheese dressing, add some blue cheese to it. If you want tarragon dressing, by all means add that. For garlic, add a crushed garlic clove. And so on. The quantities of the additions need not be precise; just keep tasting and stop adding when you like it.

Although salad dressings are a small part of an overall diet, they take up an inordinate amount of space on supermarket shelves. Why? Because these condiments are very high-profit items for their makers, who would like you to think there's such a huge difference between blue cheese and vinaigrette that you couldn't possibly do it yourself.

"Salads are ruined with bought dressings," Elizabeth David writes in her book *Italian Food*. They're usually made from water, bland soybean oil, flavorings, emulsifiers, and preservatives. Even if you want a dressing not based on oil and vinegar, such as ranch or Thousand Island, a basic cookbook will give you directions. You'll eat better, it will cost you less, and you'll free up about an acre of space in your refrigerator.

Egg Secrets

4 Things You Should Know About Buying, Cooking, and Storing This Versatile Food

Buy organic eggs. Of course, organic eggs are slightly more expensive than regular eggs, but we wouldn't be telling you to buy them unless they were better for you. The reason is they are much higher in the all-important omega-3 fatty acids, which have been shown to benefit everything from your mental health (by reducing the risk of depression) to your heart health (by reducing the risk of atherosclerosis and atrial fibrillation), says Fred Pescatore, M.D., author of *The Hamptons Diet* and a physician at Partners in Integrative Medicine in New York City.

There's more than one way to boil an egg. Do you want the control freak's method or the laissez-faire system? They both work. A lot of cookbooks want you to think there's only one way to do something—their way, of course! In some cases, that's true. If you want to beat egg whites for an angel food cake, you can't allow even a speck of yolk to get into the whites or they won't beat up into a meringue. But more often, there are several ways to do something—like boil an egg.

- *The control freak's way* is to bring the water to a boil and *then* place the eggs carefully into it. Cover the pan, and when the water returns to a boil, set the timer for 3 minutes for soft-boiled eggs or 13 minutes for hard-boiled. When the timer goes off, remove the pan from the stove and drain off the water. You'll probably be eating the soft-boiled egg immediately, but if you intend to refrigerate the hard-boiled ones, first run cold water over the eggs until they're no longer hot. (That will also make them easier to peel.)

- *The easygoing laissez-faire method* doesn't require a timer. Start by putting the eggs in the pan and covering them with cold water. Put the pan on a burner over high heat, and cook just until the water comes to a boil. Turn off the heat immediately and leave the eggs in the hot water, covered. After 20 minutes (you *can* use a timer if you want to—this is the laissez-faire way, after all) the eggs will be hard-boiled to the same degree as they are following 13 minutes of constant cooking. But you'll have helped combat global warming by saving 13 minutes of energy usage. There's nothing sacred about the 20-minute requirement; that's merely the minimum. You can let them sit in the water much longer, although eventually the whites will become a little rubbery and a greenish ring will form around the yolk. (It's harmless, but some people find it unsightly.) Eggs will be soft-boiled under this method after sitting in the hot water for 5 minutes. There's no reason for any supposed non-cook to lament, "I can't even boil an egg."

Prick eggs to make them peel easily. It's well known in Europe but not so well known in North America: Pricking eggs before boiling them makes them easier to peel. In Europe they even sell little gizmos for piercing the eggshell, but you don't need one of those.

Just take a pin and insert it about half an inch into the fat end of the egg. That lets in enough air to break the seal between the membrane and the egg white it wants to cling to. Other egg tips: Older eggs peel easier than fresh eggs. If you're making egg salad and won't be serving the eggs intact, don't peel them at all. After you've boiled and cooled them, crack them open and scoop out the egg. You're going to mash it up anyway, so why bother with all that peeling? If, on the other hand, you're planning on making deviled eggs or slices for a garnish, you do want perfect eggs.

Freeze leftover egg whites individually. How many times have you used a few egg yolks, then stored the leftover whites all together in the fridge—only to forget about them? Later, you come upon the container and can't remember how many whites are in it or when you put them there. So you toss it out. Here's a better way. Put each white into one compartment of a clean ice cube tray and freeze them. Then remove the cubes from the tray and store them in a plastic zipper bag. It's then obvious how many there are, and you can thaw them overnight in the refrigerator before using them. To lighten an omelet, add several whites to the whole eggs you use. You can even use them for angel food cake, but they won't beat up to quite as much volume as fresh ones. ◄

Cast Your Net for Sustainable Seafood

EXPERT INSTANT ADVICE

Fish is the best source of the "good" fatty acids, but buying fish and seafood, whether at the grocery store, fish market, or in a restaurant, has never been so complicated—that is, if you know what's going on behind the scenes. The fishmongers certainly aren't going to tell you.

"Wild" fish has become scarcer, and of course more expensive, as technology has enabled ever more fish to be caught by an increasingly automated fishing fleet. Overfishing has driven some formerly plentiful fish, such as Atlantic cod, to the verge of extinction.

Then along came fish farming, and for a while it seemed as if that would be the answer to, for example, the problem of declining numbers of Atlantic salmon. But even when farming solved the scarcity problem, aquaculture created new problems by possibly introducing diseases into the wild population and polluting waters. And the environmental concerns don't even address the issue of mercury contamination in the tissues of fish.

How can a fish lover sort it all out? Well, the Monterey (California) Bay Aquarium Foundation has undertaken to do it for you. It has divided many popular food fish into three categories:

- Best Choices
- Good Alternatives
- Avoid

Fish on the "Avoid" list got there either because they're so scarce or because of the methods used to farm or catch them. The list changes when changes in fishing or farming methods change, but you can keep up with it at www.seafoodwatch.org. There you can find downloadable, compact lists of fish in the various categories.

Serving Meat

9 Secrets for Getting Healthy and Tasty Results When Buying and Preparing Animal Protein

Buy grass-fed beef. Here's something the beef industry doesn't want you to know: Conventionally raised beef has more bad fat and less of the good kind than grass-fed beef. But all cattle eat grass, don't they? Yes and no. In the mass-production beef industry, cattle graze on grass for part of their lives, then they're sent to giant feedlots to pig out on corn until fat enough for slaughter. Only a small number are fed on grass for their whole lives. Irish researchers reported in 2000 that cattle fed on grass had less of the artery-clogging saturated fat in their tissues after slaughter than those fed grain, and they also had a higher proportion of omega-3 to omega-6 fatty acids. (Both are essential for humans, but omega-6 is much more common in the North American diet.) In addition, grass-fed beef contains conjugated linoleic acid (CLA), which is believed to help prevent cancer and heart disease. As if that weren't enough, the feedlot cattle also create giant manure piles that can't be absorbed by the land nearby, thus polluting water and air. Since cattle stomachs were made to digest grass, when they're fed a lot of grain they usually also have to be treated with antibiotics to prevent or treat illness. However, they get fat faster on grain than on grass; grain is cheap in America because it's subsidized by the taxpayers through the U.S. Department of Agriculture. No wonder the beef industry loves grain!

"Other white meat" is hogwash. Whoever penned the advertising slogan touting pork as "the other white meat" is clearly a marketing genius. Light coloring aside, the truth is that lean chicken is much less fatty than lean pork. A 3-ounce (85-gram) serving of broiled, skinless chicken breast provides 140 calories, 27 from fat, and only one-third of that fat is saturated. The same serving of roasted lean pork loin provides 275 calories, 189 of them from fat, half of it saturated. To top it off, the chicken serving has 6 more grams of protein than the same amount of pork.

Get Montreal's signature meat online. "Smoked meat" is available in many places in Canada, but the people who really know it say the best comes from Montreal, where it originated. And the best of Montreal's smoked meat, many say, comes from Schwartz's Montreal Hebrew Delicatessen. There are people who travel to Montreal just to eat the smoked meat at Schwartz's and consider it time and money well spent. Smoked meat is similar to pastrami but with somewhat different spices. Frank Silva, the general manager of Schwartz's, says Schwartz's didn't invent smoked meat but it has kept the same process since the deli opened in 1928. The process begins with marinating the meat, a brisket, in a special blend of spices for 7 to 10 days. That is followed by 7 or 8 hours of smoking, and 3 hours of steaming. No chemical preservatives or shortcuts are used, and that's what separates Schwartz's from the competition, Silva says. The company has refused many offers to franchise the business, but it does sell its smoked meat sliced by the pound or by the whole brisket, at www.schwartzs deli.com.

Don't expect London broil to be tender. The name has a vaguely upscale sound to it, but in reality "London broil" signifies a rather tough cut, usually from the chuck or round. London broil doesn't exist in the same sense that a porterhouse steak exists, with the term meaning a certain cut of meat from a specific part of the carcass. London broil is a term invented by a New York restaurant in the 1930s, and it remains in use because it's so useful— to the supermarkets. It's much cheaper than cuts such as T-bone, porterhouse, or filet mignon, which are instantly recognizable as steak. Flank steak used to be among those cuts called London broil, but then it became popular in its own right and the supermarkets realized they could charge more for it under its real name. Still, London broil can be flavorful, and its toughness can be mitigated as long as you know what you're up against. *Cook's Illustrated* writer David Pazmino found that he could tenderize the meat for grilling by sprinkling about 2 teaspoons salt evenly over both sides, wrapping it in plastic wrap, and letting it sit in the refrigerator for at least 3 hours, but not more than 24 hours. After the grilling, slice the meat very thinly, on the diagonal. A really sharp knife is essential.

Try rubbing coffee on your steak. Ever had coffee on your steak? Probably not, unless you've eaten at Rippe's steak and seafood restaurant in Seattle. In 2003 a chef and waiter came up with the idea of smearing Starbucks on their sirloin. It soon became a big hit, and Rippe's dubbed its creation Seattle's Signature Steak. Restaurants tend to be secretive about the recipes for their special dishes (with the exception of those that publish cookbooks, such as Chez Panisse, Moosewood, and the Silver Palate). Some home cooks make a game out of defying the restaurants and devising their own versions of their favorite restaurant fare.

Laure Dixon, a fine cook and wine connoisseur who lives in Nashua, New Hampshire, developed this version of coffee-dusted steak. She says to start with a good cut of meat and good coffee beans. (Some like espresso best.) Grind the beans to a fine powder. Then use that as a dry rub on the meat, rubbing it in with your hands. Shake off any excess. Then grill, broil, or pan-fry the steak to your preferred level of doneness. After she takes it off the heat, Laure swipes the steak across a plate containing a fine olive oil, then sprinkles sea salt all over it. (If you want less oil, just drizzle a little over the steak.) Other cooks have also attempted to re-create Rippe's steak, and you can find another version at www.supermarketguru.com.

If you have a favorite restaurant dish you'd like to duplicate, try searching the Web under the name of the restaurant or the dish. If you don't find anything, be fearless—try making it up yourself.

Dilute that serving of beef. The cattle industry would like you to saw your way through a large slab of steak for dinner. But do your arteries a favor and save the whole-steak approach for special occasions. For day-in-and-day-out dining, find ways to cook your steak with other ingredients. Examples: Slice raw beef and sauté it with peppers and onions, fajita style. Cook cut-up steak in a wok with lots of vegetables. Top a salad with steak slices. Or make shish kebab with steak cubes and veggies. You almost always eat less meat when you prepare it as part of a broader dish.

Cook your hamburgers however you want. Here's more proof that there's more than one way to do lots of things, despite what the experts say. Brothers Bob and David Kinkead, who are partners in the restaurant Sibling Rivalry in Boston, divide their loyalties when it comes to cooking burgers. Bob prefers his cooked in a pan because he says grilling gives you the taste of char, not meat. David says cooking over charcoal or wood brings out the most flavor. One thing they do agree on: Don't press on the burgers while they're cooking. That just extracts juices and dries them out.

Try healthier ground chicken or turkey. Whenever you find yourself reaching for a package of ground meat, switch over to the poultry section instead and pick up some ground chicken, ground turkey, or even some soy crumbles. All of them work just as well as ground beef for meatballs, meat loaf, or chili. However, this simple substitution can cut more than 30 percent of the calories and at least half of the fat and saturated fat in a three-ounce serving. When it's smothered in a zesty tomato sauce or flavored with seasonings, you'll never be able to tell the difference. If you are feeling a little gun-shy about abandoning the beef, use half turkey and half lean beef, or half soy crumbles and half beef.

Roast a chicken breast down. Cooked in the traditional way with breast side up, the white meat of a chicken is dry and worn out by the time the dark meat is done, but most cookbooks don't tell you what to do about it. Try flipping the bird over, as amateur (and admired) cook Laure Dixon does. Chicken cooked with its backside up and breast down produces meat that is moist and tender throughout. One small piece of special but inexpensive equipment, a V-rack, is helpful for the inverted roasting. But without that rack, you can prop up the chicken on a long cylinder of rolled-up aluminum foil. Roast in a preheated 400°F (200°C) oven until a meat thermometer inserted into the thickest part of the thigh reads 175°F (80°C). Another way to roast a chicken, favored by some cooks in the Provence region of France, is to set it on two pounds (1 kg) of garlic cloves (yes!) and roast as above. A more modest version calls for 40 cloves to be inserted into the cavity before roasting. Either way, the cooking makes the garlic much milder, and those who enjoy it can eat the cloves like a vegetable. ◁

Cookout Secrets

4 Ways to Make Your Outdoor Grilling Better Tasting—and More Fun as Well

Master the nuances of grilling. Most people never use their grills to their full potential, and restaurants that rely heavily on grilling are usually pleased not to demystify the process. There's a lot more to it than throwing on a slab of meat and trying not to burn it. Ron Rupert, executive chef at Seasons 52 restaurant in Orlando, Florida, is willing to share some of his secrets. He uses different parts of the grill for their different heat levels, and selects different woods for the subtle yet distinctive flavor they impart. For example, he uses mesquite for a slightly sweet, smoky flavor; when he wants a smokier taste, he burns oak. Also, he says, different woods burn at different temperatures. Mesquite produces a very hot fire, suitable for cooking fish, while oak burns at a temperature favorable for vegetables and meats. For a juicy steak, first sear the meat on a hotter part of the grill, then move it to a medium-hot area to allow the flavors to develop more slowly. He wows diners at his restaurant with grilled fresh vegetables (in addition to meat and fish, of course) cooked with very little added fat. The restaurant doesn't even have a deep fryer, never panfries, and rarely sautés. And each item on the menu promises to have fewer than 475 calories.

Butter up your grilled steak. When you order steak in a good restaurant, don't be dazzled by exotic spices or cooking techniques listed on the menu. There's an astoundingly simple chef's secret that provides the knock-'em-dead flavor that you can't seem to achieve when you grill steaks at home: butter. When you're grilling at home, as soon as you remove your steak from the grill, shave 1/2 tablespoon butter onto it and let the butter melt. Don't tell your guests—they'll wonder how you found the time for cooking school.

Take the spilling out of grilling. Those cute little wooden skewers were supposed to work fine if you soaked them in water first. Well, you can't soak them enough to keep them from catching fire— and then there goes the shish kebab. Round metal skewers were just fine until it came time to turn them over. You'd no sooner get the whole thing flipped over than gravity would take over, and all the stuff on the skewer would swing around too. Then there were flat skewers, which kept the food from flopping over, but they had to be bigger in order to be effective. That was fine for the meat, but the peppers, onions, and especially fragile mushrooms would often split while you were attempting to thread them onto the skewer. Kebab baskets eliminate both problems. They're a kind of long wire box with a lid and a long handle. You put the stuff into the box, close the lid, and place it on the grill or over the fire. The handle allows easy flipping.

Rediscover the campfire. Go ahead, if you want to, and buy a grill that practically duplicates your whole kitchen (including the price, if you buy one of the fanciest). But before there were grills, there were campfires, and they're still magical. You can have plenty of fun with a little fireplace in the backyard. Naturally, the grill makers don't advertise that! (Check your local ordinances to make sure it is allowed.) Here are two methods:

How I Do It A Chef Grills Ears of Corn and Lettuce

Chef Ron Rupert uses the grill not just for cooking but also as a flavor enhancer for vegetables. Here is his secret for corn on the cob, a summertime favorite. First, don't husk the corn. Place it on a medium-hot part of the grill and turn the ears as they brown. The object of this step is to cook the kernels, and that should take 20 to 25 minutes. Then peel back the husks (but leave them on the cob), remove the silk, spritz the kernels with a little olive oil, and season them with salt and pepper. Return to the grill and cook until nicely browned, 4 to 5 minutes.

Rupert even grills lettuce for one of his restaurant's signature salads. Using romaine, he first washes it and pats it dry. Then he cuts it in half lengthwise, spritzes it with olive oil, and adds salt and pepper. He cooks the lettuce briefly, over a hot fire, removing it when browned. He brushes the grilled romaine with a Caesar dressing and tops it with buffalo steak, grilled red onion rings, and corn salad.

- Dig a hole about four inches (10 cm) deep and two feet (60 cm) in diameter, and place some round stones in a circle, very close together, along the edge. A mere 10 or 15 rocks about the size of a softball will do the job—there's your fire pit.

- If you happen to have flat stones, and more of them, you can build a little fireplace. Pile the rocks on three sides and leave it open on one side to allow you to get at the fire. The stones should be piled high enough to shield the fire from the wind without cutting off the air supply. This is a simple device, not made according to a precise formula.

After you have your fire pit or fireplace, make the fire. If you're in the backyard, crumple up some paper (look for bark or dry leaves if you're in the woods). Loosely arrange small twigs over the paper, bark, or leaves to create a tepee. Add a layer of slightly larger twigs on top of that. Then light the paper. As soon as the twigs have caught fire, start piling on more twigs, using ever-larger ones as the fire gets going. When the fire will burn sticks of a couple of inches (5 cm) in diameter, pile on enough so that when they burn down, they'll create a nice bed of coals. That could take a half hour or more, depending on how big a fire you have.

Once you have red-hot coals, it's time to cook. In keeping with the primitiveness of it, find and cut a couple of nice slim branches. Sharpen one end of one with a jackknife, and poke it through a couple of hot dogs to roast over the fire. Toast a couple of rolls at the same time on the other stick. Add a piece of firewood occasionally if you don't want the fire to go out. When you've had your fill, use the sticks to toast a few marshmallows. Be sure to douse the fire completely when you're done, even if it looks as if it has gone out. The fire pit or fireplace can be used over and over again. ◂

5 Secrets for Keeping Food from Spoiling and for Using On-the-Edge Foods

Make cheese and milk last longer. Good cheese is expensive. It also gets moldy fast. Mold is fine on blue cheese, but less than delectable on cheddar. You can delay the onset by wrapping the cheese in a piece of cheesecloth soaked in whiskey, then put that in a plastic bag. Or wrap the cheese in parchment paper and then foil and keep it in the crisper drawer. To keep the side of a piece of cheese from drying out, rub a little butter on it. To keep milk or cream fresh longer, add a pinch of salt to the carton.

Soften those rock-hard raisins. You can prevent raisins from getting hard, or at least slow the process a lot, by storing them in a jar with a tight lid. But you forgot to do that, and only got to eat a handful before the 15-ounce (425-gram) box hardened into stone. It feels like a shame to toss away that food, inedible though it may be. Don't scribble "raisins" on the shopping list just yet—you can revive those hardened nuggets. Drop them into a cooking pot and add water until they're submerged. Bring the water to a boil on the stovetop and then turn the stove off. Let the raisins steep in the water for 10 minutes. Set your colander in the sink and pour your soft-and-tasty raisins into it to drain.

Save the not-yet-rotten bananas. When bananas get too ripe to be eaten whole or even to be presentable as slices, they're still fine for shakes or banana bread. If you can't use them immediately, peel them and freeze them individually in plastic wrap; thaw before using.

Make a portable root cellar. Rather than let your ginger shrivel up in the fridge or watch the carrots turn to slime in the crisper, try storing roots in a pot filled with clean sand. An unglazed flowerpot works well. Cover the roots, and pick them out as you need them. Store the pot in a cool, dark place.

Freeze the leftover tomato paste. When you just want a tablespoon or two of tomato paste, remove that from the can and drop the remainder by spoonfuls (pretend you're making cookies) onto wax paper. Put these dollops, wax paper and all, in the freezer. Once they're frozen, peel them off the paper, drop the paste pieces into a zip-seal plastic bag, and store them in the freezer. Next time you need a little tomato paste, just add a "cookie" or two to your sauce or soup. There's no need to thaw them. ◁

Beware of Buying in Bulk

Some people are so seduced by the idea of bargains at warehouse stores that they momentarily lose their common sense when shopping there. The warehouse stores won't tell you, but sometimes an item costs the same or even less in regular stores. You have to study the unit price to determine that. Why buy and store 50 cans of tuna if you can buy it a few at a time for the same price per can? Before you buy a gross of hot dogs or three kilos of grated Parmesan cheese, stop and think about how you'll store your purchases. Do you have enough room in your freezer, refrigerator, or pantry? Why buy 6 pounds (2.7 kg) of grated cheese at a bargain price if it's going to mold before you can use it all, and you wind up throwing half of it away? When you're buying just because it's a bargain, be sure it really is.

Cooking Skills
5 Easy Ways to Get You on the Road to Becoming a Fantastic Cook

Ignore the hype—you *can* cook. Cooking isn't an exotic art practiced only by cultists, although there are plenty of take-out restaurants, eat-in restaurants, delis, supermarket deli sections, and mini-marts that profit when you think that way. According to government statistics, almost half of U.S. consumers' food budget, and just under a third of Canadians', goes for meals prepared outside the home. Julia Child, the noted cook and cookbook author who brought detailed instructions for French cooking to American readers, took issue with the idea of cooking as a pastime open only to a few. "If you can read, you can cook," she wrote.

Get a back-to-basics cookbook. Julia Child's statement may not be terribly reassuring to people who have no idea where to start reading—there is an incredible array of cookbooks on the market, after all, and often they only further intimidate the novice. (We won't even get into the intimidation factor of all of those cooking shows on TV.) If you want to learn to cook, don't start with one of the just-published, hyped-up, fancy-schmancy cookbooks prominently displayed in bookstores. You need a basic,

nuts-and-bolts guide, one that will explain something as obvious to an experienced cook as "roast" or "sauté" or "braise." Here's a recommendation: *Joy of Cooking*. It has been around since 1931 and has gone through six editions in order to keep up with changing North American tastes. The older editions explain how to can vegetables and make pickles, jams, and jellies. The latest edition doesn't have those sections, but it explains the basics of many dishes from ethnic cuisines that were practically unknown in North America decades ago. There are other good basic cookbooks, but few as comprehensive as *Joy*. Once you have obtained a basic book, then just follow the advice of Alice B. Toklas, an author of another sort of cookbook—the kind that's fun to dip into to supplement the basics. "The only way to learn to cook is to cook," she wrote in 1954 in *The Alice B. Toklas Cookbook*. Toklas was a companion to the American writer Gertrude Stein, and they lived for many years in France. Toklas's cookbook has never been updated, but neither has it ever been out of print, probably because of her recipe for "Haschich Fudge," popularly known as "hash brownies." Her cookbook is an amusing mix of recipes and anecdotes from the 1930s and 1940s and is a good illustration of the notion that cookbooks don't follow just one recipe for usefulness and success.

Find out what foods your family likes. Nothing will boost your confidence in your cooking skills more than having satisfied customers—that is, family members who are happy with what they are eating. While it helps to ask everyone what their favorite dishes are, and even get them involved in menu planning, you can't always trust what people say off the top of their head when asked a broad question like "What kind of dishes do you like for dinner?" A more reliable way is to observe what dishes your family enjoys at restaurants or at someone else's house. Consult your cookbooks or surf food sites on the Web for similar recipes and surprise them by duplicating those dishes at home.

Stay current with a magazine. There are so many cooking and food magazines that you can choke trying to digest the options. So here's another recommendation: *Cook's Illustrated.* Its articles deal with basic techniques and ingredients as well as more exotic ones. They advise on the usefulness of new products, and they always explain the reasoning behind their choices. *Cook's* has no advertising or product endorsements. Finally, it's beautifully designed and well written.

Read the directions all the way through first. That sounds pretty obvious, but many cooking attempts fail if you omit this step. In the middle of a recipe, wannabe cooks suddenly realize they have to cream the butter—and it's rock-hard in the fridge. Or they don't preheat the oven to the right temperature. Or they find themselves with no chocolate when they're trying to make brownies. For Southern-style barbecue, you must start with the right cut of meat and plan on hours for it to cook, or it will be tough. If you're making an omelet, getting the pan hot makes the difference between an omelet that is easily flipped and leaves the pan cleanly, or ending up with scrambled eggs—minus the half that's stuck to the pan. ◄|

Adding Flavor
4 Surprising Flourishes That Will Improve the Way Your Food Tastes

Buy herbs and spices at a health food store. Instead of buying dried herbs and spices in those tiny bottles and cans (with the big price tags) in the supermarket, try your local health food store. Most health food stores sell them in bulk, and ounce for ounce, gram for gram, they're a whole lot cheaper than the grocery store kind. They're usually fresher, too, and many are organically grown. The per-pound (500 grams) prices, even at the health food store, can seem daunting ($15 per pound for dried parsley?), but you can scoop out a generous amount that is pretty cheap when it gets weighed up because dried herbs and spices are so light. In the sampling of spices and prices shown in the chart below, only chili powder was roughly comparable in price, although still a little cheaper at the health food store.

per ounce	SUPERMARKET	HEALTH FOOD STORE
Chili powder	$1.33	$1.19
Cinnamon (ground)	1.50	0.56
Oregano	1.24	0.75
Parsley flakes	3.32	0.94
Peppercorns	1.15	0.87

Source: Survey taken 7/12/06 at Price Chopper and St. Johnsbury Food Co-op in St. Johnsbury, Vermont

There were some differences in quality too. One of the ingredients in the supermarket's chili powder was salt, which was not included in the health food kind. (You can always add your own salt if you really need it.) The health food store chili powder had a richer spice mixture, with eight spices to five for the supermarket variety (not counting the salt). And the health food kind mentioned prominently that it had not been irradiated. Irradiation is a very common treatment in all kinds of herbs and spices.

Use wine for flavor. And say goodbye to bottled and dried mixes, bouillon cubes, and artificial flavors that the food industry would like you to use in soups, stews, and gravies. Elizabeth David writes, "If every kitchen contained a bottle each of red wine, white wine, and inexpensive port for cooking, hundreds of store cupboards could be swept clean forever of the cluttering debris of commercial sauce bottles and all the synthetic aids to flavoring." (Don't use *cooking* wine. It's not of good quality, and it's typically loaded up with sodium you don't need.) To make excellent gravy for roast meat, strain the fat off the pan drippings, add 1/2 cup wine, and scrape off the meat residue in the pan. Cook on high heat for a couple of minutes—that gets rid of the alcohol in the wine—add a little water, and cook for about 2 minutes more.

Celebrate celery. Celery doesn't get much respect. It appears most often in soups, stews, and casseroles, where, in a supporting role, it adds some of its distinctive flavor. But it's rarely the star, except in Cajun and Creole cookery, where with peppers and onions it is part of the "holy trinity." Why not let it shine? Add chopped celery—not cooked to death, but crunchy—at the last minute to creamed dishes. It adds taste, texture, and surprise. Here's another surprise: an easy relish that livens up a traditional accompaniment to pork. To a pint of applesauce, add 1 cup chopped celery and 1 tablespoon horseradish. You may like yours with more or less horseradish and celery, so feel free to adjust the quantities.

Don't be scared away from butter. Just don't use too much of it. We all know that butter has saturated fat, and too much saturated fat isn't good. But good health is less about avoiding one particular food than about your overall eating patterns. If you eat Pop-Tarts for breakfast and satisfy your daily vegetable requirement with French fries and potato chips, don't think you're protecting your health by using margarine instead of butter. The margarine makers would like you to think that, but don't let them kid you. They've made a whole industry out of fear of butter. Many great cooks—and healthy ones—swore by butter. Julia Child was ridiculed as the "cholesterol queen" for her love of butter and cream, but she remained an advocate for good butter and good food until the end, which came two days shy of her 92nd birthday in 2004. She also believed in enjoying butter (and everything else) in moderation. ◂

Gadgets and Gizmos
5 Things to Know About Buying and Using Food-Preparation Utensils and Aids

Ignore kitchen tool hoopla. A lot of manufacturers of kitchen gadgets, as well as the stores that sell them, would have you think you simply can't cook without this or that gizmo. What you never hear is that one cook's cool tool is another cook's clutter. There are fine cooks who don't have a food processor, a microwave, a blender, a slow cooker, a mandoline, a mango splitter, a gas grill, a ricer, a food mill, a toaster oven, a bread maker, a juicer, or even a coffee maker. There are other cooks who swear by any one of those items, and a whole lot more. There are cooks—good ones—who still prefer an old-fashioned, hand-cranked eggbeater to a wire whisk. When it comes to equipment, you must find your own way. Just don't think you have to figure it out all at once. If you don't want to spend a lot of money on equipment until you know what you really like, look for yard sales that advertise kitchen equipment among their wares. You can buy things for very little money, see how you like them, and either keep them or put them into your own sale.

Don't worry about wood vs. plastic cutting boards. Which side are you on, wood or plastic? The war over which type of cutting board is safest has entered a new phase: It's a draw. The battle went back and forth for more than a decade. Everyone assumed plastic could be cleaned more thoroughly, and was therefore better than wood, until some research in 1994 showed that wood retained less bacteria than plastic. More research followed, and it further confused the issue. Finally, researchers at *Cook's Illustrated* threw up their hands and declared: There isn't much difference. Just wash them with hot, soapy water, because bacteria persist on both for a long time.

Discover the double boiler. Here's a tool that's so old it never gets any hype, so it might as well be new and unknown. Cookbook author Virginia Bentley swore by a good old-fashioned double boiler. Several of them, actually, in big and small sizes. She loved them

---

SECRET WEAPON

A Brick

You don't need a special panini press, according to Jason Denton. He owns 'ino on Bedford Street in New York City, a tiny restaurant that for eight years has specialized in panini. First, he says, set the grill for about 250°F (120°C) or, if using charcoal, wait until the coals have cooled down a bit and are not too hot. Use some kind of substantial bread, such as a baguette, and slice off the domed part on top. Slice the loaf in half lengthwise. (Depending on the size, you can probably get several sandwiches from one loaf.) Put some cheese (Denton likes baby Swiss and provolone) on both sides of the bread, and the filling goes between the layers of cheese. For a filling, he uses what's in season—maybe zucchini or tomatoes with some simple cured meat. It's important not to stuff it too much, he says. Put the sandwich on the grill and weight it with an ordinary brick wrapped in aluminum foil. The brick helps everything melt together and keeps the heat even. It should be done in 3 to 4 minutes. Check Denton's book *Simple Italian Sandwiches* for a host of other ideas.

because they're guaranteed not to scorch, and they're great for keeping food warm. She liked to serve directly from them when she was entertaining. You can improvise a simple double boiler by placing a heatproof bowl (Pyrex is perfect) over a saucepan of simmering water. The bowl should sit over the water, not in it.

In with the new, but hang on to the old. Product makers will label their new-and-improved gadgets as "breakthroughs," new and better replacements for the old version that's sitting in your kitchen drawer. If you succumb to temptation and buy, don't throw out your old tool just yet. Take graters, for instance. The old-fashioned four-sided box grater, with different sizes of grating teeth, is still the best for grating tomatoes and cheeses such as cheddar. It also has small teeth that do a decent job on hard cheeses such as Parmesan. But a newer kind of grater, the rasp grater,

does an even better job on hard stuff, like Parmesan cheese, garlic, nutmeg, and chocolate. But it does a lousy job with the softer things, so hang on to that old one.

Use coffee filters for straining. Many recipes call for using cheesecloth to strain things, but David Felton, executive chef at the Pluckemin Inn in Bedminster, New Jersey, often uses paper coffee filters instead. Straining through the filters takes a little longer, but it produces a clearer liquid and they're easier to use than cheesecloth. He uses coffee filters for broth and also to strain the juice from watermelon and fresh tomatoes to use in aperitifs. The straining produces a liquid nearly as clear as water but with a little surprise to the taste buds. If you're using a cone-shaped filter, set it into a funnel and put that over a container large enough to hold your liquid. Pour the liquid into the filter. If it's taking its time about going through (it depends on what the liquid is), go do something else for a while, then pour in some more. If you're using a basket-type filter, follow the same procedure, but set it into a sieve over a jar or bowl. ◁

Picnic Tricks

7 Little-Known Ways to Eat Better and More Safely When You Pack Your Basket

Make your own soft drink, and let it cool your picnic. You'd never freeze a commercial soft drink, so all they do is give you one more thing to keep cold. But before there was Coke and Pepsi, there was lemonade. You can still make your own, using about three lemons for a quart (liter). Squeeze the lemons, which should give you about 1/2 cup juice. Mix that with 1/2 cup sugar (or to taste), and add three cups water. Voilà! The night before your picnic, freeze the lemonade in plastic milk cartons. Then use the cartons to help keep the food cool in the cooler. Drink the lemonade as it thaws.

Make potato salad with oil and vinegar. Just hold the mayo and eggs. There's no picnic food that gets more bad press than potato salad—and justifiably so, when it's made with eggs and mayonnaise, which can harbor bacteria that cause sickness. There are many delicious variations on potato salad that use oil and vinegar instead—but few cookbooks tell you that they're safe for picnics. Here's a very simple version: Boil potatoes until they're tender. Drain and dice them. Then dress them while still warm with olive oil, vinegar, salt, pepper, finely chopped onions, and/or garlic. You can eat it hot, cold, or warm.

Don't expect a cooler to keep ice cream frozen. Ads for coolers suggest they can keep just about anything cold. But don't count on one to keep frozen things from turning to goop within a few hours. "Coolers cool; they don't freeze," writes Tom Bartlett in an article in the online magazine *Slate* that ana-

lyzed the performance of six picnic coolers. However, Bartlett's top-rated cooler, the Coleman Ultimate Xtreme, priced at $49.99, kept a six-pack of beer surrounded by ice cool for four days. His favorite for the esthetics was another Coleman, the Steel Cooler. It costs twice as much, but it kept beer cool for three days and looks great. Hard coolers did a better job than soft-sided ones, but you may want a softie for other reasons. Bartlett liked the Polar Bear Soft Side Cooler, $49.95, for being easy to store and clean. He has a few cooler tips too. One: A full cooler stays cool longer than a half-full one. Pack it full in layers: ice on the bottom, then drinks, then more ice, and soft stuff such as sandwiches and potato salad on top.

SECRET WEAPON

A Checklist

Many a picnic has been less than perfect because some essential item was left behind. Make a checklist of foods and all the equipment that you need to transport and serve it. If you go on picnics often, put together a special picnic basket that contains all the basics. Leave it packed from picnic to picnic. Make sure to include such indispensables as a corkscrew, bottle opener, clips for closing bags of chips, bug repellent, adhesive strips, and antiseptic. Also pack several medium-size garbage bags for disposing of trash and recyclables when you get home.

Think finger foods ... Let's be honest: Managing forks, spoons, and knives on a picnic isn't much fun. You can make a terrific meal with foods that require only two fingers to eat! Start with the healthy nibbles: berries, cherry tomatoes, grapes, celery and carrot sticks, asparagus spears, olives, cheese cubes, crackers, and so on. Next, consult your favorite cookbook for appetizers like stuffed mushrooms, chicken fingers, or foccacia that can be eaten by hand. Need more substantial food? Sandwiches, ribs, fried chicken, and burgers all fall in the no-cutlery category. You'll be grateful come cleanup time!

... but bring lots of hand sanitizer. Bathrooms with warm water and good-quality soap are in short supply on picnics. So use the next best thing: waterless hand sanitizers. These cleaning gels kill germs instantly and dry nearly as fast. They're the perfect hand-cleaning solution, particularly if you are serving finger foods. Be sure to have a large bottle on hand.

Use lots of squirt bottles. You can buy squeezable, plastic squirt bottles for next to nothing at any restaurant supply store. Use them for mayonnaise, ketchup, mustard, barbecue sauce, salad dressings, oils, and any other condiment or cooking liquid. They are easy to pack and super clean to use. They're one of the best secret tools of professional chefs.

Keep desserts simple. For a hot summer day, there's nothing better than a slice of watermelon, a fresh-picked peach, or a bowl of cold strawberries for the perfect ending to an outdoor meal. Skip the fruit salad—and all its preparation, serving, and cleanup hassles. Or serve up your best brownies and cookies. Again, these are all finger foods that require no plates or cutlery—and that everyone will love. ◄

Restaurant Food
4 Ways to Protect Your Pocketbook and Health When You Go Out to Eat

Keep your coffee order simple. That pricey coffeehouse wants you to order your brew in as fancy a form as possible. Not only does this drive up the tab for each visit, but also stacks on hundreds of calories—from the whole milk, whipped cream, sugar and syrups. A regular cuppa joe made from good beans and with a dash of skim milk is heaven in itself, so protect your wallet and your arteries by keeping things simple.

Give gelato a try. Move over, Ben & Jerry. Gelato is an Italian ice cream that tastes great even though it isn't loaded with fat. (Gelato is 4 to 8 percent butterfat versus 10 to 18 percent for regular ice cream.) Nor is it all fluffed up with air. Cafés that specialize in gelato are popping up all over North America. Jan Horsfall, founder, president, and chief executive of Gelazzi, a gelato café in Denver, Colorado, makes his gelato fresh every day and says the quality of his extracts, cream, and eggs, makes his gelato rich and creamy. He travels to Italy several times a year to obtain the extracts. He also pairs his gelato with various liqueurs to make interesting gelato cocktails. If there is no gelato café near you and you want to try making your own, do a Web search for gelato and you'll find plenty of help.

Go when a restaurant has a downtime. Most restaurants go out of their way to attract customers at times when business is slow. Take advantage of them and you can eat for up to 25 percent less than when a restaurant is busy and the prices are at their highest. You can expect service to be much better too. Here are some examples:

- Any day of the year, early evening will usually produce "early bird specials" in restaurants.

- Lunchtime menus often offer the same dishes as in the evening for a sizeable discount. Or you can get a "businessman's special" in many restaurants.

- If you live in an area that draws tourists, the off-season forces many nearly deserted restaurants to offer specials to attract locals.

- Restaurants that have just opened often offer lower prices to attract customers, so keep an eye out for promising new restaurants.

When traveling, you can control food costs. Travel planners, local booster organizations, and food outlets of all kinds would like you to take all of your meals in restaurants when you're visiting. But you can extend your travel budget by having a few picnics instead. A trip to the local markets can furnish you with healthier and cheaper food, as well as an adventure in its own right. Buy fresh food, pack it in a sack you take for that purpose, and eat it at some lovely spot, even in the park in a city.

Also when traveling: When you do want to dine in a fine restaurant, if you eat your big meal at noon, you can do so more cheaply. ◁

Indulge in a Canadian Secret (If You Dare)

U.S. fast food has nothing on *poutine*, a Quebec concoction nicknamed "heart attack in a dish." Surprisingly, it's not at all well known outside Canada. It consists of a bed of French fries topped by thick gravy and cheese curds. It is more often eaten in restaurants than made at home, and as with any beloved dish, there are lots of opinions about how to make it.

The French fries must be large, not the skinny ones, because they support so much stuff on top. Some places have tried using cheese, not the curds, but the purists don't like that at all. And there are many versions of the gravy, as you'd expect: chicken, beef, vegetarian, and a gourmet version that calls for wine to be added to the pan drippings from roast duck and then reduced.

In Canada, *poutine* is available at restaurants throughout the country, but many authorities say the best still comes from Quebec, where it originated either in 1957 in Warwick or in 1964 in Drummondville. In Quebec, many fast-food restaurants (including the well-known American chains) offer poutine, but the purists say their versions aren't the real "mushy mess," or "pudding," as the name means in the French Acadian dialect.

part Two

AROUND THE HOUSE

That young man at the garden center is so outgoing and helpful you can't believe he's not being entirely up-front with you about how to control that infestation of aphids. It's not that he's lying; he's just not telling you about the 25-cent solution you already have at home. Contractors, decorators, repairmen, and the people who sell you appliances, clothing, and electronics all practice a similar code of silence. Well, we've managed to get a few of them to open up and let you in on their secrets. Learn about unnecessary fees and warranties, repairs so simple anyone can do them, low-cost decorating tricks, even how to get free computer security.

Decorator Secrets

3 Strategies Pros Use to Turn a Sow's Ear Room into a Silk Purse One

Learn to trick the eye with color. There's nothing quite like seeing before-and-after photos of a room transformed from dull to dazzling. The interior designers who achieve such magic are often considered intuitive and naturally creative—in fact, many do have a special knack. But most designers nurture that knack by going to school to learn hard-and-fast design rules. From these rules come their tricks of the trade. In other words, there is method to their magic. Which is where you, the homeowner, come in. You may not have been to decorator school, but you can benefit from a page out of a top designer's playbook. Follow her advice, and you might just work some magic of your own—without paying hundreds of dollars per hour in design fees.

- *Make your ceilings look taller.* Low ceilings got you down? Here's an optical illusion practiced by designers for artificially (and inexpensively) raising the roof: Add contrasting strips of fabric along the inner and outer edges of curtains. Say you've got beige curtains. Add chocolate brown fabric strips, and the ceiling will look taller.

- *Add "architectural" interest to a room.* Transform a plain-Jane room into something handsome and eye-catching with color. Paint the molding and the trim around windows and doors a shade or two darker than the walls, and paint the window sashes—the sliding parts that carry the glass—an even deeper shade. Guests will ask for the name of the designer you hired.

- *Draw the eye outside.* If you've got French doors—or another kind of glass doors—leading to an attractive yard, patio, or deck, paint them a deep, dark color to lead the eye to what's beyond.

Avoid the predictable seating arrangement. You know: sofa, a pair of matching chairs, coffee table in between. Snooze. The solution is elegantly simple. It's a trick designers call the "pull-up chair"—a nonmatching chair tossed into the mix to keep the arrangement looking fresh and unique.

Make the most of everyday items. Some of the top designers working today know that big bucks aren't a requirement for decorating creativity. In fact, having to stick to a tight budget often forces people to take chances they might not otherwise take with an expensive piece of furniture or fabric. Having to make do with everyday items can inspire some of the most attention-grabbing details in a home. Here are examples:

- *Recycle old sofa cushions.* If you're tossing an old couch, keep a couple of the pillows. Cover them in an attractive but durable outdoor fabric and use them as floor pillows for extra seating. The kids will love it, especially during Friday movie night.
- *Make a stylish porch swing.* Find an old garden bench at a flea market and cut off the legs. Attach chains or sturdy ropes and hang from hooks.
- *Customize off-the-shelf items.* Take a store-bought lampshade, for example. It's white, generic-looking, and—here's the good part—cheap. Glue a handsome red ribbon around the top and bottom edges, and you've got a personalized accessory. ◁

Clever Cover-Ups
6 Smart Ways to Transform a Room with Some Fabric or Wallpaper

Think of your sofa as your favorite shirt. In other words, cover it in a color you love to wear instead of in a neutral—what most people choose—that disappears in the room. If you choose your favorite color, one that looks best on you, the sofa will take center stage. And you'll never get tired of sitting on it.

Use bold fabric patterns in small doses. A little on a footstool or accent pillows will go a long way. It won't overwhelm, but it will still stand out. This is a good way to use an expensive fabric you love without having to break the bank buying several yards to cover an entire couch.

For large chairs, choose a small print. If you're covering a large chair, like a wingback, choose a small-print fabric. The chairs are dramatic enough. A small print helps balance that drama and looks more sophisticated.

Got kids? Choose a forgiving sofa fabric. Patterns help hide spills and crumbs. You probably know that by now. But did you also know that a fabric with a texture—a cotton velvet or some other textile with a pile—will do wonders for masking the mess? Try it. You'll worry less and enjoy more.

Dress up boring window shades. Those vanilla-colored roller shades are about as blah as it gets. But they're inexpensive, and they do their job. For a few dollars more, you can transform the shades—and an entire room in the process—by gluing a bold wallpaper print to the insides of the shades. This works best with shades 27 inches (68 cm) wide or less—the width of a standard wallpaper roll. Measure the length of the fully extended shade, and cut the wallpaper to fit, leaving an extra two inches. Roll out the shade and cover it with wallpaper adhesive using a sponge roller. Lay the wallpaper on the glue, letting the extra two inches wrap under the bottom of the shade. Use a rolling pin to smooth out air bubbles. Trim away any excess wallpaper. Because the wallpaper makes the shade a little harder to roll up and down, this trick works best on windows where you don't mind leaving the shade partially down.

Make a decorative bulletin board.

Large acoustic ceiling tiles—the kind of thing you see in office drop ceilings—make great, inexpensive bulletin boards. Go to your big-box home store. Look for the size tiles that appeal to you. Two-foot-square (61-cm-square) tiles cost about $20 for a box of four. Wrap them in the decorative fabric of your choice (leave a few inches of overlap and glue the edges to the back). You can tack these directly into your wall. Or paint a lightweight hollow-core door and attach the fabric-wrapped tiles to the door in a neat row. Lean the door against the wall, and voilà! You've got an inexpensive message board. ◂

Organizing Papers
4 Tricks for Keeping Papers and Photographs from Becoming an Insurmountable Problem

Categorize those papers. Office papers tend to pile up quickly on desktops, says Karen Lawrence, CEO of Space Matters, a home-organizing business in Richmond, Virginia. Not only do the desks become eyesores, but they result in lost documents and missed appointments. Here's a trick: Use stackable filers to sort papers on your desk into categories. Label them "Need action," "To be filed," "Read later," and "Outgoing mail."

Cast off old cards and crafts. Many people feel obliged to keep every greeting card they've ever received or every craft their child ever made. You'll enjoy these items more if you select a few and honor them by making a scrapbook, album, or wall decoration.

Weed out your photos. Instead of letting photos pile up and take over, take back your shelf space with a few simple steps. First, sort photos by person, event, or time frame (for example, "Family Beach Vacation" or "Wedding Weekend"). For each group, select the best 10 to 20 pictures, and place these pictures in an album or frame. Get rid of the rest, either throwing them away or spreading the memories by giving them away. There's no point in keeping 20 bad pictures when you have 10 good ones.

Organize and toss daily. Spend a few minutes every day picking up and organizing household paper clutter, especially newspapers and junk mail. Have special stacks or folders for bills, statements, and receipts. That way, things don't pile up and become unmanageable. ◂

Clutter Control

5 Secrets for Cutting Down on the All the Nonessentials Filling Up Your Home

Organize your home like a pro. Decluttering is big business these days. Professional home organizers know that busy people will shell out for peace of mind, which is why they charge fees of $200 to $900 per day. And while many of these professionals do good work, it's not rocket science. Home organizer Karen Lawrence offers these general tips for do-it-yourself organizing.

- Bear in mind that everything you buy is an investment of your time. Clothes must be laundered, dry-cleaned, and mended. Knicknacks have to be dusted. Toys need storing, cleaning, and fixing. As you buy items, mentally add this extra "cost" to the purchase price of the new item. You'll buy less and save money.

- Set small goals, such as decluttering one room a week or tackling one shelf or one drawer per day. If you try to organize your entire house in a weekend, you'll get so discouraged, you may quit altogether.

- Before decluttering, set aside bags and boxes labeled "Trash," "Donate," and "Belongs Elsewhere." This way, you break down a big pile of clutter into smaller, more manageable tasks.

- Sort like items together. You may be surprised that you have six black sleeveless dresses, four coolers, fifteen blue ties, or eight flashlights. Keep the best and get rid of the rest.

- Define important, clutter-producing activities, such as processing mail, paying bills, wrapping gifts, sewing or other crafts, or indoor gardening, and then create "centers" for doing these activities. Fill them with the necessary organizational tools and stay on top of the clutter. And make sure you have a wastebasket near each center.

EXPERT INSTANT ADVICE

Lazy Susan

Barry J. Izsak, founder of Arranging It All and president of the National Association of Professional Organizers, is a big fan of turntables. No, not those obsolete old record players. We're talking about storing items on a lazy Susan for easy access. "This is my favorite item for organizing kitchen cupboards and pantries," he says. There are tons of uses for them and they are very inexpensive (less than $5). Use them to organize your spices, containers, glassware, and canned goods.

Balance your closet. Clean out and organize your closet, getting it to a point that satisfies you. From now on, whenever you buy anything new—a winter coat, for example, or a pair of sandals—give away a like item, your old winter coat or your old sandals, for instance. Though your closet may need straightening every once in a while, it will remain at equilibrium, never again bursting at the seams.

Make regular donations to charity. Include furniture, clothes, and household items. Not only will you stay on top of clutter, but you'll be able to take a tax deduction for the things you donate. Keep empty boxes labeled "Donate" available. Make a run every month—or as needed—to your charity's drop-off center. Research specific charities in your area. Some groups collect old eyeglasses for children in underdeveloped countries, or barely worn interview suits for moms on public assistance.

Purge the fix-it pile. Fixing stuff is admirable. But hanging on to broken household items until you find the time to repair them burdens you mentally and clutters your garage or shop. Once a month, evaluate the items in your "someday" pile and either fix them, throw them away, or pay to have them repaired.

Have a yard sale. Whether you call it a yard, garage, or tag sale, it's a terrific way to dispose of a lot of discardable items that are cluttering up your house. Planning one is a good incentive to go through closets, cupboards, and storage boxes to gather material for the sale. ◁

Container Magic
5 Creative Ways to Use Baskets and Other Holders to Bring Order to Chaotic Items

Use the basket trick. Place a decorative basket or crate in or near the most cluttered room of your house. Place items that belong in other rooms in the basket. Anytime you exit the room, grab items out of the basket and return them to their rightful place.

Sort those loose items. Loose items, such as batteries, buttons, lightbulbs, and matches, often end up scattered in junk drawers and can't be found when you need them. Keep them at hand by labeling containers for these items.

Label laundry baskets. Save time by presorting laundry. Label bags or baskets: "Whites," "Colors," "Permanent Press," and "Dry Cleaning." You will always know when it is time to deal with a particular load, and you will never waste time separating laundry again, says home organizer Karen Lawrence.

Use paraphernalia baskets. Keep baskets or small bins on tables to store small frequently used items, such as remote controls, nail clippers, and notepads. Similarly, put a small dish on the bureau top to collect loose change and earrings, and an old mug on the desk to hold pens, pencils, and scissors. Surfaces will appear neater.

Make kid stuff reachable. Create kid storage units that are lightweight and low to the ground—rolling crates and small plastic dressers, for instance—so that children can help keep toys organized. Tape a photo or drawing of the items to the outside of each drawer or crate. ◁

How I Do It A Home Organizer's Container Secrets

A lot of what you'll hear from household organizers has to do with storage. And, indeed, proper storage is necessary for a clutter-free home. But some storage techniques are better than others. Here are dos and don'ts for storing things safely and more efficiently from Karen Lawrence:

☐ *Use cardboard for the short term.*
The basic cardboard box is ideal for moving and short-term storage. But cardboard boxes collapse under pressure when stacked. And since cardboard absorbs moisture, and moisture deteriorates cardboard, boxes aren't great for long-term storage, especially in humid attics, basements, and garages. Moist cardboard attracts insects, such as silverfish, that feed on paper. Weakened boxes allow easier access for rodents.

☐ *For long-term storage, plastic is best.*
When you use plastic containers, make sure stored items are dry before putting the lid on, because plastic can trap moisture *inside*, promoting mold and mildew growth. Also, if you are going to use plastic, use several small containers. People will often get huge plastic boxes, fill them up, and then not be able to move them.

☐ *Don't store clothes in dry-cleaning bags.*
This may seem like a good inexpensive solution for keeping clothes fresh and dust-free. But dry cleaning uses toxic chemicals, and the bags the clothes come in trap those chemicals. Also, mold and mildew can form on clothing sealed in plastic. Remove the bags before you hang the clothes in your closet—and certainly before you store clothes for the season. If you want to store them in something, use garment bags made from a breathable material like cotton.

☐ *Don't store precious photos in frames.*
If you choose to no longer display a framed photo, remove the photo from the frame and store it in an archival safe box, wrapped in acid-free tissue paper. The photo will take up much less space than the frame, which is now available for other photos. If you leave the photo in the frame, humidity will make the photo stick to the glass, and gas emissions from the materials used for framing—masking tape, cardboard, and rubber cement—may leave behind harmful residue, spotting the photo.

Housecleaning
9 Simple Secrets That Can Save You Time, Effort, and Money When Doing Housework

Use a certified germ killer. Use a cleaning product that carries the word "disinfectant" on its label when you're cleaning food-preparation areas in the kitchen such as the counters and sink. You may be impressed at how all-purpose cleaners remove visible grime, but what you're not seeing is the bacteria that are left behind, laughing at you. "Disinfectant" is a government-regulated term that means the product kills bacteria and viruses. So read the fine print of those squirt bottles.

Watch out for microfiber cleaning cloths. This isn't something the manufacturers of these little gems are going to tell you, but the authors of *The Complete Idiot's Guide to Cleaning*, Mary Findley and Linda Formichelli, will: Microfiber cloths are made out of plastic, and therefore they can scratch. Don't use them on sealed surfaces such as wood floors, marble, granite, Corian, and painted surfaces.

Clean your windows for pennies. Why should a gallon (3.7 liters) of glass cleaner, which is mostly water, cost you more than a gallon (3.7 liters) of gasoline? Because the manufacturers want you to pay for their fancy advertising campaigns. Here's how to whip up high-powered glass cleaner for pennies. Pour 1 gallon (3.7 liters) warm water into a bucket. Add 1 cup white vinegar and 1 teaspoon grease-cutting dishwashing liquid, and then stir. If you're cleaning a lot of large windows, apply the glass cleaner with a squeegee straight out of the bucket. Otherwise, pour the mixture into plastic squirt bottles and label them.

Dirty disposer? Dive in. Well, not literally. The point is to do it yourself rather than call a plumber or handyman. And don't pay for expensive foaming disposer cleaners. Disposers are easy to clean, since they provide the muscle. First, keep food waste from building up inside the disposer by only grinding small amounts of food at a time. And when you're done, run a steady flow of cold water through the spinning disposer for up to 30 seconds. Cold solidifies fatty and greasy wastes so they will be cut up and flushed down the drain. Hot melts them and smears the grease around the disposer and drainpipe.

To remove grease buildup, periodically grind a handful of ice cubes mixed with 1/2 cup baking soda. Together the powder and cubes (once again cold) will safely scour the inside of the disposer. Flush any residue by plugging the sink and filling it with 2 to 3 inches (5 to 8 cm) of water. Then run the disposer while the water drains. Grind lemon peels to freshen the smell.

Give your sink a bath. One of the most frustrating things about porcelain sinks is that they scuff if you so much as look at them the wrong way. Forget the Ajax. Instead, Linda Mason Hunter, coauthor of the book *Green Clean*, recommends an herbal bath. Steep several bunches of rosemary or thyme in hot water for a few hours, then strain. Stop up the sink, pour in the mixture, and let it sit overnight. In the morning you'll find a glistening white sink that smells like an herb garden.

Fizz your toilet clean. It's a shame you have to find room in your bathroom cabinet for a product like toilet cleaner that can do only one job around the house. Most toilet cleaners are a frighteningly caustic product, to boot. Here's the simpler path: Once a week, drop two denture tablets into your toilet and let them dissolve for at least 20 minutes. Then give your toilet's interior a quick brushing and flush. The same cleaning action that brightens dentures will leave the toilet bowl gleaming as well.

Clean your grill grate in the oven. Put away that time-consuming wire grill brush and leave that caustic oven cleaner in the cabinet. Here's the zero-effort, nontoxic way to clean the mess off your barbecue grill's grate. Simply remove it from the grill, pull the racks out of your oven, slide the grate into your oven, and set the oven on "self-clean." This same superheated cycle that incinerates everything inside a self-cleaning oven will scorch away any greasy remnants from the grate.

Clean your own curtains. Dirty drapes send some homeowners straight to the yellow pages. Too technical, they think. Then they find out that most professional drapery cleaners charge *by the pleat* to steam- or dry-clean curtains. At $10 per pleat or more, cleaning costs can add up fast. Here are some tricks for cleaning curtains yourself:

- Dust them regularly. Don't bother taking them down. Simply run your vacuum cleaner over them (from top to bottom) using the dusting brush or upholstery attachment. Focus on the tops and hems, where dust tends to gather. Avoid sucking the fabric into the nozzle by either reducing the vacuum pressure or grasping the bottom and holding the curtains tight. If you don't have the proper attachments, use a feather duster. Dusting drapes prevents dirt buildup and lessens the chances that the drapes will need a major cleaning.

- Wash the ones that can be washed. If your drapes do need cleaning, start by looking for the manufacturer's cleaning recommendations, which should be on a tag sewn inside the hem. No tag? Identify the fabric, including all trim and linings, and use that information to choose the best cleaning method. You will either machine-wash, hand-wash, or dry-clean your drapes. The delicate cycle is usually best for curtains that can be machine-washed. You never know how much the sun has weakened the curtain fibers. The same goes for the dryer—use the delicate cycle. And instead of tumbling curtains until they are dry (which could leave them in a wrinkled ball), remove them from the dryer and hang them damp. If you're lucky, you'll avoid having to iron them.

- Find an experienced dry cleaner. Few dry cleaners know how to properly handle drapes, but you won't see them advertising that fact. It's up to you to ask around. The best will measure your curtains beforehand and guarantee they will come back the same length.

Buying drapes? Check the tag. You may love those fancy silk or velvet curtains. They might even be on sale. But before you buy them, keep in mind the cost to clean them. Check the manufacturer's tag, inside the hem, for curtains that are machine washable, and you'll save big bucks in the long run. ◁

16

SCARY CHEMICALS THAT *sneak* Into Your Home

Companies using toxic chemicals in their cleaning products, building materials, and pesticides tend to focus on the benefits of their products, but they don't say much about the negative side effects. Air fresheners give off naphthalene, a suspected carcinogen. Ammonia-based window cleaners cause respiratory irritation. And some cleaners contain the nerve-damaging butyl cellosolve (also known as ethylene glycol monobutyl ether), which is absorbed into the skin. These are just a few examples of the harmful chemicals that sneak into our homes. Things are so bad, says Katie Albright of the Sierra Club of Canada, that "air quality studies show that the inside of homes is often worse than the outside." The icing on the cake? The chemical companies charge you a premium for the poisons hiding behind popular brand names.

Bad Guys

So what can be done? First, familiarize yourself with the chemical culprits, scan ingredient labels on all household products, and avoid these substances whenever possible:

butyl cellosolve

cresol

formaldehyde

glycols

hydrochloric acid

hydrofluoric acid

lye

naphthalene

PDCBs (paradichlorobenzenes)

perchloroethylene

phenol

propellants

TCE (trichloroethylene)

petroleum distillates

phosphoric acid

sulfuric acid

Good Guys

Next, keep healthy alternatives around the house. Not only will you reduce indoor pollution, but you'll save money while doing your body a favor. Here's the all-star team of effective chemical alternatives:

Baking soda. Effective mineral with mildly abrasive cleaning, whitening, and deodorizing properties. Very inexpensive. Great for carpet pet odors (page 116).

Vinegar. Derived from the fermentation of fruits or grains, vinegar has a high acid content that makes it great at killing germs, cutting grease, and dissolving mineral deposits.

Borax. A naturally occurring mineral (containing water, oxygen, sodium, and boron) with tremendously useful antiseptic, antifungal, deodorizing, and disinfectant properties. It stops the growth of mold and mildew and kills roaches (page 114).

Vegetable oil-based liquid soap. This biodegradable alternative to petroleum-based detergents can be found in health food stores.

Washing soda. Sometimes called soda ash, this mineral (sodium carbonate) cleans grease, oil, dirt, and lots of petroleum products. It is also a water softener and soap booster. Look for it in the supermarket laundry section.

Essential oils. The boiled-down essences of different plants—peppermint, lavender, and lemons, for instance—these oils can be used as natural air fresheners and to add pleasant scents to homemade cleaners. You can find some in the baking section of the grocery store.

Cleaning Valuables

4 Ways to Save a King's Ransom When Cleaning Jewelry and Other Expensive Items

Clean gold with dishwashing liquid. Jewelers are like car dealers. They sell you necklaces, bracelets, and rings and hope you bring your pieces back for service, including cleaning. But while resetting a loose diamond is beyond the skill level of the average ring owner, periodic cleaning is not. Here's how to clean that most common of jewelry items—gold. It may not tarnish like silver, but over time gold develops a dull film from lotions, soaps, and the oils secreted by your skin. To revive the luster of gold jewelry, clean it regularly in a bowl of warm water mixed with a squirt of mild dishwashing liquid. After a brief soak, gently scrub the gold jewelry using a soft toothbrush. Rinse under warm running water (careful of the drain—to be safe, put it in a wire tea strainer). Pat dry with a clean white cloth. For stubborn stains, mix equal parts cold water and ammonia. Soak the gold jewelry in the solution for half an hour. Scrub with a soft toothbrush. Rinse under cold water. Pat dry. Whatever you do, don't clean with toothpaste, which contains silica, an abrasive found in quartz, which can dull a glossy gold finish.

Wipe pearls often to keep them clean. A pearl's value is largely determined by color, luster, and the thickness of its fine coating, or nacre. Because pearls are highly sensitive to chemicals and salts, it's important that you wipe down your pearls after you wear them, using a slightly moistened, very soft cloth such as chamois. This removes harmful substances such as perspiration, perfume, and makeup that can penetrate the pearls' porous surface.

(As a preventive measure, always apply perfume, makeup, and hair spray *before* you put on your pearls.) To occasionally clean more thoroughly, use a mild bar soap such as Ivory and lukewarm water to create light suds. Dip your cloth in the suds and gently wipe the pearls. Rinse with clean water and dry on a soft cloth. Never soak pearls. And never hang them to dry, since that might stretch the string. Remove stubborn solids from their surface using your fingernail. Since your fingernail has a hardness of 2.5 or less on the Mohs' scale, and pearls register from 2.5 to 4.5, you probably will not scratch them.

Precautions with Gold and Silver

☐ Avoid getting chlorine on your gold or silver jewelry at any cost. Both of these precious metals react to this common chemical and will deteriorate over time if exposed to it. Remove your gold or silver rings and bracelets when cleaning with chlorine bleach. And take them off before jumping into the pool or climbing into the hot tub.

☐ Although some jewelers recommend cleaning gold or silver jewelry with toothpaste, it's best not to. Some toothpastes contain harsh abrasives that can dull the metal's finish or scratch a stone.

☐ Don't soak jewelry with precious stones for more than a few seconds. The water can dissolve the glue that holds the stones in place.

☐ Silver reacts to salt, to acid foods like mustard and ketchup, and to sulfur-containing foods like eggs and mayonnaise. Don't use a silver serving piece with any of these foods and clean it right away if it touches them.

Skip the polish when cleaning silver. It's toxic and it smells bad. Instead, Mary Findley and Linda Formichelli recommend this low-tech cleaning approach: Put a sheet of aluminum foil in a plastic or glass bowl and sprinkle with salt and baking soda. Fill the bowl with warm water and add the silver. The tarnish actually migrates to the foil, leaving your silver clean. Dry and buff.

Swish away unreachable grunge. Okay, so you probably won't toss your grandmother's grungy old crystal decanter, but you may banish it to the top shelf, where it's as good as gone. Same with that dirty, narrow-necked coffee carafe. Before you go shopping for new pieces to display in your home, try swishing a mixture of rock salt and vinegar around the inside of these containers. The salt will gently scour the surface while the vinegar will help remove stains, especially lime deposits. For wine stains, try swirling a small amount of warm water, baking soda, and rock salt. Or dissolve a denture-cleaning tablet in the vessel and let it stand overnight. The next morning, rinse with clean warm water.

Cleaning these narrow-necked objects is one thing, but drying them is another challenge. Instead of waiting forever for the thermos, vase, or decanter to dry in your dish rack, drain the water and use the following trick to remove the last of the moisture: Wrap a paper towel around the handle of a wooden spoon so that the towel extends slightly beyond the end. Stick the towel-wrapped spoon into the decanter and let it rest on the bottom overnight. By morning the towel should have absorbed most of the condensation. ◄

Insect Pests
3 Ways to Get Rid of Annoying Bugs in Your House Without Expensive Toxic Pesticides

Shoo away flies with basil. How's this for a great way to get rid of flies *and* guarantee your family fresh pesto throughout the years? Put several basil plants around your kitchen. Flies hate basil, so they'll stay away. Not only will your kitchen be flyless, but it will smell like summer all year long.

Turn away ants with vinegar. Instead of spending big bucks on some toxic insecticide, keep ants away from your household surfaces with vinegar. Fill a clean spray bottle with a 50/50 solution of water and white vinegar. Spray anywhere you see ants infiltrating—along baseboards, on kitchen counters, in moist bathrooms. Unlike poisons, the vinegar is 100 percent harmless, and a quart costs pocket change.

Stop roaches with boric acid. Don't pay upward of 20 bucks for a one-pound (500-gram) can of roach powder at your hardware store, when you can buy the same thing—boric acid—for a fraction of the price. A white powder used as a laundry whitener and disinfectant, borax is also lethal to roaches. You can make your own roach-control powder by mixing equal parts borax and flour, and then sprinkling the mixture where you've seen roaches—along the base of basement walls, in jar lids placed in cabinets (even though it is relatively safe to use around the house, do not place the borax where children or pets can get into it). The starch in the flour attracts the roaches. The mixture sticks to their legs. They track it back to their nests, where it kills them and other roaches. ◄

Personal Care Items
3 Tricks to Keep Hair-Care and Grooming Gear Working Smoothly

Take it easy with curler cleaning.
If you use harsh cleaners on your hair curlers, you risk having those damaging chemicals transfer to your hair. Instead, make your motto "Hair today and hair tomorrow," using this money-saving cleaning technique. For curlers that are submersible in water—plain rollers, Velcro rollers, foam-coated wire sticks—fill your bathroom sink with warm water, mix in a couple teaspoons of your own shampoo or facial cleanser to create suds, and let them soak. (If it's gentle enough for you, it's gentle enough for your curlers.) Gently comb out any hair stuck in the curlers. Then wipe with a rag to remove caked-on films. Rinse and either dry with a clean towel or air-dry.

For stubborn stains, such as hardened setting lotions or gels, mix up a solution of 1/4 cup warm water and 1 tablespoon liquid fabric softener. Gently scrub the solution in with a vegetable brush. Rinse and dry.

For nonsubmersible electric curlers, clean with a rag or brush and the fabric softener solution. Rinse by wiping the curlers with a damp rag, and then dry.

Brush up on hairbrush cleaning.
The first trick with maintaining brushes is to remove the hair often, instead of waiting until it is thickly matted. Every so often, wash them in an economical and effective cleaning solution—2 teaspoons shampoo with 1/4 cup vinegar in a sinkful of warm water. Remove any loose hair, soak the brush for several minutes, and use a wide-toothed comb to remove the remaining hair stuck in the brush (pulling it through each row of tines on the brush). The solution will loosen any built-up oil and dirt, as well as gunked-on hair gels and sprays. Scrub the brush clean using a nailbrush. Rinse with warm, running water. Let the brush air-dry.

Soak razors in mineral oil. Razor manufacturers want you change razors as often as you change shirts, of course, but a simple trick will prolong your razor's life. Pour some mineral oil into a shallow dish and soak it for a few minutes. The mineral oil will halt the corrosion that dulls the cutting edge. When the soaking time is up, dip the corner of a cloth in rubbing alcohol and wipe off the oil. ◁

Controlling Odors

5 Low-Cost Ways to Prevent and Remove Offensive Smells Around the House

Dust away that carpet funk. There's nothing worse than odors trapped in the fibers of a rug or carpet—especially when they're from pet accidents. You may think a professional rug cleaner is the only solution. Think again. Sprinkle baking soda on the odor-causing stain. Let it sit all night, and then vacuum it up the next day. Repeat until the odor is gone.

Skip fancy brand-name fresheners. Chemists are out there in corporate labs right now cooking up the next air freshener scent, while marketers are busy concocting all the selling points to get you to part with your money to have it. But air fresheners don't really freshen the air. They mask smells, and experts say they can actually irritate the lungs. Instead, look for products that actually kill the bacteria that cause odors. Or try the money-saving tricks described below.

Control cooking odors with vinegar. Boil 1/4 cup vinegar per 1 quart (1 liter) water. The rising heat carries the odor-neutralizing vinegar particles to the same surfaces where the smoke and grease landed.

Bleach a foul-smelling garbage can. Scrub the inside with a nylon-bristled brush and this solution: 1 cup bleach, 1 gallon (3.7 liters) water, plus two squirts of dishwashing liquid. Rinse with the garden hose. Air-dry, and sprinkle inexpensive borax in the bottom of the can once it's dry to prevent the growth of odor-causing molds and bacteria.

Use onion and air for a musty basement. In the short term, cut an onion in half and leave it on a plate in your basement. The onion absorbs musty odors. To solve the problem, start by ventilating. Since the musty smell comes from mold and mildew, which thrive in dank, dark environments, you want to get the stale air moving. Open windows and doors, use fans to circulate air, and use dehumidifiers to remove the air's humidity. Next, don protective eyewear and a dust mask, and kill the odor-producing growth with a solution of 2 to 4 tablespoons bleach per 1 quart (1 liter) water. Using a spray bottle, spray any surfaces that won't be harmed by the bleach, such as cinder-block walls and concrete floors. Scrub with a nylon-bristled brush. ◁

SECRET WEAPON

Activated Charcoal

We all know that an open box of baking soda will keep refrigerator odors at bay. But what do you do if you are faced with a strong, persistent, and unpleasant odor in your fridge or freezer? Just head off to the nearest pet store or five-and-ten and buy some fine activated charcoal in the aquarium supplies section. Spread some in a shallow pan and put the pan on a refrigerator or freezer shelf. The charcoal will not harm your food. After about eight hours, put the charcoal in a 350°F (175°C) oven for 20 minutes to reactivate it. By reactivating the charcoal, you can reuse it many times. In a pinch, you can also use cat litter or fresh (unused) ground coffee to absorb fridge odors.

Tools and Supplies

8 Savvy Tips for Using Tools to Best Advantage and Making Them Last a Lifetime

Get the right tool for the job. Charles Cox, a Pennsylvania-based stationary engineer (boiler operator) and freelance handyman, thinks he knows why homeowners shy away from doing their own household repairs. "They either don't know what tool they need or they don't want to buy it," he says. "So they rely on professionals." His example: a leaky faucet. A homeowner fails to free the old, corroded handle from its stem and gives up, calling a plumber and paying more than $100 for the house call. A quick trip to a hardware store, however, and the homeowner could have bought a tool known as a faucet-handle puller for less than $10. This simple screw tool forcefully lifts the frozen handle without scratching its finish. Then, with old parts in hand, the homeowner could have found the right replacement parts at the hardware store. A 25-cent washer might possibly have done the trick. The point? Trust the right tool to save you money.

Spring for a decent set of screwdrivers. Some things are great to keep around generation after generation. An old jackknife. Your grandfather's workbench. Slotted screwdrivers aren't one of them. After prolonged use, flat-head screwdrivers tend to wear down. Their blades grow thin and rounded at the corners. Pretty soon, you're stripping screws and ruining woodwork with slips and gaffs. If they have sentimental value, keep them around for prying open cans of paint. But do yourself a favor and buy a set of new, high-quality screwdrivers—or a screwdriver with interchangeable heads. And if it's too late, and you're stuck trying to remove one of those stripped screws, run a hacksaw blade through the screw slot to make it straighter and deeper.

Save paint longer. Too often, homeowners leave leftover paint in its original can. Labels fall off, cans rust, air leaks in, and the paint goes bad. Instead, store paint in glass jars. Not only can you instantly tell the color of the paint inside, but jars are more airtight than cans. To further tighten the seal—and make sure the lid doesn't stick—wrap a couple of layers of Teflon tape around the jar threads before sealing them.

Clean paintbrushes better—and less often. How many times have you gotten lazy and thrown away a perfectly good paintbrush because you didn't want to face the mess of cleaning it? If you're painting with oil and will be again the next day, you don't have to clean it. Just remove the excess paint from your brushes and rollers and then wrap them tightly in aluminum foil or plastic wrap. This will keep them from drying out. If you're using a water-based paint, and your brush or roller just won't come clean, don't toss it. Many of today's water-based paints contain resins similar to those used in oil-based paints to improve adhesion, gloss, and durability. After cleaning and rinsing the brush or roller in water, try a second rinse in paint thinner or turpentine to completely clean it. Afterward, wash with clean, soapy water to remove the thinner.

Find studs for less. Wall studs, of course. Instead of some expensive stud-finding gadget that may or may not

How I Do It A Handyman Keeps Tools to an Easy-to-Carry Minimum

Some people can fix anything. You may or may not be one of them. But if you follow fix-it pros around, you'll quickly learn that efficiency is one of their key traits. They don't waste their energy—and they don't lug around more tools and equipment than they need. Most can get by on a small, broadly useful selection. Handyman Charles Cox is a case in point. He does many of his jobs with five basic tools. Keep these five tools in a plastic tool tray, and you'll be prepared to tackle most minor repairs.

Channel lock pliers

An adjustable wrench that will give you a firm grip on anything from a pipe to a loose nut. Put a little duct tape on the teeth to keep it from scarring metal.

Interchangeable screwdriver

Different sizes and types of heads fit into the end, making this easier to keep up with than a handful of different screwdrivers. It's great for here-and-there jobs (but grab the cordless driver and let the batteries do the work for everything else).

Adjustable wrench

Why try to keep up with a tumbling mess of wrenches, when one adjustable wrench fits all?

16-ounce (500-gram) claw hammer

From tacking up picture hangers to pulling rusty nails from old salvaged wood, the claw hammer is an absolute must.

Continuity tester

The electrician's basic diagnostic tool, a continuity tester is a battery-powered device with a lightbulb, a probe, and an alligator clip. With the power off, you can use this tool to detect shorts in sockets, electrical appliances, and extension cords. If you can do light electrical work, such as replacing a faulty switch, you'll save a bundle. With a little practice, adequate safety precautions, and a continuity tester, you can do it.

work, turn your electric razor on and run it along the wall. You'll hear a change in the vibration as you cross a stud with it.

Don't get stuck on duct tape. Ready for some shocking news? Duct tape is not perfect. Although the manufacturers of duct tape would like you to believe this silvery cloth tape can fix any problem (even remove warts!), the truth behind the hype is that it's not all it's cut out to be. Oh, it's fine in a pinch, but duct tape is almost always a temporary solution. Even the pros who work on heating and air-conditioning systems will tell you it's not the best way to attach ducts. It deteriorates and turns to powder over time. And that's on metal, the surface best suited for duct tape.

When used on glass and plastic, duct tape can peel away within months, especially when exposed to sunlight. Duct tape does not stick well on wood either, and it can destroy fine wood finishes, leaving behind a gummy, hard-to-remove residue. And duct tape should never be used on live wires as a substitute for black electrical tape.

Clean your belt sander. Belts always seem to gum up prematurely, before the sanding surface is worn down. And replacement belts can cost four or five bucks each. Instead of tossing them when they gum up, try this trick: Secure the sander upside down (clamp it or have someone hold it) and press the rubber sole of your shoe to the belt. It will come clean, allowing you to use it much longer. Sales reps will wonder why their sanding belts are gathering dust on the hardware store shelf.

Keep your tools from getting rusty. Moisture in the air invites rust, and if the moist air gets into your toolbox or tool drawer, it corrodes the tools. And if you are like most of us, you store your tools in an often damp garage or basement. One good way to keep the air in your toolbox dry is to drop in some packets of silica gel, sold at hardware stores and craft shops. You can often get them for free in the packing of new products. Once the silica gel becomes saturated, renew the packets by placing them near a lit 60-watt lightbulb for 15 minutes. Another effective moisture absorber that will keep the contents of your toolbox rust-free is a handful of mothballs. You can also use a 1-ounce (30-gram) cube of camphor, sold at local pharmacies. Because camphor loses its effectiveness after about six months, you'll have to replace the cube twice a year. ◀

Hiring Help
4 Tricks for Getting the Best Job for the Money That You Shell Out to Repair People

Hire a qualified electrician. A handyman can be a real help when it comes to tackling small jobs you don't have time to complete, or skilled jobs you just don't feel comfortable attempting. You may even be tempted to give your handyman small wiring jobs or other electrical work. Before you do, however, make sure he is licensed to do electrical work (if local code requires it) and that his work is up to snuff. "You get the wrong guy messing around with your electrical wiring—someone who doesn't know what he's doing—and you're in trouble," says Jim Abbott, owner of Handyman Matters in Toronto, Ontario. The mistakes, which can be dangerous, are hidden behind Sheetrock walls or within electrical panels. Look for red flags, such as light switches and outlets in strange places. "I've seen it," Abbott says. "A guy runs out of wire and puts a switch at eye level or an outlet halfway up the wall."

Ask your handyman for a guarantee. "A lot of handymen give their customers the tailgate warranty," says Jim Abbott. "They drive away in their pickup truck with your cash in pocket, and all you see is their tailgate disappearing. That's it. That's your warranty." Instead, ask them if they'll guarantee their work for up to a year. If they will, get it in writing. If they won't, take their reluctance as a red flag.

Choose your plumber, then your fixtures. If your plumber is charging you by the hour to install new bathroom or kitchen fixtures, here's a sure way to save money. Ask him what brand he likes best. Chances are this will be a common, dependable brand that he's very familiar with. Choose models made by this brand, and he'll install them more efficiently, saving time and money by not having to struggle through detailed instructions about what washers go where and what size wrench he needs to tighten everything. Also, he's more likely to install products correctly if he's already done it countless times before, and that will save you repair costs in the long run.

Shorten that repair visit. Any repairperson who is paid by the hour will happily lounge around your house chatting up a storm or watching you get organized. The clock is ticking, after all, and that kind of work is oh-so-easy. With a little forethought, however, you can make sure that every minute of a repairperson's visit is nose-to-the-grindstone productive.

- Discuss all of the details of the job over the telephone—while the clock *isn't* ticking. This also ensures that the worker will arrive with all of the necessary tools and materials.

- Clear away any obstructions in advance of the repairperson's arrival, and make sure there's proper light for the worker to see by.

- Check the house over for all tasks that this particular repairperson could handle—thus saving you service charges in the future.

- Tell the worker not to bother cleaning up. Cleanup is never done to your specifications anyway, is it? The worker will be out your door in a minimum of time—and your bill will be the minimum as well. ◂|

How-To Secrets
4 Little-Known Tricks That Make for a Successful Do-It-Yourself Job

Quiet that slamming screen door. Forget trying to track down a professional handyman, and then paying big bucks for him to drive out and fix your noisy screen door. Here's the easy way to achieve silence of the slams: Apply a few small beads of clear silicone caulk along the jamb in a few places where the door hits. Prop the door open for a few hours to make sure the silicone dries before you close it again.

Keep pictures straight. There's no telling what an interior decorator would charge you to solve the annoying and recurring problem of pictures that won't stay level. Follow this nifty trick and you won't have to find out. Push straight pins into the backside of the frame, one at each bottom corner, and then clip off the heads, leaving about a quarter inch sticking out of the frame. Hang the picture. Straighten it with a level. Gently push the bottom corners so that the pins prick the drywall, securing the frame in place.

Be your own plumber with plastic pipes. You might find it less daunting to do your own plumbing work if you use PVC pipes instead of copper pipes. PVC is cheaper, and there are no torches and soldering involved. All you need are the plastic pipes and glue. Here are a couple of trade secrets for working with PVC:

- Before cutting, measure the length you want, mark it with a pencil, and then wrap tape around the pipe. Using a pencil, follow the edge of the

A Guide to Money-Saving
Easy-to-Do Repairs

Avoid paying an electrician $100 for two drops of oil to quiet a rattling fan.

As the owner of Handyman Matters, Jim Abbott has fielded his share of homeowner calls. After a while, he says, you start to see patterns—recurring problems that homeowners could avoid *if they only knew better.* Maybe after reading Abbott's advice, you will know better the next time ...

... your bathroom fan starts rattling.

Sure, that rattle is annoying, but even more troublesome is the thought of paying an electrician to come to your house and fix it. Fear not. According to Abbott, many exhaust fans are a snap to repair, a fact that escapes most homeowners, who don't want anything to do with a hardwired electrical fixture. But instead of being hardwired into your ceiling or wall, many fans simply plug into a *box* that's hardwired. That means that if you can stand on a ladder, pop off the fan cover and remove a few screws, you can safely remove the fan. (Be sure to cut power to the fan by flipping the circuit breaker switch before you begin work.) Once you've removed the fan, put a couple drops of oil on the fan shaft. Chances are that will stop the rattling. And you will have avoided paying an electrician 100 bucks for two drops of oil. If not, then take the fan to an electrical supply retailer or home-improvement store and buy a replacement fan that plugs into the same housing. You'll still save money.

... you feel a draft.

Another common caulk-related problem has to do with air leaks. "The way a lot of houses are built these days, you'll have a 2 x 4 wall with a brick veneer on the outside," he explains. "People will caulk around the outside of their windows, which seals the windows to the brick. But the brick is outside the vapor barrier. Brick veneer is designed to breathe. It's even got weep holes to let moisture escape. So caulking the windows to the brick does not tighten up the house." Instead, to stop drafts, caulk gaps around the *inside* of your window frames.

... your kitchen or bathroom caulk goes bad.

Abbott sees it all the time. The silicone caulk around a kitchen sink begins to deteriorate. Water seeps into the fiberboard or plywood beneath the countertop laminate and the counter starts to swell and rot. "The next thing you know, you have to replace the whole countertop." Same goes for the bathroom. If the caulking around the tub or shower fails, water can ruin drywall and, over time, cause dry rot in wood floors and framing. The solution is to prevent expensive damage with a little inexpensive maintenance. Remove the old caulk, clean and completely dry the area, and apply new caulk. "Even if you're not comfortable working with silicone caulk," says Abbot, "paying someone $100 to do the job could save you thousands in the long run."

tape around. Remove the tape, and you're left with your cutting mark.

- Avoid gluing fittings backward. Once the glue dries, the pieces are stuck, and mistakes become do-overs. Try this trick to make everything come out right. After cutting your sections, dry-fit them in place, making sure the fittings face the right way and lengths are correct. When everything looks right, make a mark across both pipe and fitting with a thick colored wax pencil. When you take them apart to apply the glue, you'll be able to line up the pencil marks again quickly and easily for a perfect fit.

Your drill doesn't need fancy attachments.
The electric drill is by far the most popular power tool in our homes, and manufacturers sell all kinds of add-ons to help you drill holes that are straighter and of proper depth. Here are three tricks that eliminate the need for these extras:

- To drill a hole to a precise depth, you don't need a special collar to stop the bit. Just mark the depth on the bit with a piece of masking tape.

- To drill a vertically straight hole, you don't need a frame that holds the drill perfectly upright. Just nail two short scraps of wood together at right angles to use as a guide. Just be sure the scraps have square factory-cut edges.

- To drill a horizontally straight hole, again you don't need a frame. Just slip a washer on the bit before you put in the drill chuck. The washer will slide forward or backward if you are not drilling straight. ◁

Bath and Kitchen Improvements
6 Pitfalls to Avoid When You Are Upgrading Your Plumbing and Ceramic Tiles

Check your toilet trap.
Some toilet makers cut corners to lower costs. Sometimes they cut curves as well—trap curves. When buying a toilet, make sure the trap (the S-shaped tube underneath the toilet that the water goes down when you flush) is fully glazed. Like the outside of the toilet, the inside of the trap should be shiny and smooth. Otherwise, toilet paper will get caught on the sides of the tube and clog your toilet. Very inexpensive toilets may seem like a bargain—how different could toilets be, after all?—but the unglazed traps will prove that all toilets weren't created equal.

Look for a lifetime faucet warranty.
Some manufacturers brag that their kitchen and bath faucets come with lifetime warranties. But it's up to you to read the fine print. Look all the way at the bottom of the page for those tiny asterisked footnotes. There you may find that certain aspects of a faucet—the finish or valves—are covered for only one to five years, not for life. And since valves can total 25 percent of the cost of a faucet, you want to make sure the valves are also covered for life.

Don't fall for a cheap faucet.
Hidden beneath the gleaming exterior of kitchen and bath faucets is the truth about how they were made. Cheaper faucets are metal shells covering copper tubes. More expensive faucets are cast brass, which means the brass has been poured into a mold and the faucet is all one piece.

Buying one of the more expensive faucets may save you money in the long run. Eventually water will poke tiny holes in the copper tubes of the cheaper faucets. This can occur very quickly if the water is acidic (lots of chlorine), leading to the need for a new faucet in as few as three years. The cast brass will last much longer. Next time you march down the plumbing fixture aisle, go armed with this insider info, and you'll be better prepared to make a wise purchase.

Check that brass finish. Brass fixtures can make a beautiful addition to your bathroom or kitchen, but looks can be deceiving. Some brass is coated with a lacquer finish that regular cleaning with bathroom chemicals will remove, leaving you with a tarnished brass showerhead. Make sure the product description of the brass fixture mentions PVD (physical vapor disposition). Brass finished using this process means that the coating will not come off and your brass will not tarnish. PVD is a must for exterior door hardware, which is often exposed to corrosive salt air near the coast and acid rain. PVD-finished brass may cost a bit more, but it will maintain its bright good looks a lot longer.

Save money by using porcelain tiles sparingly. Some contractors and tile store sales reps like to push porcelain tile, touting the fact that its through-and-through color consistency means that chips hardly show up. Ceramic tile, on the other hand, features a surface color and a differently colored inner core (usually terra cotta). If it chips, they'll say, the inner color stands out. Of course,

they'll downplay the fact that porcelain tile costs more and that they earn more when they sell it. The benefits of porcelain tile are real, but sometimes unnecessary. Before you buy, think about how much foot traffic a room will get. Hall bathrooms, where guests will be wearing heels and boots, might need porcelain. Bedroom bathrooms, where people walk around with slippers on, might be fine with ceramic.

Test a tile pattern with photocopies. Having trouble visualizing how those fancy tiles will look when installed as a backsplash for your kitchen counter? Or you need to figure out which pattern will work best? You don't want to be disappointed when those decorative tiles that looked so great in the showroom turn out to be just the wrong thing for your kitchen, or to discover that the pattern you envisioned just won't work. To avoid either of these, make color photocopies of the tiles and tape them to the wall. You can rearrange them until you get the right look. ◁

CHOOSING THE *right* Mattress

Mattress sales mean big bucks for retailers. The bedding department for furniture stores is typically one of the highest profit-margin areas. But few high-value consumer products defy quality rankings more than mattresses. One reason is that so much of what makes a mattress comfortable—size, coil type, firmness level—depends on the preferences of the individual. Comparing one model to another just doesn't work. Another reason has to do with the way the industry operates. Bedding manufacturers don't have consistent model names. Store A may sell one manufacturer's top-of-the-line model in a blue damask cover and call it "Joyful," while store B may have the same model covered in green and call it the "Mayflower," while store C may cover that mattress in white satiny ticking and call it the "Crescent."

There are objective criteria, such as material and construction quality, says Missouri author and veteran furniture retailer Michael Fugate. Here's his advice on the four basic types of mattress coil systems:

The Bonnel coil system	The continuous-wire system	Individually wrapped coils	Offset coils
A system of hourglass-shaped coils tied together by thinner spiraling wire. The maximum number of coils in this system, often found in lower-priced name-brand mattresses, is 364 in a full-size mattress.	As the name suggests, this is made from a single wire, often more than 200 yards (180 meters) long. These are most commonly found in Serta mattresses. While the continuous coil tends to be strongest, it does not necessarily offer the most support.	Sometimes known as Marshall or pocketed coils, these are encased in fabric. These are found in Simmons and Sealy mattresses. One advantage: Because they're not connected, one sleeper's movements don't affect another sleeper in the same bed.	Like Bonnel coils, these are hourglass shaped, but the coils are squared off on top and bottom for maximum support. Some Sealy mattresses use this system.

Whatever the type of system, coils should be tempered with heat or electricity for long-lasting springiness. The edge should have a sturdy wire or foam border for stability and to keep the edge firm. The higher the coil count, the more stable the mattress is. Most mattresses feature 300 to 800 coils, with 500 to 800 considered firm. But mattresses with lower coil counts can feel firm if the coil wire is thicker. (Wire thickness is referred to as the wire's gauge. The higher the number, the thinner the wire. Look for a minimum of 14-gauge coil wire and 6-gauge border wire.) While firm, these low-coil-count mattresses can grow lumpy more quickly.

Buying Mattresses

5 Secrets for Getting a Great Deal That Will Give You Many a Good Night's Sleep

Be wary of mattress comfort guarantees. When it comes to buying most things, money-back guarantees are typically a good thing. But do you really want a mattress that someone may have used for several weeks? Straight off the bat, you should know that major bedding manufacturers do not allow retailers to return mattresses just because they didn't feel good. So any retailer offering you the chance to return a mattress after you've given it a test run is almost certainly putting returns back into inventory and selling them as new. Just the thought is enough to keep you up at night.

Buy box spring and mattress in a set. Box springs and mattresses that come in sets are built and fitted for one another. Separate units can cause problems. And since box springs absorb up to 50 percent of the impact, using a well-fitted box spring can prolong the life of your mattress.

Avoid box foundations. Unlike box springs, these plain wooden platforms covered with fabric have no springs. They are usually meant to make a cheap mattress feel firmer and can actually cause the mattress to break down more quickly. Without box springs, the mattress ticking, padding, and other upholstery can wear out more than twice as fast.

Don't assume a firm mattress is best. There's been a change of thinking when it comes to mattresses. Studies show that the long-held belief that firmer mattresses are best for people with back pain may not necessarily be true. Chiropractors say your spine should look the same when you're lying down as it does when you're standing. If you sleep on your side, a too-firm mattress may not have enough give to let your shoulder and hips sink into the mattress. Your body will be unnaturally compressed. Instead, you should look for a mattress designed to conform to the spine's natural curves and to keep the spine in alignment when you lie down. The mattress should also distribute pressure evenly across the body to help circulation, decrease body movement, and minimize the transfer of movement from one sleeping partner to the other.

Skimp on the kids' mattresses. Yes, you read that right. Mattress manufacturers and retailers know how young parents dote on their children. They prey on this tendency to provide "the best that money can buy" by offering high-priced bedding designed expressly for children. Top quality is fine when it comes to car seats, fresh food, and other things directly related to your child's health and safety. But almost any moderately priced bedding will give children proper support. So why buy the most expensive mattress for your six-year-old, when he will eventually outgrow it—if he doesn't destroy it first by bed-wetting or trampolining? ◁

Furniture Fixes

7 Amazingly Easy Tricks for Giving New Life to Your Old Pieces of Furniture

Revive your wicker. Wicker furniture can be a challenge to clean. But that's no reason to pay a professional. Stephen Berne, a Vancouver-based antique chair restorer who is especially knowledgeable about chair caning, Danish cord, and wicker repair, offers these insider tips:

- Use a vacuum cleaner with a brush attachment to lift dust, dirt and lint from within the woven reeds.

- Wipe wicker with a clean cloth moistened with paint thinner (first try a little thinner on an inconspicuous spot to make sure it does not harm the finish). For stubborn stains, lightly rub with a green pot scrubber moistened with paint thinner.

- To bring up the sheen on wicker, apply furniture wax with a clean cloth.

Tighten that sagging chair seat. Like any seasoned craftspeople, furniture restorers have their tricks. Here's one that will save you money the next time your wicker chair seats stretch and droop. First, make sure the chair is made of some natural material, such as rattan or bark (and not paper rush). If so, then turn the chair upside down and wet the bottom for a minute or two by wiping it with a clean sponge dipped in warm water. Once the bottom is soaked (the top should remain dry), then right the chair. When the woven seat dries, it will be tighter.

Repair frayed woven chair seats. If you have a chair with a woven paper rush seat (wicker made of twisted paper), you probably already know that the paper has a tendency to tear in front, where legs constantly rub it. Here's a quick cosmetic fix: Squeeze a bit of white craft glue underneath the torn strands, and tape it with masking tape to hold it in place. When the glue is dry, remove the masking tape, and no one will ever know the strands are broken.

Mask wood furniture scratches. Furniture refinishers would prefer to have your business, but you can save hundreds of dollars by hiding scratches using one of several inexpensive methods. Drop by the hardware store, and pick up a putty pencil or scratch polish. Make sure it matches the color of your wood finish. Apply as directed, and presto! The scratch disappears, not your money.

Follow the antique furniture golden rule. Do as little as possible to change the original construction and finish of your antiques. By stripping a finish and putting on a new finish, you can drastically reduce the value of antique furniture. If a chair is a little loose and creaky or a table's lacquer top is cracking, that's okay.

Protect fussy antiques without the fuss. Contrary to what the makers of those lemon-fresh, spray-on furniture polishes claim, you don't need fancy chemicals to clean and protect wooden chests, desks, tables, and chairs, even if they are your prized possessions. In fact, those products can do more harm than good. "Some sprays have additives that will never come off," says Nancy

Rosebrock, conservation manager at the Biltmore Estate in Asheville, North Carolina. "They crosslink chemically over time and become insoluble. A lot never completely dry, and they attract dirt, darkening the finish." And that, she says, can decrease the value. Instead, Rosebrock suggests a simple regimen of preventive care and cleaning for your wood furniture:

- Protect the wood from moisture. Use coasters, wipe up spills, and avoid cleaning with water.
- Dust regularly with a soft, dry white cloth.
- Wax once a year with a furniture wax, such as Johnson paste wax—but only if the wood's finish is intact. The paste wax, which protects the finish without penetrating the wood, keeps dust from binding with the surface the way car wax makes water bead. Pick a wax that matches the color of the wood (for instance, a lighter wax for maple and a darker one for walnut). If the wood finish is cracked or rubbed away, skip the paste.

Steam out a dent. A dent on a wooden surface can often be fixed by swelling the compressed wood fibers back to their normal size using moisture and heat. Prick the varnish finish of the dented area several times with a fine pin so that moisture can penetrate into the wood. Then cover the dent with a pad of wet cloth, put a metal bottle cap on top of the pad to spread the heat, and apply a clothing iron on a high setting for a few minutes. Be careful not to scorch the finish. Afterward, when the wood is completely dry, fill the pinholes with a thin coat of fresh varnish. ◁

Saving Energy
6 Special Things to Know About How to Reduce Your Consumption of Costly Utilities

Do the math on your home's energy usage. Here's a quick and easy way—without the costly expert advice of a energy consultant—to figure out if you could save money by taking more energy conservation measures. Tally up your fuel and electric bills for the past 12 months. Divide their total by the square footage of your home, not including garages and unheated basements. What do you get? Most homeowners pay 60 to 90 cents per square foot ($6.50 to $9.50 per square meter) per year in fuel and energy costs. If your rate falls within this range, there are many cost-effective ways to dramatically reduce your bills. If your rate is higher than this range, don't waste a moment!

Stop premature bulb burnout. It's as annoying as it is costly to have a ceiling fixture or lamp that needs a new lightbulb every month or two. The lightbulb manufacturers would just as soon you did nothing about it—nothing, that is, except keep buying new bulbs. But premature bulb burnout is a symptom of a bigger problem. The typical 60-watt incandescent bulb lasts 1,000 hours. At 10 hours a day, that's 100 days or a little more than three months. If you notice bulbs burning out well before the estimated life expectancy printed on the bulb carton, you may have a problem. Here are three possible causes, along with quick-and-easy solutions:

- *Poor ventilation.* If attic insulation covers a recessed fixture, it can overheat the fixture, burning out the bulb. The fix: Clear away the insulation to allow the fixture to properly ventilate.

- *Excess wattage.* If you're using a high-wattage bulb in a small, enclosed fixture, such as a lamp globe, the excess heat could snuff the filament. The fix: Remove the bulb and replace it with a lower-wattage one or a compact fluorescent.

- *The shakes.* Vibration, like heat, can make a filament fail sooner than it should. The fix: If your lamp or fixture is in a high traffic area, near a slamming door or on a ceiling beneath a floor that gets constantly trampolined by excited kids, replace the incandescent bulb with a compact fluorescent, which doesn't have a filament.

Cut your electric bill. Saving energy is a hot topic these days, so it's not surprising that marketers have jumped on the bandwagon, trying to lure gullible consumers into buying all sorts of bogus gadgets and other products supposedly meant to save them money. The U.S. Federal Trade Commission recently settled charges against marketers who claimed their "liquid siding" product drastically reduced home energy bills. You *can* save money by conserving energy. And you can do it without a major capital outlay. Here are two surefire ways to cut back on your electric usage and slash monthly bills:

- It's important to know that 20 percent of the average electric bill goes toward lighting. Save $60 a year in electric costs by replacing your five most frequently used incandescent light fixtures with Energy Star bulbs.

- Unplug those rechargeable batteries. Few people realize what a drain battery chargers for cell phones, laptops, toys, kitchen appliances, and power tools can be. If you have finished charging the item, unplug it. Otherwise, it's just sitting there costing you money.

Reduce heating and cooling costs. Half of your utility bill (electric or gas) goes to heat or cool the home. The easiest and cheapest thing you can do to reduce your heating or cooling bills is to clean or change furnace and air conditioning filters frequently. If you don't, the unit works harder, doesn't cool or heat at full capacity and may cause premature failure. At about $5 for a filter, it doesn't make sense to put it off (some filters can be vacuumed and replaced for no extra charge). Also be sure to close your foundation vents in winter if your home has a crawl space.

Don't use the fireplace. No matter how much your real estate agent may tout the romance and charm of a fireplace in your home, don't ignore this doctor-certified fact: The typical household fireplace chugs pollution into your living areas and sucks heat out—that's right, most draw away more heat than they provide. If someone in your home has asthma or other lung problems, resist the temptation to build a fire. If you can't do without, explore the new high-tech enclosures that are designed to radiate heat and keep fumes out of the house.

Analyze fridge-use claims skeptically. Appliance companies and retail salespeople love to tout the energy-saving advantages of newer, more efficient refrigerators. They claim that the fridge is the biggest energy hog among household appliances. And that the energy efficiency of refrigerators and freezers

Sealing Ducts for *Savings*

According to the U.S. Department of Energy, American homes lose up to 20 percent of the air that moves through their duct systems due to leaks, holes, and poorly connected ducts. And the same holds true for Canadian homes. Not only will faulty ducts make it more difficult to keep the house comfortable (no matter how the thermostat is set), but your utility bills will take a bigger bite out of your paycheck. All the more reason, say the home heating and air-conditioning contractors, to hire them to seal your ducts. But the money you spend on having a contractor work on your ducts might offset any savings you'll see in the future.

Unless the ducts are hard to reach, chances are you can seal them yourself, saving those contractor fees while making your home more comfortable, more energy efficient, and safer. Here's a step-by-step approach, beginning with a few expert tips for recognizing poorly performing ducts.

Signs of duct problems

- ☐ High utility bills in summer and winter.
- ☐ Some rooms are difficult to heat and cool.
- ☐ Stuffy rooms never seem to feel comfortable.
- ☐ Little or no air flows from registers.
- ☐ Air filter gets dirty quickly (needs changing more than once a month, which is a sign of leaks in return ducts).
- ☐ Streaks of dust at registers or duct connections.
- ☐ Lack of insulation on ducts in attic or crawl space.
- ☐ Tangled or kinked flexible ducts in your system.

How to seal ducts

1. Reconnect any disconnected ducts.
2. Seal air leaks using mastic (a gooey, highly effective adhesive that dries to a soft solid) or metal tape. Mastics and tapes should be UL 181 approved. Never use duct tape, which doesn't last nearly as long (see page 118).
3. Make sure connections at vents and registers are well sealed where they meet the floors, walls, and ceiling. Use spray foam to seal the gaps.
4. If your ducts are uninsulated or the insulation is torn or showing gaps, first seal any loose ducts and then add proper insulation.

Insulate attic or crawl-space ducts using material, such as fiberglass batting, rated at least R-6.

has improved dramatically over the past three decades. All true. A typical new refrigerator with automatic defrost and a top-mounted freezer uses less than 500 kilowatt-hours (kWh) per year, whereas a typical model sold in 1973 used more than 1,800 kWh per year. But how many people need to replace a 1973 fridge? Many homeowners with much younger models step onto the appliance showroom floor, urged on by fashion, prestige, boredom—and what they've heard about energy savings.

But you might find the math getting fuzzy when it comes to figuring out just what those savings are. According to the U.S. government's "savings calculator," at recent average national electricity rates ($0.086/kWh), with a midsize, auto-defrost top-freezer model, an Energy Star model would save $7 a year in electricity over another model made from 2001 to 2006. For the same refrigerator made from 1993 to 2001, the average savings would be $32 per year, still not enough to justify buying a new fridge. If your current fridge was made before 1990, the savings are substantial—from $130 to $227 per year. You might have other reasons to buy a new refrigerator— you're remodeling the kitchen or you need a larger fridge—but given the scale of energy savings, it only makes good financial sense to trade in your old fridge if it's truly old. What's a good rule of thumb? Since U.S. efficiency standards first took effect in 1993 (and in 1995 in Canada), requiring new refrigerators and freezers to be more efficient than ever before, it makes sense to upgrade if your refrigerator is a pre-1993 model. Anything younger than that depends on other factors— looks, size, whether you're remodeling or not. If you do upgrade, bear in mind that the most efficient full-size models carry the Energy Star label, meaning they exceed the government standards by 15 percent or more (full-size freezers must exceed government standards by 10 percent and compact refrigerators and freezers by 20 percent). ◅

SECRET WEAPON

Extra Insulation

Since heat rises, a good deal of the heat lost by a house is through the attic. So even though your attic is already insulated with batts or loose fill between the joists, it often pays, especially in older homes, to add another layer of insulation. It doesn't cost a fortune, and it's a job that most homeowners can do themselves, using rolls of fiberglass insulation available at any home center. Run the new insulation over the tops of the joists at right angles to the existing insulation. This covers any gaps in the first layer and insulates the heat escape routes created by the joists. When adding new rolled insulation, work from the eaves toward the center using a piece of plywood as a platform to kneel on. You can cut the insulation using heavy-duty scissors. Three precautions: Use unfaced insulation; if it has facing, slash it every few inches so that it won't trap moisture. Don't block vents in the eaves. And don't cover recessed lighting unless it's marked IC (for insulated ceiling).

Windows Secrets

3 Things You Should Consider If You Have Old Drafty Windows That Are Not Energy Efficient

Think twice before replacing windows. Purchasing replacement windows for your home may not be the money-saving venture that window companies claim that it is. Some companies claim a 35 percent reduction in energy bills. Energy Star, the internationally recognized energy stamp of approval, estimates that Energy Star windows that replace single-pane windows can save homeowners $110 to $400 per year for an average home, depending on the region. That may sound like a lot of money, but when you consider that replacement windows typically cost more than $450 per window ($5,000 to $25,000 per home), the savings just don't add up.

However, Harvey M. Sachs, Ph.D., director of the Buildings Program at the American Council for an Energy-Efficient Economy (ACEEE), says that in most houses, windows account for less than 15 percent of the total heat loss. So even if you replaced all the windows with perfect insulators, you would save at most 15 percent. At those rates, it would take years to recoup the cost of the windows through energy savings. "Getting new windows is really a lifestyle option," says Sachs. New windows may look better, but "it may be more cost effective to do other upgrades."

Make your current windows weather tight. Adding caulk, weather stripping, and a storm-window alternative is often the most cost effective way to fix old windows. Not only will filling gaps stop drafts, making you feel warmer in the winter, but tightening up your house means your furnace or boiler does not have to work as hard to keep your house warm, and your air conditioning doesn't have to work as hard to keep it cool. Here are some low-cost tips for sealing up windows without spending an arm and a leg to replace them:

Caulking. If your windows are a little drafty, easy-to-apply and inexpensive caulk (about $3 per 10-ounce [290–ml] tube) can effectively plug gaps around window frames and sills. For a house with 15 windows, at half a tube per window, the total cost could be less than $25.

Weather stripping. The quality and thickness of foam weather stripping varies (as does the cost, from about $6 to $19 per 20-foot [6-meter] roll). Attach it below the bottom sash, between two sashes and other places to stop those icy wind tunnels. Depending on the type of weather stripping used, the cost to seal 15 windows might run you $90 to $285.

Storm window alternatives. Storm windows aren't that much less expensive than replacement windows (and sometimes they still let in drafts). The least expensive storm-window alternative is the plastic film that seals with a hair dryer. It costs less than $10 per window for the kits (and even less if you buy your own roll of clear plastic and two-sided tape). The drawbacks? You can't open a window if you need to, and you have to reapply them each winter. But the energy savings just may be worth the inconvenience.

Another alternative is window glass film, which is applied directly to the glass. Window film has come a long way in recent years and is no longer associated with bad tinting jobs. It the summer, it reduces solar heat and in the winter it preserves indoor heat. You can get it professionally installed for between $5 and $10 per square foot ($50 to $105 per square meter).

If you do buy windows, get the right ones. If you plan to buy replacement windows, make sure you don't get snookered into buying a cheap window that will have to be replaced again in the near future—or the wrong type of window for your needs. Always look for the Energy Star label. Energy Star is an internationally used designation that government agencies give companies that meet strict energy requirements. Here are six key facts you'll need in order to buy the best windows for your climate conditions:

1. In addition to the Energy Star label, look for the National Fenestration Rating Council label. The NFRC is a nonprofit collaboration of window manufacturers, government agencies, and building trade associations founded to establish a fair, accurate, and credible energy rating system for windows, doors, and skylights. Its label means the window's performance is certified.

2. The lower the U-value, the better the insulation. In colder climates, a U-value of 0.35 or below is recommended. These windows have at least double glazing and a coating that reduces heat transfer through the window.

3. In warm climates, where summertime heat gain is the main concern, look for windows with double glazing and spectrally selective coatings that reduce heat gain. You don't need a U-value below 0.35, so don't pay extra for it.

4. In temperate climates with both heating and cooling seasons, select windows with both low U-values and low solar heat gain coefficient (SHGC) to maximize energy benefits.

5. Select windows with air leakage ratings of 0.3 cubic feet per minute or less.

6. Window quality means nothing if windows leak around the frame. Look for a reputable, qualified installer. ◁

Energy Conservation Myths

You hear a lot on television and in the popular press about energy conservation. Some of it is worthy advice. Some of it is flat wrong. Here are four widely touted energy-saving myths that you should know the full facts about:

Just having a programmable thermostat won't save you energy. You have to program it properly.

Programmable thermostats save you money

Well, they actually do—but only if you program them for savings. Many people mistakenly think that these computer-chip-driven electronic devices *automatically* calculate efficient temperatures. But they don't. You must program them to lower the thermostat temperature at night or during the day when you're at work. Do that, and you'll save an average of 15 percent on your monthly bills.

Ceiling fans cool a room

They don't cool the room, but they do cool the people in it by creating a windchill effect on the skin. That's a good thing, allowing you to raise the temperature of your air conditioner thermostat or turn the AC off altogether. But where people go wrong is leaving those fans on when they leave the room. Instead, treat the fan like a light and turn it off. Otherwise, it will waste electricity.

Computer screen savers save energy

Screen savers prolong the life of your monitor by displaying a moving image to prevent a fixed image from being burned into the phosphor of the screen. But they do nothing to save power. Instead, they burn up electricity. Your computer may have an energy-saving mode. To activate it, go into your operating system software's control panel and explore your computer's power management options.

It takes more energy to turn a computer on than to let it idle

This may or may not be true with a car (depends on how long you idle it), but it's certainly not true with a computer. Shut your computer off at night or when you will be away from it for a long period of time.

Selling Your House

3 Lists of Tricks That Will Help Increase the Value of Your House in the Eyes of Buyers

Boost your curb appeal. You've heard it before—that sprucing up out front can help lure busy buyers into your home. But curb appeal is so important it bears repeating. Here's a step-by-step approach:

1. Walk the perimeter of your house, removing all garbage cans, wood-piles, and leftover building materials (wood, cinder blocks, and bricks).

2. Clean and sweep gutters. Check for roof moss and dry rot.

3. Prune bushes and trees. Remove all dead plants or shrubs. Keep plants from blocking windows. Remember: You can't sell a house if buyers can't see it.

4. Weed and mulch all planting areas.

5. Keep lawn freshly cut, fertilized, and watered.

6. Clear patios and decks of all small items, such as small planters, pots, charcoal, barbecue grills, toys, and tools. (Put them in a shed or storage unit.)

7. Check exterior paint—especially the front door and trim, the first detail a potential buyer will see. Clean, scrape, and repaint if necessary.

Boost your home's interior appeal too. The real estate trend known as staging started in some of the swankest neighborhoods in California and Florida and is spreading across the country. Staging specialists, often combining Realtor know-how with an interior designer's eye, make minor changes to your home in order to appeal to poten-tial buyers. Staging takes the concept of improving your curb appeal inside the home and pushes it even further.

The key principles of staging include decluttering, cleaning, and "neutraliz-ing." "It's not about replacing expensive items like windows and floors. It's about looks," says Kevin Reid Shirley, a Washington, D.C.-based Realtor and staging specialist. "It's about making what you already have irresistible." Statistics show that the work of stagers helps houses move faster and often boosts the selling price.

Stagers might make formal design ideas, recommend outside vendors (painters, haulers, and furniture rentals), oversee the process, and do the final showcasing of the home such as rearranging furni-ture and accessorizing. Some include the fee in their nondiscounted commis-sion rate. Others charge flat or hourly fees in the thousands of dollars.

Save those fees while enjoying the advantages of staged home by using Shirley's advice:

- *Think of your home as a product.* It must be priced right and look better than the other homes in your mar-ketplace in order to be competitive.

- *Prepare to pack early.* When you sell your home, you're going to have to move. When you move, you're going to have to pack. Most of the princi-ples of staging just mean that you're going to pack up some of your things early. If you need room to store extra

6

THINGS YOU SHOULD
know
About Real Estate Agents

Although you can sell or buy a home on your own, it's tricky, and most of us opt to use the services of real estate agents. While these pros can be very helpful in finding the right buyer or locating the perfect house, you have to remember that they are in the game to collect a commission. Here are some things that you should keep in mind when dealing with real estate agents.

1 Licensed real estate agents aren't as qualified as their pay scale might lead you to believe. In California, for example, all you need to get an agent's license is one three-unit college course and a passing grade on the state's three-hour, multiple-choice test.

2 They might not be showing you all the listings, only the ones that pay the highest commission. In the U.S. these days, many listings pay 2.5 percent rather than the traditional 3 percent commission to the buyer's agent. That half percentage point can mean losing $1,500 on a $300,000 home. Make sure your agent is showing you all listings, the ones that pay 3 percent and the ones that pay 2.5 percent.

3 Agents sometimes delay putting a home on the multiple listing service. That way, they can show it to their clients first in an attempt to rake in both the seller's and buyer's commission.

4 Open houses are not a great way to sell houses. But they are a great way for agents to snag new clients. So that open house you're busting your butt over might not be worth the trouble—at least to you. For the same reason, agents include very few details in the ads they run for your house. They want as many people as possible to call. Even if your home doesn't suit the house hunters, the agent now has their names as potential clients.

5 Agents don't always push for the highest price. Sure, they're working for commission, but sometimes a quick and easy sell for $190,000 is better than waiting for $200,000. That $10,000 difference is a lot of money to you ($9,400 when you subtract the total 6 percent commission), but at a 3 percent seller's commission, it comes out to only $300 for the agent.

6 You can back out of the deal. Though it's rare, some sellers change their minds after they've received offers on their homes. Maybe their job situation or their children's school situation changed. Maybe they have reasons for not wanting to sell to a particular buyer (they're going to demolish a beloved home and put up condos). If the offer is equal to or better than the asking price, the agent may claim that you owe the commission anyway, since the buyer has met the terms of the agreement. But there are other conditions that still must be met, such as inspections, appraisals, and obtaining financing. You can use these as grounds to back out.

possessions, use the garage or rent a storage unit.

- *Neutralize your home.* Buyers decide to buy or not to buy a home in a matter of minutes. If they spend even a few moments admiring your personal belongings, such as photographs, heirloom china or tchotchke collections, that's a distraction and invaluable time wasted. "We want them to be able to envision the space with their furnishings and belongings there," Shirley says. "By removing these personal items, you allow potential buyers to imagine their belongings in the space."

- *Clear surfaces.* Remove all unnecessary objects from tabletops, desks, and shelves. Keep decorative objects on the furniture restricted to groups of 1, 3, or 5 items (odd-numbered groups look better). Work extra hard to free up kitchen counter space. Remove messages, magnets, and pictures from the front of the refrigerator. In bathrooms, remove unnecessary items from countertops, tub, shower stall, and commode top. Keep only the most necessary cosmetics, brushes, perfumes, and such in one small group on the counter.

- *Thin out crowded rooms.* Rearrange or remove some of the furniture in your home. Less furniture makes the rooms appear larger.

- *Simplify busy walls.* Take down, reduce, or rearrange pictures and objects on walls.

- *Organize closets.* Pack up and remove all seasonal clothes from your closets. That will make your closets appear bigger. Disorganized closets tell buyers that your home does not have enough storage space.

- *Patch, paint, and clean like crazy.* Spackle wall holes and cracks. Apply a fresh coat of paint to rooms that need it. (Neutral wall colors, such as tan, taupe, beige, and cream, paired with bright white trim, lend a clean, classic, and spacious look to rooms.) Clean carpets and drapes if they need it. Clean windows to invite natural light and enhance views. If an object can't be cleaned or repaired, repaint it or replace it.

Last-Minute Cleanup

EXPERT INSTANT ADVICE

When you get the call from your real estate agent that potential buyers are just 15 minutes away, here's an 11-point hit list of last-minute touches.

1. Quickly wash the dishes, or at least put dirty dishes in the dishwasher.

2. Make the beds.

3. Wipe the counters.

4. Empty the garbage.

5. Hide dirty clothes in the washer or dryer.

6. Do a quick vacuum of high-traffic areas.

7. Turn ceiling fans on low.

8. Open all curtains and blinds, unless otherwise advised.

9. Turn on all lights and lamps.

10. Close garage doors.

11. Make sure all toilet lids are down.

- *Forget the potpourri or fresh-baked cookies.* Those common tricks fall flat. The best two fragrances home buyers can smell in your home are Pine-Sol and paint! The perception is that a clean home is a well-maintained home.
- *Decorate dead space.* If you've got unused rooms or finished basement space, help buyers envision how they might use the space. Turn that extra bedroom (the one you use as a closet) into a home office. Set up a desk and computer, even if you have to borrow props or buy them for cheap at a local thrift shop.

Let them see light. If you're selling your home, remember this: What really impresses buyers, at least on a subconscious level, is how bright, airy, and spacious a home is. So here are the secrets for reinforcing this impression:

- Remove a few pieces of furniture from each room and rearrange the remaining furniture for a sparse look.
- Pull two-thirds of the clothes out of every closet and store them away. You want a visitor to peek into the closet and think, Yup, plenty of room in here!
- Open all curtains and blinds, wash all windows, and put high-wattage bulbs in all lamps.
- If you have any dingy, stained, or cracked walls, repair them and repaint in a light color. ◄|

Buying a House
2 Simple Secrets That Could Save Thousands When You Are Looking for a New Home

Buy the house before making other major purchases. Salespeople will gnash their teeth when they read this, but hold off on making any major purchases if you're also about to buy a new house. Taking out a loan for a new car, for instance, could radically change your financial picture from the point of view of a mortgage bank. You could be turned down for a mortgage if the bank isn't sure you can handle the payments.

Don't talk about renovations. Your natural, genial nature could cost you thousands of dollars when it comes to buying a house. So for once in your life, turn off the charm. Most people who are selling a home have a lot of themselves invested in the property and they feel better knowing that the next owner will appreciate the abode they're giving up. If you fall into a long-winded conversation with a home's seller about the paneling you want to rip out or the tree you intend to cut down, the offended seller will be less likely to drop his price during negotiations. If you must meet the seller, keep it brief and cordial—but say nothing about your plans for the property. ◄|

THE TRUTH ABOUT
vinyl siding

Polyvinyl chloride (PVC) is the most popular siding material. Lots of money and energy on the part of the manufacturers, distributors, and salespeople go toward pushing vinyl siding, as it's commonly known. The marketers prey on the universal homeowner dread of exterior maintenance. Yet while vinyl may be a viable option for some people, it's no miracle product. Listen to what the vinyl salesman says, and then think about what he's leaving out. Here's what he may not be telling you.

Vinyl siding is made from a toxin

While vinyl siding on your house will not likely lead to health problems, PVC is known to cause cancer in humans. Fires in vinyl-clad homes are more dangerous because of the toxic fumes produced by the burning plastic.

Adding vinyl siding is not necessarily a home improvement

Often owners of older homes in need of repair turn to vinyl as a solution. But installing vinyl over wood that is already water damaged can simply mask a minor problem, turning it into a major problem with time. Moisture trapped beneath vinyl will accelerate rot, promote mold and mildew, and invite insect infestations in leftover wood siding and framing. Even in new homes, vinyl siding can act as a moisture trap.

Vinyl siding is not so easy to clean

Over time, vinyl siding grows dingy with dirt and mildew. Marketers often say cleaning it is as easy as spraying it with a pressure-sprayer. But pressure-washing vinyl is a no-no, since the high-powered water can seep in between cracks and get trapped behind the panels, leading to the above-mentioned rot. Power-washing can also rip vinyl panels right off the wall. And you can't freshen vinyl up with a coat of paint. More likely, you'll have to scrub the entire house with warm, soapy water.

Vinyl siding is not maintenance-free

Every siding material requires maintenance. Period. Vinyl installation requires lots of caulk around windows and doors and at corners. Exterior caulk eventually shrinks, cracks, and mildews. Gaps open up, and water enters. Time for maintenance. Also, the vinyl siding pieces are secured to the house by a nail or staple. As the vinyl contracts and expands with the temperature changes, these fasteners can loosen and strips can buckle (especially if they're secured too tightly). High winds can loosen or remove fasteners. Time for maintenance. As vinyl ages, it fades and grows brittle—even more brittle in cold weather—and can crack and shatter when struck by a ball or limb. You can't (or shouldn't) paint faded vinyl. And since vinyl cannot be patched (like wood can), you have to replace an entire panel to fix one crack. All together now: Time for maintenance.

Vinyl siding does not increase an older home's value

More and more people around the country are coming to appreciate historic homes as one-of-a-kind antiques in their own right. As a result, old home values are rising—but not if they have lost their historic charm. While vinyl siding may look like "authentic" wood, installation usually calls for the removal of much of the original wood siding and artistic exterior trim—moldings, scrollwork, gable shingles, and decorative attic vents—that people love.

Vinyl siding will not cut your energy bill

Thin and flimsy, vinyl is not a good insulator. The addition of foam backing beneath the panels will do next to nothing to add energy efficiency to your home. In older homes, experts estimate that if the original wood siding is removed to make room for the new vinyl siding, the net effect would be a loss in energy efficiency.

Vinyl siding will not last forever

The slogan of the siding industry is that "vinyl is final," and its ads imply that vinyl siding is permanent. But don't you believe it. Sure, vinyl will last a long time, a very long time. But vinyl siding is just not as durable as wood or masonry siding. As vinyl starts to noticeably fade and dull, it becomes less attractive. At the same time, the longer you have the siding, the more likely it is to be damaged—accidentally hit by a ball, a branch, a mower or snow blower, strong hail, or wind-blown debris. This means replacing an entire panel with a bright new mismatched panel. At this point, to preserve the value of their property, many homeowners opt for the ultimate act of maintenance: replacing the siding.

The Good Earth

7 Ways to Create a Rich, Fertile Environment for Your Lawn and Plants

Don't bother to test your soil. If you only listened to the "experts" in gardening magazines, you'd fork over some green to a soil lab before you ever forked compost onto your garden. But some gardening professionals think this can be a waste of money. Garden center manager Connie Smith, for example, has never tested soil. In general, she says, if you are diligent about adding compost, manure, and peat to your soil, it will achieve the required pH balance and essential minerals. If you want to learn more about the general nature of soils in your area, the extension agent at a nearby university, or an expert at a local garden center, will tell you what to expect and make recommendations for additions to your soil.

When is testing soil a must? If you're having problems growing a plant that should succeed in your area, especially if your neighbor's plants do well with the same sun exposure, you might have an issue with your soil and a test could help point to a solution. Also, you may want to test your soil first if you plan to dump fertilizer on it every year: You may be wasting money and pouring unnecessary chemicals into your garden when all it needs is a dose of lime or a load of manure.

Get your mulch for free. Mulch is essential stuff for retaining moisture and inhibiting weeds, but the owners of your local garden or home center will be laughing all the way to the bank if you buy it by the bag. Fortunately, arborists and tree trimmers are often looking to give away their wood chips—otherwise, they have to pay a landfill to take them. Call a local arborist and ask if you can get a load of chips dumped in your driveway at the end of the day's work. Many are happy to oblige. Also, check with your town's parks or public-works department, because it often puts wood chips in a publicly available stash where you can load up for free. If you don't have a pickup, place a large piece of sturdy plastic, a painter's drop cloth, or even an old bedsheet in the backseat or trunk of your car, pile the chips inside, then pull it out at home with the help of a friend.

Beware, however, of making mulch from the chips of diseased or insect-infested trees. Always ask about the source of the chips before taking them.

Whack those leaves into instant mulch. To quickly turn your raked leaves into mulch, dump them into a large trash can and lower your Weed Whacker into it. This process will reduce your leaves to a tenth of their former volume. They'll be easy to pack up and dispose of if that's your wish. But ground-up leaves make excellent mulch too. Your garden store manager will shake his head with dismay when you start passing up the bags of shredded root.

Use compost instead of fertilizer. North Americans spend literally hundreds of millions of dollars a year on bags of dirt. Sacks of so-called designer soils sell by the truckload each spring. However, you can get all the benefits of these products, as well as expensive fertilizers, by making your own compost. Work the compost into your garden soil before planting, and spread 1/2 inch to 1 inch (1.25 cm to 2.5 cm) compost over

the garden every winter after the harvest. Your soil will be more fertile, easier to work, and have better drainage.

Build a simple backyard compost bin. To compost with lawn trimmings, leaves, and other yard waste, you need a big bin, and big bins equal big bucks if you buy your composter at a garden center or through a catalog. But landscape designer Jennifer Appel has a simple plan for a backyard bin that anyone can build. All you need are a few simple supplies:

- A used wooden pallet, available just for the asking from supermarkets and warehouse outfits
- Two 8-foot 2 x 4 (2.4-meter 38 x 89-cm) studs
- 15 feet (5 meters) of galvanized chicken wire or hardware cloth, 3 feet (91 cm) wide. Choose the finer-mesh hardware cloth if you'll be composting kitchen scraps and other small items.
- A square of breathable landscaping fabric, cut to fit the top of the pallet

Place the pallet on a smooth, level surface near your garden. Saw the 2 x 4s in half, and nail one piece to each corner of the pallet to create four posts. Starting at one corner, staple the wire mesh to the posts, wrapping it around the edge of the pallet to form a box. Instead of stapling the mesh to the final post on the front side of the box, secure it with picture hooks or a twist of picture-frame wire. That way, you can swing open one panel of the mesh for easier access to the compost.

Staple the landscaping fabric over the top of the pallet, and load in your composting materials. Use a mix of carbon-rich waste (sawdust, wood chips, and leaves) and nitrogen-loaded waste (non-meat food scraps, grass clippings, and manure). The open slats in the pallet under the pile will help bring air to the compost from below, reducing odor, but turn the pile with a pitchfork or shovel every week or so to make sure it gets enough oxygen. Within a month, you'll have some nutritious compost ready for the garden, and the marketing mavens at the "designer soil" companies will be going back to the drawing board.

Make a low-cost kitchen composter. You'll be more likely to compost kitchen scraps if you have a composter that's closer to the kitchen sink than that pile way out in the garden. But judging by the glossy gardening catalogs, you'd think you have to spend a pile of money as big as a compost heap to get a good kitchen composter. Instead, head down to a supermarket or home store to pick up a 30-gallon (114-liter) plastic garbage can. To make the can compost-ready,

use a power drill with a 1/2-inch (125-mm) bit or a hammer and a large nail to punch holes in it. Starting near the bottom of the garbage can, place the holes 4 inches (10 cm) apart in a ring around the side of the can. Then move up the side of the can 6 inches (15 cm) and drill a new ring of holes. Continue this pattern until you reach the top of the garbage can. Put a few drainage holes in the bottom too. Place the can outside your house in a location convenient to the kitchen and on the way to the garden. Use a bungee cord with hooks at each end to secure the lid against scavenging animals, and turn the contents at least once a week. And throw that gardening catalog, with its expensive composters, into the recycling pile.

Brew your own compost tea. What's compost tea? It's a liquid that's formed by steeping compost in water until the resulting brew is rich in nutrients and beneficial microbes. More versatile to use than compost, the tea can be used to

How I Do It A Nursery Owner's Trick for Preventing Hand-Tool Loss

Indiana gardener and nursery owner Gene Bush has a nifty solution for keeping garden hand tools handy—and preventing them from getting lost in leaves and mulch. Bush mounted an old-fashioned mailbox by the gate to his garden, and he keeps a set of hand tools in it, so they're always ready when he spots a weed that needs digging or a shrub that needs pruning. Bush puts an oiled rag in a zip-sealed plastic bag inside the mailbox, so he can wipe down the tools when he's done with them. Whenever he takes a tool out of the mailbox, he flips up the red flag—this means a tool is out (rather than mail is in), and it reminds him to replace the tool when he's done instead of losing it in the mulch.

feed plants of all kinds, replacing expensive fertilizers. Garden stores will sell it to you by the gallon, and numerous machines can be purchased to brew the tea, but it's easy to make your own with a few basic supplies.

The simplest method is to suspend a cheesecloth bag of rich organic compost in a bucket of water or a watering can for two to three days. Carefully remove the bag and its contents, then use the brew to feed your plants immediately.

You'll get far more microbial growth—and thus more benefit for your garden—if you take a few additional steps. Microorganisms will only grow if they get an adequate supply of oxygen, and an aquarium pump and hose are just the ticket to deliver it. Get a 5-gallon (19-liter) plastic bucket and place it near an outdoor electrical outlet. Attach one end of the plastic hose to the aquarium bubbler, and place the other end in the bottom of the bucket. Fill about one-fifth of the bucket with rich compost. Now fill a second bucket with water and let it stand overnight to let the chlorine in the tap water dissipate. Otherwise the chlorine will kill the microorganisms in the compost. Add the chlorine-free water to the compost, filling the bucket to within 6 inches (15 cm) of its rim. Then add 2 tablespoons unsulfured molasses to the mix as food for the microbes. Turn on the aquarium pump so it bubbles through the mix, and let it brew for two or three days, stirring occasionally. When you're ready to use it, strain the tea through cheesecloth into the second bucket, and return the solids to the compost heap. Apply the tea to plants immediately. ◁

Outdoor Plants
9 Ways to Make the Most of Your Flowering and Foliage Plantings

Don't pay retail for plants. Why pay top dollar to a garden center when you may be able to find plants that are every bit as healthy at other outlets? Arboretums and botanical gardens often hold plant sales, as do neighborhood and high school gardening clubs. Though your local nursery owner won't be happy, your purchases will go toward a good cause.

Give the gift of perennials. You could pay top dollar to give a potted plant to a friend for a birthday or other special occasion. Or you could keep your money and find beautiful plants in your own garden to use as gifts. Many perennials need to be divided every couple of years as they grow. Flowers that grow from bulbs, such as tulips and lilies, are the easiest to divide. After these plants flower, gently lift them from the ground, pull off the little bulbs that have formed alongside the original bulb, and replant these in potting soil. Voilà! A living gift for your best friend.

Ask a neighbor to divide perennials. Although garden centers don't like to talk about it, many of those pricey perennials they stock on their shelves are available for free in your neighbor's garden. Ask if he or she has any perennials that need to be divided—offer to help with the labor in exchange for taking some home for your own garden.

Smaller can be better. Nurseries and garden centers would love to sell you the biggest plant they can, since they can charge top dollar. But if you're buying flowering perennials, choose a 1-quart (1-liter) container of plants over a 1-gallon (3.8-liter) container. Young perennials tend to grow quickly, and within a single season they will catch up in size with those larger plants you could have purchased at a considerably higher cost.

Beware of fast-growing invasive plants. Some common garden varieties may become all too common in the garden if you aren't careful, warns Denver botany professor Greg McArthur. Although garden centers may try to sell you on easy-to-grow plants (knowing that a fast-growing plant makes for a happy customer), some plants spread aggressively and can be very hard to get rid of once they are introduced in a garden. These include ground covers such as periwinkle (*Vinca minor*); flowering plants like fleabane and other asters, broom, forget-me-nots, hollyhocks, verbena, yarrow, and daisies; and other plants such as ferns, mints, and strawberries.

Moreover, some of these plants may leap the garden fence (or, more likely, send roots underneath it) and invade your neighbors' plots or nearby open space.

Such invasive species can seriously alter the local plant environment. Most of these plants have their place in a garden, but make sure to keep them in their place by pulling up shoots wherever you don't want them, or by planting such varieties only in defined areas such as pots, containers, beds bounded by pavement, or raised beds.

"Drought tolerant" doesn't mean "don't water." Beware of the self-appointed xeriscaping expert who says all you need to do is plant the right varieties and then throw away the hose. To get a proper start on life in your garden, drought-tolerant plants need regular watering for the first year after you plant them. After that, as long as you've planted varieties suitable for your zone, these plants should be able to live on the local rainfall in all but exceptional drought conditions.

Wildflower mixes may be wilder than you expect. Seed companies make those boxes or bags of premixed wildflower seeds seem like the answer to all your prayers. Just scatter them on the ground, add water, and a beautiful meadow full of wildflowers will magically appear. But be careful. According to Susan Aldrich-Markham of the Oregon State University extension service, those mixes may contain invasive species that are inappropriate for your area.

Some plants that are considered desirable, decorative varieties in one part of North America may turn into harmful weeds elsewhere, in places with different growing conditions. One researcher planted the seeds from 19 wildflower mix packets, and all 19 contained species that were invasive somewhere in North America. Eight plants were considered noxious weeds in at least one U.S. state or Canadian province.

How do you make sure your wildflower garden is safe and appropriate for your area? The best method is to select packets of seeds for individual wildflowers, rather than mixes, so you can choose your own blend and be sure what you're planting. If you opt for a seed mix, Aldrich-Markham recommends buying from a local company, because the more widely a mix is distributed, the more likely it is to hold inappropriate seeds for a given area. Make sure the packet lists all of the varieties of seeds it contains, and look up any plants that are unfamiliar. It's a bit more work, but you're better off doing the legwork in advance than planting a meadow from hell.

Squirt rosebushes with this secret formula. Longtime gardener Rita Carey from Squamish, British Columbia, works at a garden center, but that doesn't stop her from recommending this homemade, environmentally friendly spray for rose pests and diseases. Here's her recipe: In an empty 1-gallon (3.8-liter) milk jug, mix 1 1/2 teaspoons baking soda, 1 tablespoon vegetable oil, 1/2 teaspoon liquid dish soap, and 1/2 cup white vinegar. Fill the jug the rest of the way with water and add the mixture to a sprayer. Spray all of the leaves and stems of your roses at least once a week during growing season.

Go low-tech for drip irrigation. For watering flower beds and other plantings, drip irrigation is the best method—it's extremely water-efficient, and the slow, deep watering is great for plant health. But landscape contractors mentally tote up another boat payment when they sign up for your big drip-irrigation job. Maybe you don't need the expense of a full installed system—here's a simple way to give plants a deep soaking with no expense at all. Save up plastic 2-liter soda bottles and 1-gallon (3.8-liter) milk bottles. Punch a small hole in the bottom of each, then fill each container with water. Stand each bottle next to a plant, and it will slowly release the water. For trees, use 5-gallon (19-liter) collapsible water carriers designed for camping, with their valves set on the slowest drip. With this method, you'll leave the contractor high and dry. And even if you do have a centralized drip-irrigation system, these portable irrigators are extremely useful for watering isolated shrubs, trees, and flowers. ◁

SECRET WEAPON

Stirrup Hoe

Longtime gardener Glenn Deines is a retired blacksmith and welder in the farming town of Platteville, Colorado, and he knows his tools. His favorite device for his home garden is the stirrup hoe, which is just about twice as efficient as a traditional hoe. The stirrup hoe looks like, well, a stirrup attached to a wooden handle. The metal blade digs and cuts in both directions, pushing and pulling, and it's particularly effective in compacted earth, like the paths between garden rows. Since you don't swing a stirrup hoe like a regular hoe, it's great for working in tight spaces between rows—more accurate and less damaging to plants. Also called circle hoes and loop hoes, these tools are easily found at garden and hardware stores.

Container Plants
6 Secrets for Making Your Potted House and Patio Plants Flourish for Less

Don't line pot bottoms with pebbles. Anyone telling you to fill the bottom inch or so of indoor plant containers with pebbles is just trying to sell you a load of fancy stones. It's a waste of money, and it's not good for the plants, says Phil Goodin, head of a Denver-area high school's Plant Lovers Club. Although the conventional wisdom used to be that pebbles or shards of clay pots in a container improved drainage, plant experts now say such stones occupy space the plant roots need and may encourage growth of fungus. Instead, you want a solid column of soil right down to the bottom of the container. If you're worried about soil washing out of a pot's drain hole, cover the hole with a scrap of window screen or a single pot shard before filling the pot with soil.

Try some of those free containers. That fancy-schmancy garden store would just as soon you didn't think about it, but you probably throw away scores of items every year that are perfect for container gardening. Popcorn tins and plastic ice cream buckets make particularly good outdoor flowerpots. All you have to do is drill holes in the bottom of them for drainage. If the exterior of the container is not to your liking, a can of spray paint will change that quickly.

Keep your plants alive when you're away. How do you care for plants while you're away from home? One common solution is to pay someone to water your indoor and outdoor container plants. But you can greatly reduce the need for watering by taking a few steps before you leave home.

- Always use a potting mix with moisture-retaining polymers (or add polymers to the mix). These compounds retain water for later use by thirsty plants.
- When you're headed off on vacation or a work trip, move your plants out of direct sunlight—behind windows with sheer curtains is a great spot.
- Turn down the thermostat in winter to keep the interior of the house cool.
- Move pots and containers close together, so the plants will provide each other with shade and humidity.
- Place sensitive plants inside tents made from white plastic trash bags—place a bag upside down over each plant, using stakes as "tent poles" to keep the plastic off the foliage. Cut a few small holes in the plastic to allow oxygen to reach the plant.
- To conserve water in outdoor containers, move them to a location sheltered from the wind and cluster them together.
- You can also bury potted plants to their rims temporarily and mulch around them.

The neighborhood kid who was counting on making a little extra money won't be happy with these water-saving techniques, but, on the other hand, your lawn will probably still need mowing when you get back.

Vegetable Gardening
7 Tricks for Growing Incredible Edibles in Your Veggie Patch

Salvage your dried-out plants. If your plants do dry out completely while you are away, you can revive them when you get home by soaking the containers in a tub or kiddie pool. Use warm (not hot) water, and submerge the pots until bubbles stop appearing from the soil. Remove the pot and drain any excess water.

Put an IV drip on that plant. You can pay $100 or more for electronically controlled devices that automatically water your plants while you're away from home. Or you can use the low-tech, inexpensive, and just as effective method recommended by nurse Jennifer James: Hook your plants up to an IV drip. Plastic intravenous solution bags can be refilled with tap water by removing the spike at the mouth of the bag. Hang a bag above a plant and set the dial to slow drip. Only medical professionals can buy intravenous equipment, so ask a friend who works in the field for used bags and feeder lines.

Use a rope to water your plants. Another solution for watering while you're away takes advantage of the capillary action of natural fibers. Place your potted plants next to a tub of water, then cut natural-fiber clothesline or other rope in lengths that will reach from the tub to each pot. Anchor one end of each cord in the tub with a rock or brick, and coil the other end around the soil atop each pot. Water will flow across the rope to the plants. ◁

Be careful of hardiness zones near borders. Knowing the hardiness zone for your area is critical to choosing the right plants for your gardens and landscaping. These zones are predominantly based on the coldest temperature during winter and on the dates of the first and last frost. The zones are numbered, and plants are generally labeled with these numbers so you'll know which ones are most likely to thrive in your area. But here's a fact that could trip you up if you aren't careful where you buy: Although both Canada and the United States use a numbering system for their zones, the scales are different. For example, the zone for much of northern Montana is 3b, but the same zone over the border in southern Alberta is 4a, even though they share virtually the same climatic conditions. If you shop in the border states or provinces or, even more critically, if you order plants by mail or from the Internet, it's crucial to know which zone system the vendor is using. Otherwise, you might find that your new plants are immigrants with the wrong documentation.

Try vegetables with training wheels. If you're worried that you've got a black thumb, start with green beans, tomatoes, and radishes—and herbs such as basil, rosemary, and thyme. Sure, the experts will get bigger yields, but these can't-miss plants guarantee plenty of luscious fresh vegetables during your first season, and you'll be encouraged to try more vegetables next year.

Jump-start spring with a movable greenhouse. Fancy garden stores will be happy to sell you a spiffy prefabricated greenhouse for starting seedlings or protecting plants from early or late frosts, but it won't come cheap. Fortunately, it's easy to make your own portable shelter for young plants, says longtime gardener Enga Lokey, who lives in sunny Australia but says winters are plenty cold there. All you need to buy is some clear plastic sheeting, four 18-inch (46-cm) lengths of rebar (steel reinforcing rods used for concrete), and some concrete-reinforcing mesh. The mesh looks like wire fencing, typically comes in 5-foot (1.5-meter) widths in rolls or panels, and is available from hardware stores and lumberyards. To cover a garden bed that's 4 feet (1.2 meters) wide, cut the mesh to a 6-foot (1.8-meter) length with wire snips or a pair of bolt cutters. Bend the mesh into an arch form, then anchor it at each corner over the bed by driving the rebar pieces through the mesh like tent stakes, using a hammer or small

sledge. Now dig a trench 4 to 5 inches (10 to 13 cm) deep along one side of the resulting tunnel, lay one edge of the plastic sheet in this trench, cover it with soil, and anchor it further with rocks. Pull the plastic over the archway, and anchor it at the ends and on the other long side with rocks, bricks, or a piece of lumber. Use clothespins to gather the loose plastic and keep it from flapping in the wind.

This simple shelter will protect seedlings from cool breezes, keeping the temperature inside several degrees warmer on frosty nights, and it's sturdy enough to resist a snowfall, Lokey says. Always open up the plastic during sunny days or the plants inside will get too hot. When the danger of frost is past, put away the structure or move it to cover some newer seedlings. The same structure can be used to protect plants from frost in the fall, or even to keep producing salad greens all winter. You won't feel like you need to take out a second mortgage to buy a fancy greenhouse.

Protect seedlings with a homemade cloche. The French invented the glass cloche, or bell jar, to protect seedlings from frost. You can buy beautiful cloches today, but why not save your centimes and make them yourself from plastic 2-liter soda bottles or 1-gallon (3.7-liter) milk jugs? Using a sharp knife, carefully slice the entire bottom from the bottle. Place the bottle over the seedling, leaving the cap off for ventilation. Bury the lower edge of the bottle in the soil to anchor it

How I Do It A Veggie Grower's Surefire Seed Mix

Nancy Deines has been gardening in eastern Colorado for half a century, and one of her favorite tricks for the vegetable garden is mixing carrot seeds with radish seeds. She spaces the seeds evenly in the row, starting early in the growing season and continuing to plant every few weeks until midsummer. Here's the beauty of it: Radishes are among the quickest vegetables to sprout from seed, and the fast-growing seedlings will mark the row within a week. As the radishes are harvested, they break up the soil next to the maturing carrots, allowing them to grow thicker and deeper. And the carrots will be easier to pull when it comes time to harvest.

Another hint from Nancy: The best-tasting carrots are the ones pulled right after the first frost.

in place, or poke a stick into the ground next to the seedling and place the bottle over the stick. With the money you've saved, buy yourself a nice bottle of French wine.

Try this simpler method for supporting tomato plants. Trellises or cages work well enough for holding up tomato vines, but they are not always cheap and you have to find a place to store them. As a result, many commercial growers have adopted the "Florida weave" for supporting tomato plants, and there's no reason home growers shouldn't use it too. To construct the Florida weave, drive a steel fence post or sturdy wooden post at each end of the row of tomato plants and at every second plant between. Now tie polypropylene twine, which doesn't stretch, to the post at one end of the row about 10 inches (25 cm) off the ground. Run the cord to the second stake, and secure it by wrapping it a couple of times around the stake at the same level.

Continue to the end of the row, keeping the cord tight, then return back up the row on the other side of the stakes, securing the cord at each post. The tomato plants' stems should be held between the two taut cords. As the plants grow, add new layers of twine about 10 inches (25 cm) apart. Prune suckers to remove the weight that must be supported and encourage productive growth. You won't need those old tomato cages anymore, but maybe you can make a few bucks by selling them at a yard sale and put it toward seeds for the following season.

Keep those fresh garden vegetables coming in the fall. The grocer starts rubbing his hands with anticipation as the first frosts approach, knowing that home gardeners will soon be forced to return to the veggie aisle in numbers. But you can extend your growing season for weeks if you plant the right vegetables and take a few simple steps as autumn approaches.

Broccoli, cauliflower, peas, spinach, and many other greens can be planted in midsummer for a fall harvest, and root crops such as beets, carrots, parsnips, and turnips will stay fresh in the ground through the fall and into winter. (Mulch over the tops of these plants to prevent the ground from freezing around them.)

To keep plants producing as long as possible, continue to water regularly, keep picking fruit before it goes to seed, don't get lazy about weeding as the summer wanes, and cut back overgrown foliage near the garden so your vegetables get enough sunlight.

Often the first frost of the season is only a warning sign, and if you protect your plants, you'll get another two or three weeks of warm growing weather before regular frosts set in. Cover tender plants with lightweight blankets, sheets, newspapers, or even buckets or tubs. Remove these covers as soon as the temperature rises above freezing the next day. This way, your greengrocer will keep tapping his fingers on the counter and waiting for you to come shopping.

Hang those green tomatoes. If sub-freezing weather is forecast and your tomato vines are still loaded down with green fruit, pull the entire plant out of the ground and hang it upside down in a cool, dark place, such as a basement or garage. The fruit will ripen, and you'll enjoy homegrown tomatoes for another couple of weeks while the trucks full of rock-hard out-of-state tomatoes unload at the supermarket. ◁

Your Lawn
6 Tricks to Help You Create a Lush Low-Care Sea of Green in Your Yard

Build up the low yellow spots.
The makers and sellers of pest and fungus treatments would love you to believe that every yellow or dead spot is the result of a sinister invader that can be eliminated with frequent use of their expensive products. But some yellow spots are simply the result of low spots in your lawn, especially if they appear after heavy rain. Grass can suffocate or rot in standing water. Try spreading a layer of compost over the yellow spot to raise it up to the level of the surrounding ground. Within a week or two, new grass will likely sprout to fill the patch.

Quit bagging up grass trimmings.
If you have the kind of mower that shreds grass and drops it right back onto the lawn, you can reduce the recommended amount of lawn fertilizer by at least a third—and possibly even half. The salespeople at your garden center would tear their hair out if they knew you were onto this secret, but a mulching mower will save you having to spread pounds and pounds of chemical fertilizer every year.

Save a bundle on lawn aeration.
It seems that every year a swarm of eager workers roam around the neighborhood posting handbills and ringing doorbells, insisting that you need to aerate your lawn—right now! If you don't keep track, you might do it three or four times a year. Relax. Most lawns only need aerating once a year to improve the drainage and breathability of soil, and it's important to do it at the right time for your area and grass type. Some

grasses do better with aeration at the beginning of the growing season, and some prefer it at the end.

You don't have to pay someone else an arm and a leg to do your aeration. It's not rocket science, and it's no more strenuous than mowing a lawn. Just be sure to mark your sprinkler heads and any buried cables first. Ask several of your neighbors if they'd like to go in on an aeration party, then chip in to rent a machine. You can hire the machines at hardware stores for half a day for about the same amount that you'd pay to have a single lawn aerated. You can take turns using the machine on each of your own lawns, or pay a strapping teenager to do them all in a morning. Either way, you'll come out ahead.

Treat your lawn to a healthy tonic.
You don't have to pay big bucks to the fertilizer makers to spruce up your lawn with a shot of healthy nutrients. Many homeowners have had great success with homemade lawn "tonics" made from simple products that might already be on your pantry shelves. The recipes vary, but most share these common ingredients:

1 can non-light beer

1 can non-diet soda pop

1 cup ammonia

1 cup liquid dish soap

1 cup molasses or corn syrup

1/2 cup mouthwash

What do these ingredients have to do with promoting a healthy lawn? The beer, soda, and molasses stimulate bene-ficial microbes. The ammonia is a source of nitrates, the main ingredient in most fertilizers. The soap helps spread the solution evenly and bind it to the blades of grass. And the alcohol in mouthwash deters some pests. Mix these ingredients in the reservoir of a 10- or 20-gallon (38- or 76-liter) hose-end sprayer, and apply it to your lawn every three weeks or so. Water well after application. Your lawn will be lusher and need less water, and the big oil companies that supply the raw materials for many fertilizers will have lost another customer.

EXPERT INSTANT ADVICE

Reseeding a Lawn

Whether you've got a small bare patch or half a lawn to reseed, it's best to do it in the late summer or fall, when cool temperatures will give the grass a good start.

1. Rake off any dead grass and debris. Loosen the soil in the bare patch to a depth of 1 inch (2.5 cm). If the grass was killed by dog urine or a chemical spill, douse the area thoroughly with water several times to dilute the harmful chemicals.

2. Spread 2 to 3 inches (5 to 7.6 cm) of compost over the area, then smooth it with the back of a rake so the compost is level with the surrounding soil.

3. Mix the seed with an equal amount of damp sand a day before you sow it. The moisture will jump-start the process of germination. Scatter the seeds evenly with the sand; that way, they'll stay in place on the ground, even on a windy day.

4. Cover the seeds with a thin layer of compost, then water the area gently, being careful not to wash the seeds away.

5. Keep the area moist with a fine spray of water two or three times a day until the seeds germinate, then water regularly along with the rest of your lawn.

How I Do It   A Mowing Pro's Guide to Creating a Beautiful Lawn

Yard-maintenance companies will tell you that only their experts know how to mow a lawn beautifully every time. But with these expert mowing techniques recommended by Bill Klutho, gardening guru at the John Deere tractor company, you can have a lawn as smooth as the fairways at Pebble Beach, without paying the "greens fees" demanded by lawn professionals.

☐ *Alternate your mowing route.* Lawns that are mowed the same direction every time develop unsightly stripes that may grow back irregularly. To avoid creating a pattern that lasts all season, alternate mowing one direction across the lawn the first time and then perpendicular to this direction the next time.

☐ *Mow early.* For the best cut, mow in mid to late morning, when it's cool but the morning dew has dried off.

☐ *Take your time.* Don't speed through mowing, because you may miss spots. While you're mowing in a wide-open area, stay in control by keeping your mower on a medium speed setting. Throttle down to lower speeds when you're turning corners and trimming borders for a closer cut.

☐ *Adhere to the one-third rule.* For a healthy lawn, never remove more than one-third of the grass blade at one time.

☐ *Don't cut your grass too short.* Grass about 3 inches (8 cm) tall usually looks better, encourages a deeper root system, and helps prevent weeds from invading.

☐ *Keep your blade sharp.* Sharp lawn mower blades produce a well-manicured lawn, and clean cuts promote better grass health. Use a mill bastard file or a grinding wheel to sharpen the blade, maintaining the blade-surface angle that came from the manufacturer.

☐ *Water infrequently but deeply.* In most parts of North America, lawns need about an inch of water per week during the growing season.

Deter lawn-damaging raccoons. If you wake up in the morning to discover small round holes in your lawn or even large patches of turf mysteriously rolled up, it is probably the work of raccoons or skunks, who visit at night and dig in search of worms, grubs, or other insects that live in your lawn. They are especially likely to show up after a rain, when the water forces their prey close to the surface. Some pest control experts would have you believe that the only viable solutions to this problem are expensive ones: installing a secure or electrified fence, setting out traps, or undertaking an elaborate grub-elimination program with toxic insecticides. But the solution is quite simple. Just go to the store and buy a couple of boxes of moth crystals and sprinkle them over your lawn. This will help persuade the raccoons, who have very sensitive noses, to dine elsewhere. Also, to avoid attracting them, make sure your garbage cans can't be knocked over and have lids that are securely closed, with a bungee cord if necessary.

Dogged by yellow-spotted grass?

If you have a dog and your lawn is covered with yellow or brown circles, the dog's urine may be the culprit. In serious cases, the spots may require reseeding or new sod. The problem is the nitrogen in the urine: Although nitrogen is a key ingredient in most fertilizers, the concentration in undiluted urine is too high for the grass, and it dies from the stress of its own growth. It's a myth that female canine urine contains some substance that causes the die-off. The likely reason female dogs cause more problems is that they tend to urinate all at once on a flat surface, rather than marking as males do, thus concentrating their impact in one spot.

What to do? Some books and websites claim that changing the pH in a dog's urine by altering its diet will reduce the damaging effect of the urine. Veterinarians say, "Hogwash!" Changing the pH content of dog urine has not been shown to affect its impact on grass, and making a dog's food more acidic or alkaline in an effort to change pH can be dangerous, possibly leading to bladder stones or infections. The only way to remedy the problem is to dilute the dog's urine, and there are two ways to do that. The most effective is to pour water on the spot on the grass within 8 hours of a dog urinating on it. Less effective but also helpful is adding water to the dog's diet, through feeding it wet food or moistening dry food with water. The dog will relieve itself more often, but the concentration of nitrogen in the urine will be lower. ◅

Landscaping
7 Little-Known Tricks for Turning an Ordinary Yard into a Dream Setting

Landscape with clipboard and shoe leather.
Before hiring a designer or spending a small fortune on new plants, take a walk around your neighborhood with a clipboard and a digital camera, recommends landscape designer Ryan Peif from Greeley, Colorado. Make a checklist of the types of plants you need in your landscaping—flowers, ground covers, shrubs, and such—then take note of the plants you like or dislike in each category around the neighborhood. Equally important, observe what grows well in yards and gardens with the same sun exposure as your own—the soil type and growing conditions in your neighbors' gardens are likely to be very similar to your own. If you see a plant you don't recognize, take a photograph or ask your neighbor for its name. You're not trying to mimic that beautiful garden at the Jones's house down the block—you're picking the best of the best from an entire row of gardens.

Now, armed with your checklist and the photos of plants you might like, head to a garden center and start shopping. The experts there will help—for free—with advice on when to plant each variety, how big they will grow, and how many plants you need to fill a given space. You're well on your way to a beautiful landscape, and without the overhead of a landscape designer.

Use a free landscape consultant.
If you go to a residential landscaper and give him carte blanche to come up with a plan for your yard, dollar signs will immediately pop into his eyes. So why

not start the process with the services of a free consultant instead? In the United States, the local Cooperative Extension office will provide free pointers and free literature to help you establish the look you want, based on the character of your neighborhood, the climate you live in, and the care required to maintain the plantings and features you want to include in your yard. You can find your local extension office in your phone book's federal government listings, under the Department of Agriculture. Enlist the Cooperative Extension's help in drafting a detailed plan for your yard, and *then* approach a landscaper if you need further professional help. You'll be in much more control of the landscaping budget when you know what you're talking about.

Try the low-tech method for laying out landscaping. Many professional landscapers use specialized computer software to help their clients visualize exactly how their landscaping will look—and to tweak the design until it's just right. But guess who's paying for the fancy computer gear? If you're designing your own landscape, you can use this low-cost way to visualize the outlines of paths, beds, and walls. Buy some brightly colored clothesline or similar lightweight, highly visible cord. Lay the cord along the lines of your paths and beds. Now you can check out the way it looks from different vantage points around your house, deck, and street. It helps to have a partner who can adjust the lines as you make suggestions. When you're happy with the layout, use water-soluble athletic field marking spray (available at many hardware stores) to mark the lines. Place dots every couple of feet along the lines, a couple of inches inside the planned path

or bed. Double-check the position from your different viewing points, then paint a solid line. This is where you'll dig.

Scope out new garden centers. Identify the neighboring yards that you admire, and ask the people who live there where they shop for plants and supplies. Then visit the garden center they recommend, but leave your checkbook or credit card at home. Ask lots of questions about your garden's problems and needs without any obvious intention of buying anything. If the staff gives you ample attention and answers your questions coherently and completely, you'll feel happy coming back with your wallet. It's the quality of information the staff provides that marks the main difference between a great garden center and your average home and garden store.

Keep the grass. Your nursery and landscape store would prefer you didn't think about it, but decks, outdoor fountains, and even flower beds are generally more work for the homeowner than simple grass. Decks need resealing periodically, fountains need their water skimmed and filters cleaned, and flower beds require weeding, deadheading, mulching, and more. Square foot for square foot, mowing a regular lawn is a comparative breeze.

Wait and save on plants and supplies. Your garden center sure wishes you'd pay top dollar by stocking up in the spring, when demand is high for plants and supplies. But if you have the space to store items like potting soil, manure, and fertilizer, you'll save a bundle if you buy it in the fall, when merchants are trying to move out their inventory. Planning a big landscaping job for next year? Order your fencing, stones, and other materials in the fall, and store them over the winter for big savings. Bulbs are usually planted in the fall, so they won't be discounted, but this is also usually the best time of year for planting trees, shrubs, and many perennials, and some garden centers may be overstocked on these plants as winter approaches. Landscaping contractors, too, may be eager to squeeze in a final job after most people have stopped thinking about their lawns and gardens—they may be more willing than usual to dicker on price.

Add a simple water feature to your yard. Although a small pond, burbling stream, or splashing fountain is often a highly desirable addition to a landscape, building these features can be expensive and fraught with problems. But there's an easy way to add water and life to your garden that doesn't involve moving parts or a pricey contractor. All it takes is a kids' plastic wading pool, says Indiana nursery owner Gene Bush.

Using Bush's plan, you can use a wading pool to build a self-contained bog that's perfect for water-loving plants such as irises and marsh marigolds.

- Choose a site where the new plants will look natural—the border of a wood or near a pond or ditch, for instance.
- Excavate a hole to the depth and diameter of the kiddie pool. Test the pool's fit in the hole, and remove or add dirt until the pool sits flat on the bottom of the hole and its top rim is level with the ground or lawn.

- Using an awl or a sharp knife, punch holes around the sides of the pool 4 inches (10 cm) below the rim, to allow some drainage during periods of heavy rain. Install the pool in the hole and pack dirt around the sides firmly.
- Now fill the entire pool with a mixture of one half coarse sand and one half peat. Level the surface, then use flat stones or pavers to cover the plastic lip of the pool. Flood the pool with water, and you're done.

It's ideal to construct your kiddie-pool bog in the fall, allowing it to settle over the winter, and make final adjustments or additions in the spring before planting. Any plants that love wet feet will thrive in your new bog, including cow parsnips, irises, creeping Jennie, and many more. To maintain the garden, all you need to do is ensure it stays wet, Bush says. By midsummer you'll have a beautiful new addition to your yard, and you won't have lined the pockets of a landscape designer. ◁

Getting Healthy Plants at a
Discount Center

Garden centers and nurseries would like you to believe you're a fool if you buy plants from discount hardware outfits, supermarkets, and department stores, but in many cases these discounters buy plants from the same distributors as the premium garden centers do. The difference is in what happens after the plants go on display at the store—generally, plants will receive more expert care and constant attention at a garden center, and so they'll stay healthier.

How do you avoid buying a lemon of a lemon tree at a big-box retailer? Fortunately, plants don't have very good poker faces—they show how they're feeling, and if you know what to look for, you can buy healthy plants wherever you shop. So here are five things to watch.

General surroundings

Take a quick look at all of the plants on display. If they generally look good, they're probably getting decent care. If half of them are drooping or brown, head somewhere else, even if the plants you want look healthy.

Roots

If roots are bunched up and growing profusely out of the drainage holes, the plant is pot-bound and likely stressed. Conversely, if the plant lifts easily from the pot, it may have just been repotted, and its roots won't be ready for the garden. With trees or shrubs, the root-ball should feel solid inside the burlap covering.

Overall appearance

The leaves should be green and shiny, not wilting or yellow and brown. The plant should be full and bushy, rather than tall and lean. Stems should be uncracked and scar-free.

Buds

Look for budding rather than flowering plants. Budding plants will transplant easier.

Pests and disease

Inspect the entire plant carefully, especially under the leaves, for any pests or signs of disease.

If the plant passes this entire inspection with flying colors, it likely will thrive in your garden, no matter the pedigree of the purveyor.

Yard Care

6 Maintenance Tricks That Every Home Gardener Should Be Aware Of

Lay off the fertilizer with new plantings. Novice gardeners may be tempted to fertilize newly planted trees or shrubs right away—and unscrupulous fertilizer sellers will egg them on. But fertilizing stresses new plantings severely, because the plants will produce too much stem and foliage growth without the root system to support that growth. Instead, wait several months after planting before applying fertilizer. If everyone knew this, fertilizer company stocks might sink a bit, but plants would be thankful.

Save money on plant-food refills. Those liquid plant-food sprayers that attach to the end of a hose are super-convenient, but they come with a hidden cost. When the bottle of plant food is empty, the manufacturer is betting you'll buy another bottle as a refill … and another … and another, thus padding the company's bottom line. Manufacturers promise a miracle with their liquids, but just because Brand X came in the bottle doesn't mean you can't refill it with the less expensive Brand Y or your favorite recipe for homemade liquid fertilizer. These bottles often carry a warning label that says something like, "Empty bottles cannot be reused." That's because there's an insert in the neck of the bottle specially designed to make a snug fit with the sprayer end. But here's the trick: In most cases it's easy to gently pop out this insert with a screwdriver or a pair of pliers. Now refill the bottle, tap the insert back into place, and hook up the sprayer. If you're careful, you can reuse the same bottle many times.

Here's a good recipe for homemade liquid plant food: Mix 1 tablespoon Epsom salts, 1 teaspoon baking soda, and 1/4 teaspoon ammonia, then add this to 1/2 gallon (2 liters) warm water. Dilute this mix with another gallon (3.7 liters) of water, and spray your plants with this brew once a month. It's also good for houseplants.

Leave branches in place to root out stumps. Digging out the stumps of big shrubs and trees is nasty work, and you might be tempted to dig out the checkbook instead and pay a landscaping company to do the dirty work for you. But if you know one of these pros' favorite secrets, you can leave some green stuff in your wallet. When you have to remove a shrub or tree that has sturdy branches, don't cut it all the way to the ground before digging out the stump. Instead, remove most of the trunk and branches, but leave two or three stout limbs attached to the stump, spaced around the circumference. Now, when you start digging, you can use these branches as levers, giving you major mechanical advantage for working the stump and roots out of the ground.

Steer clear of trees with that "weed and feed." Your local home center might like you to believe that the "weed and feed" mix on sale this week will solve all your lawn problems, but it can cause new problems if you apply it carelessly. Many trees, shrubs, and ornamental plants can be stressed or even killed by such fertilizer, and weed-killer mixes applied to the lawn above their

How to Apply Herbicides Safely

Sometimes you have to use an herbicide to control a virulent weed. But one drop of herbicide on the wrong leaf could kill a plant you love. To reduce this risk as much as possible:

- Always consider every alternative to chemical weed controls before spraying. The best defense against weeds is a healthy garden and lawn, with mulch covering any bare ground or empty spaces.

- Before applying any herbicide, check local restrictions. For example, one popular herbicide ingredient, 2,4-D, has been banned in some localities.

- Spray first thing in the morning or in the evening, when it's cool and there is no wind. Some herbicides (those containing 2,4-D, 2,4-DP, and dicamba or MCPA, MCPP, and dicamba) will turn to vapor and move through the air as the day warms. It's safer to use these chemicals in the evening so the weeds will have more time to absorb them before the temperature rises.

- When you are mixing herbicides, remember that stronger is not necessarily better—it may just be adding cost and putting your other plants at more risk without increasing effectiveness.

- Adjust the nozzle to a medium to coarse spray, and keep the sprayer low to the ground to reduce drift of airborne chemicals.

- Use a 2-foot (60-cm) square of cardboard as a shield to protect your good plants.

- Always wear eye protection and gloves.

root zones. Certain plants are extremely sensitive to mixes that contain dicamba or phenoxy herbicides, including apple, box elder, catalpa, dogwood, forsythia, honey locust, lilac, Siberian elm, and sycamore. Keep the spreader well away from such trees, and treat specific weeds only as needed.

Be careful using weed barrier cloth. Landscaping fabric and other artificial weed barriers are effective options to herbicides—to a point—but they may also cause new problems and still fail to prevent weed growth in the long run. In many cases, it's a shortcut not worth taking, says professional gardener Susan McCausland from Boulder, Colorado. The best place to use barrier cloth is under gravel or rock borders, walkways, and other places where few or no plants are growing.

In garden beds, especially in wet climates, weed barriers may cause numerous problems: They can hold too much moisture, suffocating some plants. They can promote the growth of molds and fungi, and they may cause roots to grow shallower. Moreover, since most people mulch over weed barriers, they soon create a new layer of topsoil as the mulch decomposes, and the weeds that move into this fresh soil will be even harder to remove because their roots will intertwine with the barrier fabric. Even if you don't mulch over the fabric, organic material and seeds will eventually blow in, and weeds will take root.

Plastic barriers are the worst: They block oxygen and moisture from reaching the soil, and they become brittle and disintegrate, making them very difficult to remove. Fabric landscaping or agricultural sheeting is better, because it breathes. The best barriers are those that can be removed each season, so the soil can breathe, or that decompose into the soil, such as burlap or newspaper. Landscapers and garden shops will try to tempt you with this one-stop solution to weeds, but the real way to fight weeds, McCausland says, is to craft healthy soil with compost and mulch and to pull weeds regularly so problems don't get out of control.

Try these homemade hose guides. If you read gardening catalogs, you'd think you're not a good gardener unless you pay for fancy hose guides to keep the hose from wrecking your favorite plants or tipping over lawn furniture as you drag it around the lawn. But it's easy to make your own guides and install them anywhere a hose might snag. To start, buy the required number of 18-inch (46-cm) lengths of rebar. These are available precut at gardening centers. Drive these rods into the soil with a hammer or hand sledge. To prevent injuries, never leave the end of the rebar exposed; instead, cover the bar with one of these attractive choices:

- Paint a PVC pipe, 1 inch (2.5 cm) in diameter, an attractive color or pattern, and cut it just long enough to cover the rebar. The hose will spin the pipe as it rolls past.

- Cut bamboo or copper tubing to the appropriate lengths and use these as rollers.

- Find two ceramic pots that are about 4 inches (10 cm) tall and have a drainage hole in the bottom. Slide the two pots, the first facing down and the second facing up, over the rebar. The two stacked pots will create an hourglass-shaped roller. If the drainage hole is a little too small to fit over the rebar, widen the hole by twisting the rebar into the opening until it slides easily through. ◁

Pest Control
8 Special Tricks for Sending All Those Plant-Eating Critters Packing

Learn more before you spray. Beth Smerek, a bedding plant specialist at a Boulder, Colorado, nursery, advises that most insects are beneficial or neutral to your plants, and when beneficial insects (such as those that eat pests) are killed, a dependency on chemicals is created. Before killing everything that moves the minute you notice some holes in the leaves, bring an affected leaf or picture of the problem to a reputable garden center or an extension agent and find out what is wrong. Then you can choose the treatment that will attack that problem specifically. Smerek adds that it's safer to use chemical treatments on indoor plants, because the indoor environment is completely artificial and contained, and thus the chemicals won't affect creatures other than the target pests.

Kill slugs with beer or coffee. You can buy expensive and toxic slug repellents, but natural methods are cheaper and just as effective. Slugs, it turns out, have a fatal vice: They like beer too much. Fill an empty tuna or cat-food can with beer and bury it in your garden soil up to its rim. Overnight, slugs will move into the beer and drown. You can throw out the entire can in the morning and replace it with a fresh batch. Not a beer drinker? Slugs hate coffee—or at least caffeine—just as much as they like beer. Researchers have found that a solution of 1 percent to 2 percent caffeine will kill slugs. That's much more than the average cup of coffee contains, but coffee still might act as a deterrent. Spray foliage with the brew or sprinkle the grounds around your plants. (Many coffee shops give away grounds to gardeners for free.) If nothing else, coffee grounds make a good addition to the soil, especially for plants that like acidic soils.

Kill slugs with salt. If you're not squeamish, you can deal with slugs you spot in the garden by hand. Sprinkling salt on the critters will kill them, and you can throw them into the trash. Or you can put a board or two on the garden soil, and slugs and snails will take shelter in the damp shade beneath them. Pick up the boards and scrape the creatures into the trash. To make your garden less inviting to slugs and snails, always water it in the morning. If the soil is dry at night, the critters will be less active.

Use newspapers to control earwigs. Frustrate the insecticide salesmen with this no-poison, low-tech solution to earwig control. In the evening, roll up sheets of wet newspaper and lay them around the garden. At sunrise, earwigs will crawl inside the wet pages to take shelter. Collect the papers before they dry out, bugs and all. Don't throw the newspapers into your trash cans, or the earwigs will soon escape and make their way back to the garden. Either burn the papers and bugs, shake the earwigs into a toilet or sink and flush them down the drain, or tie up the papers and bugs tightly inside a plastic bag—with absolutely no openings—and put them in the garbage can.

Don't rely on marigolds to keep pests away. Those cheerful yellow and orange flowers are often sold to gardeners with the promise that they'll deter pests from attacking vegetables, but marigolds' effectiveness against pests is limited. They only work well as a defense against nematodes in the soil, says veteran gardener Beth Smerek. Still, the blossoms are pretty in the garden, so go ahead and plant them. They can't hurt!

Repel aphids with a citrus-rind spray. Soap solutions are usually the recommended method for dealing with aphids. But the makers of insecticidal soaps don't tell you that some of them may harm your plants as much as, or more than, the little bugs. Here's an approach to try before you spray. Ironically, even though aphids love citrus trees, they don't like ground-up citrus rind. Grate the rind of one lemon or orange and combine it with 1 pint (500 ml) boiling water. Let it steep overnight, then strain through a coffee filter to remove the bits of rind. Add the mixture to a spray bottle, and spray the aphids on the leaves of the plants. Make sure to spray underneath the leaves, where many aphids gather. Reapply every four to seven days as long as the aphid problem persists.

Make your own insecticidal soap spray. If citrus spray doesn't work and you need to turn to soap to get rid of aphids, there's no need to buy a commercial product. Add 2 teaspoons liquid dishwashing detergent to 1 pint (500 ml) water to create an insecticidal soap solution. Now, whether you make it at home or buy it at the store, always test the solution on a few leaves before applying it broadly. Spray a few leaves on each species of plant you'll be treating, then wait a day to see if the leaves curl or spot. If not, you can treat the entire affected area. As with the citrus solution, you'll need to spray every four to seven days.

How I Do It An Expert Gardener's Favorite Organic Pest Controls

Although she runs a major garden center, Connie Smith is not a fan of toxic chemical controls for garden pests. The vast majority of pest problems can be corrected with inexpensive organic solutions, Smith says. Here are her four favorites:

☐ *Soap spray.* Great for aphids, mites, and other soft-bodied insects. Choose a commercial variety or brew your own: 2 teaspoons dishwashing liquid, a few drops of vegetable oil, and 1 gallon (3.7 liters) water. Do not use soap sprays in drought or hot weather, or you may damage leaves, and always test them first on a few leaves.

☐ *Horticultural oil sprays.* These smother eggs and developing pests. Use light oils year-round, except in temperatures over 85°F (29°C). Use dormant oils before plants leaf out.

☐ *Sulfur or lime sulfur spray.* Use to control fungus such as powdery mildew and various blights. It's especially effective on fruit trees, berry bushes, and roses. In general, this spray should be applied during the dormant months or very early in the growing season, as buds begin to swell. Do not apply in temperatures over 90°F (32°C), and never use within two weeks of applying horticultural oil.

☐ *Bt (Bacillus thuringiensis).* This is bacteria, usually sold in a spray, that is used as a last organic resort to control caterpillars and some moth larvae. A different form is used to kill mosquito larvae.

Smith says the first three sprays will solve 80 percent of common garden pest problems, with no harmful residues or other long-term issues.

Get rid of grubs and Japanese beetles for good. If you have a problem with grubs eating your grass and plants, chances are you also have a problem with Japanese beetles, because the grubs are most likely the larvae of the beetles. You can solve both problems by just killing the grubs so that they don't develop into beetles. Although gardening outlets are quick to sell fast-acting toxic chemicals to kill the grubs (and a lot of other less harmful insects), there is a perfectly fine natural remedy that will get rid of them for years to come. Called milky spore, it causes the grubs to contract a disease that kills them. Other beneficial organisms are not harmed. The only problem is that you have to be patient. Milky spore is slow acting—after you spread the granules on your lawn, it can take a year or more for the spore to become established in your soil. But once the spore is established, it keeps working for a decade or more. There are reports of a single treatment lasting 40 years. Milky spore is not cheap; a single can of the granules runs about $40, but considering the length of the benefit, it's a real bargain. ◄

Animal Pests

5 Strategies for Making Destructive Four-Legged Visitors Unwelcome in Your Yard

Stink that groundhog out with cat litter. A groundhog (woodchuck) has taken up residence in a burrow that's conveniently next to your backyard garden. The pest control company wants a couple hundred dollars to remove him. Even if the cost doesn't give you pause, then the traps or poisons that some of them use will—particularly if you have kids or pets. What the pest control company won't tell you is that it's easy to stink a groundhog out of his home—for zero cost. Each day when you scoop out the cat boxes in your house, dump that foul-smelling debris down Mr. Groundhog's hole instead of throwing it into the trash can. After a few days of this treatment, the groundhog will pack up and move. Once he's gone, pour rocks into all of the entrances to the burrow so no other animals will decide to move in.

Protect your garden from deer with eggs. A family of deer can wreak havoc on your yard.

They breakfast in vegetable gardens and munch ornamentals and fruit trees at night while you sleep. What to do? Put the shotguns away. Save your money by saying no to high-tech gadgets like strobe lights and noisemakers, expensive repellents, and tall, ugly fences. For a fence to be effective, it must be a full 8 feet (2.4 meters) high—11 inches (28 cm) taller than Shaquille O'Neal. Instead, arm yourself with eggs. Deer hate the taste and smell of raw eggs, which is why many popular commercial repellents feature stinky egg solids as the main ingredient. Here's what you do: Crack half a dozen eggs into 2 quarts (2 liters) water. Mix well, until all the yolks are broken and blended with the water. Sprinkle the raw-egg mixture on the leaves of the plants you want to protect. The mixture should remain effective until the next rain. Reapply after that.

There are other odors that deer don't like: Try hanging cheesecloth bags of stinky socks, deodorant soap, or human hair in the garden. (You can get hair at a salon or barbershop.) The smell may make wary deer steer clear of your garden.

Choose plants to keep deer away. Deer also don't like to brush against certain aromatic plants. So try planting artemisia, lavender, and Russian sage as a natural fence line. Or, if you can't get the deer to stop eating the plants they like, consider replanting with plants that deer dislike. These include such popular plants as begonias, cosmos, daffodils, foxgloves, irises, marigolds, peonies, snapdragons, and zinnias, along with shrubs and trees such as boxwood, holly, juniper, lilac, pine, and spruce.

Fence rabbits out of your veggie patch. Numerous sprays and powders are sold to deter rabbits from the garden, but many of these are not safe for use on garden vegetables. A rabbit-proof fence is the best protection for your vegetable garden. Use chicken wire, and make sure the fence's bottom is buried by at least 6 to 12 inches (15 to 30 cm), otherwise the rabbits will tunnel underneath it. The fence needs to extend at least 30 inches (76 cm) above the ground.

Try other rabbit deterrents. Because a fence is an unattractive addition to many gardens, you may want to try a few low-impact deterrents against voracious bunnies:

- Remove brush piles and other hiding places for rabbits. Clean up spilled birdseed from feeders.
- Post realistic-looking rubber models of snakes or owls in the garden, or cut an old hose into snakelike lengths and coil them among your plants.
- Hang dog hair in cheesecloth bags or distribute it among the plants to frighten away rabbits. Strong-smelling soaps are also said to deter rabbits.
- You can buy coyote or fox urine to spread among plants, fooling rabbits into thinking a predator is nearby.

Remember, rabbits are not dumb bunnies. Eventually they will figure out they're safe from each of these deterrents, so you'll have to mix up your methods to keep them on their toes. ◁

Gardening Tools
7 Easy Ways to Get a Handle On the Tools That You Use to Care for Your Garden

Spritz your tools to repel dirt. The secret weapon against messy tools is the cooking oil spray you keep in the kitchen cabinet. Spray a coat on a shovel or trowel before using it, and clay soil will slide right off. Spray the blades and underside of your lawn mower, and wet grass won't stick to them. Another trick for clean tools? Keep a bucket of sand in the garage or shed, and plunge a spade or hoe into the sand before putting it away. The sand will scrape off any dirt or other mess that has stuck to the blades.

No need for fancy kneepads. Here's a low-cost alternative for gardening kneepads: Use a scrap from an old closed-cell foam camping mat. This will protect your knees just as well as the fancy models in gardening catalogs. It's tough, shock absorbing, and easy to clean with soap and water. If you or your kids don't have an old pad to cut up, check with your local Boy Scout troop or a university outdoor program. The pads get torn and are often replaced. Your garden shop manager will be on his knees begging you for business when he hears about this.

Make tools easy to spot. Don't lose your tools among your flower beds, shrubs, and grass. Exposure to the weather could harm them, and they could pose a danger to passers-by as well. To keep your hand tools from disappearing, paint the handles bright red or orange, making them more visible, a trick dating back to at least the 19th century. A couple of wraps of bright electrical tape will serve the same purpose. Either way, you won't be ringing the cash registers down at the garden center as soon as you might otherwise.

Make a simple tool stand between garage studs. Before investing in a high-priced rack for your garden tools in a shed or garage, look at the walls: If the walls are framed with exposed 2 x 4 (38 x 89 cm) studs, anyone can build a stand for garden tools in a matter of minutes. All you need is some 1 x 4 (19 x 38 cm) pine, some scraps of old 2 x 4, and some nails.

- For long-handled tools—such as shovels and rakes—cut a length of 1 x 4 so that it spans a couple of studs and nail it into place about 36 inches (90 cm) above the floor.
- For shorter-handled tools—an axe, for instance—nail another length of 1 x 4 between two studs about 24 inches (60 cm) above the floor.

- For both sets of tools, nail another 1 x 4 across the bottom of the studs to form a foot piece that will keep the lower end of your tools from sliding out.
- Finally, to help keep the tools upright, cut short blocks of 2 x 4 as spacers and nail them between the 1 x 4s and the garage wall at both the top and bottom. Two blocks in each cavity between studs usually works fine.

Voilà! Slide your hoe or rake behind the 1 x 4s, handle first, and it will be held in place for quick access.

Give trimmings a saucer ride. How do you move weeds, pruned branches, rocks, and the like from your garden? Hoity-toity gardening catalogs would have you believe you need to spend a small fortune on a pushcart. But, in

Give Your Lawn Mower a **Tune-Up**

When the lawn mower starts running a bit rough, don't run to a repair shop and pay an exorbitant minimum charge and steep hourly rates. Maybe all you need is a single new spark plug. Even the least handy homeowner can keep his lawn mower in tip-top shape with this simple annual tune-up. Each mower is a little different, and you should consult your owner's manual for the specifics of your machine. But these basics apply to every mower.

☐ Before you work on a lawn mower, always remove the wire going to the spark plug so that there is no way that you can accidentally start the mower.

☐ Clean the underside of the mower thoroughly, scraping off dried-up grass clippings with a putty knife. Unplug any air vents and channels.

☐ Unscrew the spark plug with a deep-socket wrench that fits the hexagonal nut. Install a new plug of the exact same type, being careful not to cross-thread it (setting it in askew, so the threads get damaged as you turn it). Tighten gently.

☐ Unscrew the engine cover and vacuum up any dirt and grass clippings.

☐ Unscrew the oil dipstick and carefully tip the mower onto its side, allowing the dirty oil to drain into a pan, such as an old pie tin. (Some mowers have an oil drain plug that can be removed with a wrench, so the oil can be drained without tilting the mower.) Check the owner's manual for the correct oil type, and pour in new oil until the dipstick reads "full." Clean up any spilled oil with a rag.

☐ Unscrew the air-filter cover, remove the filter, and discard it. Clean the filter area thoroughly with a rag and an old toothbrush. New paper air filters are simply reinserted with the pleated side facing out. Foam filters should be soaked in clean, new motor oil; squeeze out the extra oil onto a rag, then insert the foam filter into the proper position. Replace the cover.

Before storing a mower for the winter

Run it until the gas tank is empty. Disconnect the gas line and, if possible, lift off or unscrew the gas tank and clean it by putting half a cup of fresh gas inside and swishing it vigorously. Do not store gasoline in any container over the winter; always use fresh gas in the spring.

Parts for popular mowers are available at hardware and yard-supplies shops. And you won't pay a repair shop's markup to get them.

addition to their expense, carts and wheelbarrows are heavy and unwieldy, especially on hills. They're often overkill for everyday tasks. The solution? A flying saucer sled. Attach a rope to a handle of one of these round, steel or plastic sleds, and you'll have a sturdy sledge that pulls easily across grass and paths. If you have kids, come winter, this is one garden tool that will still find plenty of use!

Put old golf gear to work in the garden. You can buy all sorts of carts and racks to wheel around the garden with your rakes and trowels. But you can skip right past that page of the gardening catalog if you have an old golf bag on wheels. Long tools fit neatly in the main compartment, and hand tools can be clipped to the outside. The pockets hold seeds, shears, and other smaller items. And if you discover any tees inside one of those pockets, they can be put to use too. Wooden or plastic tees make great color-coded markers for newly seeded gardens.

You can't move the holes off a golf course, but you can borrow the idea for use at home. Take a 10-inch (25-cm) length of PVC pipe that's 1 1/2 inches (38 mm) in diameter and bury it so it stands vertically in the ground at the edge of your vegetable plot. Now you have a caddy to hold your rake, hoe, or shovel at the ready: Just turn the tool upside down and slide its handle into the pipe. Strategically locate these tool caddies around your yard and garden.

Coil a hose without mechanical assistance. You can buy all sorts of hose reels and carts—some of them are so elaborate they look like machines the

fire department ought to be operating. If you handle your hose right, you can coil it easily without the fancy gizmos. A hose with longitudinal stripes helps you coil the hose without twists—just keep the stripes running straight as you coil and uncoil. Unkink a hose by pulling one end across the lawn; the weight of the hose will help pull out those twists, and you can judge by the stripes when it's straight. Leave a balky hose in the sun for an hour, and it will be much more pliable and easy to coil.

Inexpensive wall hangers—decorative or plain—make fine places to coil a hose. But if you want to recycle something from home, try these alternatives:

- Cut down an old plastic trash can until you have a tub about 18 inches (46 cm) deep. Punch drainage holes in the base, and coil the hose inside.

- Spin the hose around an old automobile wheel lying flat on the ground. You can dress up the wheel with a coat or two of green or white metal paint to look good in the garden.

- Turn a large old terra-cotta pot upside down and wrap the hose around it.

- To store a hose in winter, drive a stout nail into the wall or a stud in a garage or shed, hang one side of an old bicycle inner tube over the nail, loop the other end through a coiled hose, then pull that end up to hang it over the nail.

Before storing a hose for any length of time, screw the two ends together so that bugs can't nest inside. ◁

gardening Aids

Who says you can only use proper tools in the garden? These common household and workshop objects, including a couple of items normally considered candidates for the trash bin, can be put to work as gardening aids in surprising ways.

Kitchen tongs

Take a pair of kitchen tongs outside with you when it's time to trim back any prickly vines, limbs, or rosebushes. The tongs will allow you to hold or bend the branch painlessly while you snip with the other hand.

Sandpaper

Keep a sheet of fine sandpaper or emery cloth handy in your toolshed. When rust appears on your pruning saw blade or some other metal tool, rub it away with a light sanding. Follow up with a light coating of oil—for instance, from a rag carrying a touch of motor oil or olive oil.

Old hose

A length of old garden hose will help you keep tool edges sharp and prevent accidental cuts. Use heavy shears or a utility knife to cut the old hose to the length of the tool edge (on a saw or shovel, for instance). Then slit the hose lengthwise down one side to make an opening for your tool edge. Slide the edge of the tool into the hose, and secure it with twine or a bungee cord.

Ice pick

Speaking of old hose, if a garden hose that's still in use has sprung pinpoint leaks, go to your toolbox and pull out the ice pick. Heat the point of the ice pick over a candle flame until the tip glows, then touch it carefully to the leaky spot on your hose, letting the surface melt and seal.

Carpenter's belt

Adapt your carpenter's belt to the great outdoors. When you're able to carry all of your little gardening implements around your waist—twine, hand tools, measuring tape, and such—you'll save yourself a score of trips to the shed during one day's work.

Soap bar

Before you dig your hands into that soil, scrape your fingernails across a bar of hand soap. The soap that collects under your nails will create a dirt barrier, preventing that embedded, impossible-to-clean rim of dirt underneath. When you wash your hands, the soap barrier will dissolve.

Coffee grounds

Once your coffee grounds have "done their job" inside the house, put them to work outside too. Sprinkle them in your garden, where they will decompose and add nutrients to the soil.

Paper cups

If your seedlings are vanishing from the flower bed overnight, you need a shield to protect them from pests such as cutworms and slugs. Cut the bottom off a paper cup and place the cup over your seedling to keep the hungry critters at bay.

Clothesline

To make a more comfortable grip on your trowel or another garden tool, wrap the handle tightly in cotton clothesline, then cover the clothesline with several wraps of duct tape. Long-term, the bulkier, softer grip will be easier on your hands.

Buying Clothes

11 Strategies for Finding Flattering Garments at a Reasonable Price

Buy next year's attire now. To save loads of money on your clothing purchases, go shopping toward the end of the selling season. For instance, buy your spring and summer duds in July or August rather than in March, when prices are highest. This will mean some planning and forethought—you're going to get most of the wear out of these new clothes *next* summer. But the payoff is enormous.

So when exactly are the selling seasons for clothing? Michael Laimo of Mercury Beach-Maid, a New York City sportswear wholesaler, says that there are two major selling seasons that apply both to men's and women's clothing:

- Spring/summer: March through the end of August.
- Fall/winter: August through February.

However, women's clothing also has "transitional seasons," which are influenced by weather:

- Summer into fall: August through October (dark clothing with short sleeves).
- Winter into spring: March through April (long sleeves and bright colors).

Invest in one great garment. From those slick magazine ads, you might get the idea that you have to spend a mortgage payment on a single outfit if you want to look stylish. Not so, says Los Angeles clothing designer Bobette Stott. Here's the key to controlling your clothing costs: Buy one key piece of high-quality clothing that you will dry clean and fuss over. This garment should last you for years. For a man this item could be a jacket, a good sweater, or a sport coat. For a woman, it could be a great blouse, a jacket or a nice cardigan sweater. Mix and match your high-quality garment with inexpensive, washable clothing that you replace every couple of seasons. With this approach, you will be investing only in one exquisite, showcase piece of clothing—but it will lend its class and style to anything else you wear.

Avoid "one size fits all" clothing. The idea of "one size fits all" clothing sure sounds attractive: You can't go wrong, right? Buy it, and you know it will fit!

Actually, most manufacturers who label their clothing this way are pulling the wool over your eyes. You will usually find this designation on lower-priced clothing, mostly on tops for teenagers. Here's what manufacturers are up to: It's easier—and therefore cheaper—to mass-produce and inventory a garment when it's all in one size. But the only garments that are truly "one size fits all" are some socks, which are made of fabric that's stretchy enough to adapt to a broad range of foot sizes. Otherwise, when you see "one size fits all" on a garment, keep shopping. Look for higher-quality clothing that will last a long time.

Buy online to get deep designer discounts. The clothing market is swamped with garments that vendors need to unload. This is good news for you, because it means you can buy almost any designer clothing online at a big discount. When you shop at a brick-and-mortar retailer, you are footing the bill for the store's rent, employees' salaries, cushy carpet, and fancy display racks. Online vendors are no-nonsense, product-shipping businesses that do not have all of the overhead and decorative trimmings.

So here's how to get exactly the designer clothing that you want at a fraction of the price: Go to your local department store or boutique. Try on the duds that you like, write down the designer's name, a description of the garment, and the size, then go home. Fire up the computer and conduct an online search for the designer. If the garment you are looking for has been in the stores for just two or three months, you will be able to buy it online for 50 to 75 percent off the retail price.

SECRET WEAPON

RN Number

Garment manufacturers often ship their trendy new styles straight to discount stores at the very same time that they ship them to high-priced department stores, says Stott. The trick is that the manufacturer may package and label the clothing differently for the two stores. How can you tell if the discount-store item is the same, or a cheap knockoff?

Here's the secret: Every piece of clothing is tagged with a code that identifies the garment's manufacturer, no matter what the packaging says. You will see the letters "RN" followed by several numbers on the tag. So jot down the RN number of the garment you like at the department store and see if it matches the number of the garment in the discount store. If the numbers are the same, the manufacturer is the same.

Use these strategies and your clothes will always be on sale. Many of us are programmed to take store pricing at face value. If you see a pair of trousers on the rack priced at $48, well, that's what it's going to cost you to take them home, right? No. The truth is that clothing stores are so desperate to move their merchandise these days that you can take home just about any garment at a discount—if you know how to go about it. Here's how to take advantage of a clothing store's flexible policies:

- Take a full-priced garment to the checkout counter and ask them to hold it for you until it goes on sale. Many stores will accommodate you, and you will be assured that they won't sell out of your size.

- Go ahead and buy the item you want at full price, but keep the receipt in an envelope in your car. Two weeks later, drop into the store with your receipt in hand. If your garment has gone on sale in the meantime, go to the register and ask for credit.

- Make friends with one of the salespeople at your favorite clothing store. This clerk will be able to alert you to upcoming sales, and will keep an eye out for the kind of clothing you like. Selling clothing has become difficult enough that he or she will work like the dickens to get you to buy merchandise.

- If you're making a big purchase at a department store, go ahead and get the extra discount they offer for

---

WHAT **CLOTHING RETAILERS** DON'T WANT YOU TO KNOW ABOUT Pricing

You know the shopper's mantra, "Never pay retail," right? In case you've ever doubted this bit of wisdom, here's an inside glimpse of how retail pricing works for clothing.

It's impossible to know precisely what a particular retailer paid for the garments on display, but the pricing process works like this: Say a shirt comes in with a suggested retail price of $60, preprinted on the hang tag. Early in the selling season, the retailer will put that shirt on display for that price. Out of all of the people who end up buying

that shirt, only 10 to 20 percent of the buyers will pay this original price.

Once you factor in sales and coupons, the price of the shirt starts creeping lower and lower. By the end of the selling season, that shirt is marked down to about $20, which is about what the retailer paid for it. But don't feel bad for the retailer—the store's bean counters have their eye on the *average* selling price of the shirt through its entire sales cycle. The retailer is happy if that average hits twice the wholesale price.

So the next time you consider buying clothing that's not on sale, ask yourself: Isn't it worth waiting a month or two if I can get this garment at a 60 or 70 percent discount?

---

accepting a store credit card. The card will qualify you for future discounts too. But be sure to pay the balance off immediately so you don't have to pay finance charges; store credit cards often have exorbitant interest rates.

Buy classic jeans. When you buy a pair of jeans, put on a pair of blinders so you won't be distracted by all of those trendy styles that involve fading, weird cuts, peculiar colors, and even intentional rips. Manufacturers love it when you fork over cash for this trendy clothing because such jeans go out of style in a heartbeat—and then you have to buy a new pair in whatever the new style is. Instead, buy classic five-pocket blue denim jeans. These will last you for years, and even when they do fade, you won't mind, because they will look totally natural.

Check the nap. Your suit looks funny, but you just can't put your finger on why. Not all manufacturers pay attention to the direction of the nap of fabric—the way the fibers lie—particularly garment makers in developing countries. When you're buying a suit, says Ingrid Johnson, a professor of textiles at the Fashion Institute of Technology in New York City, here's an easy way to test whether the fabric was cut running the same way in both pieces: Run your hand across the fabric in the suit jacket and then in the same direction across the skirt or pants. For instance, you might stroke from top to bottom on a sleeve of the suit jacket and then top to bottom on the skirt. The fabric may feel rough or it may feel smooth—either is okay. But you want to be sure it feels *consistent* on each

piece of the suit. If it doesn't, find another suit.

Color-test duds before buying. When you buy a garment in a store, conduct two quick checks to make sure the coloring in the fabric is high quality: Slip on a pair of sunglasses (the brown-tinted variety work best) to make sure the colors in the clothing still match. Then walk the garment over to a window and check that the colors match in daylight too.

Why bother? Though shoppers rarely hear about it, manufacturers spend a lot of time fretting over a quality issue called metamerism, says Johnson. You see, good manufacturers and retailers make sure that colors of a garment match in all light sources. Here's the problem: A garment may have a few different materials all in the same color—say, a jacket exterior, the cuffs, and the piping. Those different pieces need to all match whether the light source is incandescent, fluorescent, or natural light. If you buy a garment and it doesn't pass this test, you have a right to return it.

Be especially careful when you buy clothing in an off-price outlet. That "bargain" garment could be marked down because it has a serious color problem.

Slip into something old. Open up the yellow pages and jot down the addresses of vintage clothing stores in your area. If you care about the way you dress, it pays to prowl such stores regularly, says Birgit Mueller, an Emmy Award-winning television costume designer. First of all, clothing from the 1950s and 1960s is usually better quality than

5

QUICK FIXES FOR
wardrobe malfunctions

1 Tape up unruly clothing. Slip a few strips of double-stick tape into your purse for use in emergencies. Originally devised for keeping toupees in place, a bit of tape with adhesive on both sides will get you out of any number of dilemmas, says television costume designer Birgit Mueller. If your cleavage is hanging out of your blouse, a couple of strips of double-stick tape will keep your exposure to a minimum. If a button pops off or a hem falls apart, this stuff will secure your clothing until you can have it mended. And if you have to wear a new pair of pants but you haven't had time to hem the cuff yet, two-sided tape will rescue you once again.

You can buy double-stick tape at beauty-supply stores, drugstores, costume houses, wig shops, or in the lingerie sections at department stores. A pack of 50 one-by-three-inch (2.5 x 7.5 cm) strips sells for about $5.

2 Steam that shine away. You've just ironed your dark trousers, and now there are embarrassing shiny spots on the fabric. Don't fret, says clothing designer Bobette Stott. These spots aren't unusual, especially if your garment is made of a wool blend. Here's her cure: Mix 1 ounce (2 tablespoons) distilled white vinegar with 5 ounces (145 ml) water. Dip a clean cloth into the mixture and blot it onto the shiny spots. Then fire up your steam iron and pass it a few inches above the fabric. The steam will help the vinegar break up the shine. Hang the garment to dry, and it's ready to wear.

3 Race against the spot. The more quickly you treat a stain, the better your chances are of removing it. If at all possible, take the garment off immediately and blot at the stain with a paper towel or a clean cloth and try to remove as much of the stain as you can. Then either squirt laundry pretreatment onto the spot and wash it, or take it straight to a dry cleaner.

Remember that heat, like time, is working against you in this race. Never put a stained garment in the dryer, and never store it in a warm area.

4 Blot, don't rub, a stain. Have you ever seen a restaurant patron take a napkin and rub furiously at a stain on her blouse? Big mistake. Rubbing at a stain will only damage the fabric. Instead, moisten the napkin with water and blot at the stain to draw it off. Many people swear by using club soda this way, and the bubbling does provide a little assistance in releasing some new stains.

5 Staple that patch. The quandary is an old one: You start out sewing a patch onto a uniform thinking you have it perfectly situated. But by the time you've stitched its entire perimeter, the patch has somehow contrived to wriggle a few degrees out of kilter. So to keep your patch on an even keel, just staple it to the shirt where you want it, then sew the edges down. When you're done, use a staple remover to straighten the prongs of the staple and pull it out of the fabric.

modern garments. Such classic clothing keeps coming back into style, too, so it's a good investment. You'll be guaranteed a unique outfit—there's zero chance that you'll run into someone else at a party wearing the same dress. Also, vintage clothing is a particular boon for petite people, since clothing was sized much smaller then than it is today.

Shop to hide your bulge. Want to disguise that "spare tire" building up around your midsection? These wardrobe tricks will help:

- Don't wear corduroy, velvet, or any other material with a nap (raised fibers). This adds bulk to your shape and makes you look wider.
- Avoid satin or any other shiny material, which will accentuate bulges.
- No plaids.
- Wear loose, dark fabrics that hang well—preferably silk or high-quality rayon.

Buy wrinkle-free, satin-weave cotton. Nobody wants to go to work in a dress shirt that looks like you've slept in it. Textile expert Ingrid Johnson says that there's actually a special kind of cotton that resists wrinkles—but chances are that a store clerk will have no idea how to identify such a garment for you. Satin-weave cotton, which is more common in women's clothing than men's, feels smooth under your fingertips. But to be sure you're getting satin weave, here's a quick and simple test, says Johnson: Grab a handful of the cotton fabric, squeeze, then let go. Does the fabric hold those wrinkles? If so, that's conventional cotton. Does the fabric spring back relatively wrinkle-free? If so, you've found satin-weave cotton. ◁

Cleaning Clothes
6 Ways to Keep Your Garments Looking Good Longer

Don't clean your clothes out of habit. Many people believe that you should wash a garment every time you wear it. But that's a waste of effort and detergent. When you get home from work, change into your T-shirt and jeans, then evaluate your work duds before you toss them into the hamper. If your clothing passes this five-point check, you can put it on a hanger, air it out for two hours, then return it to your closet:

- *Does it need repair?* Any rips, missing buttons, falling hems, or broken zippers?
- *Does it need a dry cleaner's care?* Tough stains, particularly oily ones, should be taken to the dry cleaner within a day. If you wait weeks, your odds of getting the stain out are reduced dramatically.
- *Does it need to be laundered?* If the garment shows any of the routine smudges and dirt that come out in the wash, drop it into the hamper.
- *Does it pass the sniff test?* Yes, steel yourself and sniff the armpit of that shirt.
- *Does your* body *need to be washed?* If the answer is yes, then chances are the clothes that were hanging on that body need to be washed too.

Lighten up on laundering and soap. Detergent companies don't want you to know this, but most of us are chronically overwashing our clothing. We're wasting time and money (and detergent!), and we're wearing out our clothes faster. In reality, most clothing only needs a touch of spiffing up. Do your regular wash using half the package-recommended amount of detergent, and set the washing machine at the lightest setting. When you have clothes that are truly filthy, use the full measure of detergent and a longer setting.

Ease up on the laundry extras.

Household product manufacturers try to sell us all kinds of special washing aids, but clothes don't really need those dryer sheets and that fabric softener. The fabled "static cling" is not as horrible as the TV commercials will have you believe. If you do encounter garments that cling to each other because of static electricity, just dampen your hands and brush them across the material to kill the electrical charge. Towels will absorb water better if they are not doused in fabric softener; cleaning cloths work better without softener too.

Determine how clean your dry cleaner's facility really is.

If your clothes come back from the dry cleaner with a funky odor, your first move should be to take off the plastic covering and hang them up in the open—preferably outside on the back porch. There are two possible reasons for this odor, says Brent Newbold, who owned a laundry for more than 20 years and is now chief financial officer for Holy Cow cleaning products:

1. The cleaner didn't dry all of the solvent out of your clothes. Not a big deal. It will evaporate now.
2. The impurities weren't filtered out of the dry-cleaning solvent, and you have dirt from someone else's clothes stinking up your garments. Yuck!

So let your clothes hang in the open for two hours, then give them the sniff test. If they're still stinky after a couple of hours, your problem is with impurities, not solvent. Go to another dry cleaner.

"Clothes should smell clean and fresh if the dry cleaner is running his plant correctly," Newbold says.

Preserve your heirloom gown correctly.

The prom or your wedding is a warm memory, and now you want to preserve the gown you wore. Many dry cleaners will gladly charge you $150 to $500 for special protective packaging called "heirlooming." Typically, the gown is thoroughly cleaned and then sealed in plastic and arranged inside a nice, windowed box. But if this service is not done correctly, that precious gown could be ruined. Asking these two questions will help ensure that your gown will be properly protected:

How I Do It A Costume Designer's Stain-Removing Secrets

You don't get to be an Emmy Award-winning costume designer without learning to think quickly on your feet. Here are Birgit Mueller's in-a-pinch fixes for stained clothing:

- ☐ For an oil stain, sprinkle the spot with baby powder, let the powder absorb the oil, then brush the powder off.
- ☐ To clean up a dribble of solid food, makeup, or lipstick, wipe with a piece of velvet. Keep a handkerchief-size square of velvet in your purse for emergencies.
- ☐ Use a piece of white chalk to cover a stain on a white shirt.
- ☐ To remove an ink stain, spray the spot with hair spray, then launder.
- ☐ To remove a red wine stain, blot it with gin, then launder.
- ☐ To remove the odor of sweat from a shirt, mix 1 ounce (30 ml) vodka with 2 ounces (60 ml) water in a squirt bottle and spray it onto the armpits. "We used to use that trick on movie sites in the desert," Mueller says.

- Do you perform this service yourself or do you send it out? If your dry cleaner sends your gown out for servicing, that's actually a good sign. Some specialists in the business really know what they're doing. However, some dry cleaners buy heirlooming kits from suppliers so they can do the job on-site, and some of them may cut corners on preparing your gown.

- Will my gown be vacuum sealed? For long-term protection of the gown, all of the air must be removed from inside the packaging. Otherwise, the garment will turn yellow and deteriorate. If your dry cleaner is doing the work on-premises, ask whether he owns his own vacuum-packing equipment.

Dry-clean your suits less frequently.
Your dry cleaner won't tell you this, but most people bring their suits in to be cleaned way too often. New York City fashion coach Susan Sommers often hears clients complain, "My suit looks like hell after only one season." When she asks how often they dry-clean their suits, the answer is inevitably, "Every two or three times I wear it." That cleaning schedule is just too frequent!

If your suit is just a little wrinkled, use a steamer on it to relax the fabric—or have the dry cleaner press it for you. If you get a spot on your suit, try removing it with a disposable fabric-cleaning wipe before you take it to the dry cleaner. Try to dry-clean your suit only once per season. ◁

How Good Is Your Dry Cleaner?

The quality of work varies drastically from one dry cleaner to another. So if you're considering taking your best clothing to an unfamiliar dry cleaner, what assurance do you have that your duds won't be ruined?

Laundry expert Brent Newbold suggests giving him a little audition. When you want to use a new dry cleaner, take him just three items to clean:

- ☐ A cotton shirt.
- ☐ A light-colored linen shirt or blouse.
- ☐ A light-colored silk garment.

These three offer just enough variety for you to evaluate a dry cleaner's work. When you get your clothing back, here's what to look for:

Color. Did the garments come back their original color, or is there a dull tint to them? If the latter, then the dry cleaner is skimping by not cleaning his filters regularly. You see, a dry cleaner's chemical formula is used again and again. After it's used to remove the impurities from a load of clothing, the dry cleaner runs the chemical through a carbon filter to remove those impurities before it's ready for the next load. When the dry cleaner tries to get too much mileage out of a filter, the impurities build up in the cleaning chemical and leave your clothes looking dull. This will be particularly evident in the light-colored clothing. Also, if your cleaner has too much moisture in his cleaning solvent, it will draw color out of silk garments and fade them.

Fabric feel. Does the garment look and feel the way it did when you first bought it? If the dry cleaner has correctly added sizing to the garment, it will have a like-new body. Otherwise, it will feel limp—like an old rag. Because it requires more heat than any other fabric, linen is one of the most difficult for a cleaner to "finish" properly with pressing and sizing. A good cleaner also uses special products to keep your silk feeling soft and supple.

Pressing. Is the pressing neatly done? Each garment should look perfect and ready to wear. A good dry cleaner hires experienced pressers who know a zillion tricks of the trade for giving every garment a clean and crisp look. Rookie employees—or employees with too big a workload—will do a sloppy job. The cotton shirt is a good test of pressing quality because it's a common item that many cleaners do not press well. If you want to throw an extra pressing challenge at the cleaner, turn in a pleated skirt or pleated pants along with the garments listed above. Pleats require extra time and effort, and the cleaner's staff should double-check afterward that the pressing was correctly done.

Buttons. Are there broken or missing buttons? Good dry cleaners will bend over backward to replace missing or damaged buttons for free—even when the problem is not the cleaners' fault. They will retrieve a loose button from the button trap in their machinery, find a replacement in their in-house supply, or even trek to a garment shop or button supplier to find the right match. If all of those measures failed, Newbold used to offer to change an entire set of buttons on a garment to a new set for free. "A repeat customer is worth his weight in gold. You want people to say, 'Wow!' " he says.

Besides examining the garment, you should also consider the facility's turnaround time. A conscientious dry cleaner will have your clothes done within two hours if you're in a hurry. If you're told the wait is three days, go somewhere else.

Storing Garments
5 Guidelines for Wrinkle-Free Clothes and Orderly Closets

Strip off the plastic bags. Never store your clothing in the plastic bags that come from your dry cleaner. Clothing needs to breathe, and the moisture that gets trapped inside that dry cleaner bag can damage your garments. If you want protection for garments that you put in storage, go to a discount store and buy a breathable cotton garment bag.

Get out-of-season clothes out of your way. One problem with snatching up all of those department-store "bargains" is that your closet gets packed tighter than a tuna can. This is a problem, because your clothes need room to hang freely if you want them to come out of the closet fresh and wrinkle-free. There is one key maneuver for freeing up closet space:

- Find a place where you can hang spillover clothing from your closet. This might be in an empty guest-room closet, a hall closet, or a hanging bar in the laundry room. Every spring and fall, rotate the out-of-season clothing out of your bedroom closet and into your remote closet. Then bring the newly in-season clothing into your bedroom closet.

- If you are rotating your clothing out like this every six months and your clothes are still jam-packed in your everyday closet, rotate them into and out of remote storage four times a year instead of two. Keep only this season's clothing in your bedroom closet. Or keep only one month's worth of clothes in your closet. This means some clothing hanging in remote storage will actually be in season. That's okay—it will be put in rotation next month.

- Review your everyday clothing needs. If you wear casual clothes five days a week, don't store your fine clothes (suits and sport coats, for instance) in your closet. Put them in the remote location with the out-of-season clothes.

Get rid of clothing you don't wear. As you are rotating your clothing, examine every item. If there's anything you haven't worn in a year—no matter how cute it is, no matter what fond memories it might evoke—get rid of it. You can't afford to have it cluttering up your home. Think hard about your lifestyle. If you are like most of us, you own much more clothing than any one human needs. Buy less and get rid of more. There's no need to open your wallet every time you encounter an incredible bargain.

Know the right ways to keep moths at bay. Unfortunately, the bug-repelling powers of cedar closets and chests are grossly overrated. Sure, a moth will run when it gets a strong whiff of cedar—but we bet you didn't know that that pungent cedar-y smell will peter out after a year or two. Reviving the scent requires sanding off the surface layer of the wood, and almost nobody bothers with that. "When you can no longer smell the cedar, the moths can't either," says textiles professor Johnson. By the same token, if a dry cleaner asks if you want to pay to mothproof garments that are going into storage, tell him, "No, thanks." Dry cleaners mothproof clothing by adding a liquid to the cleaning solvent they use, but the secret is that this treatment only lasts for a month or two.

The better way to store those wool and silk garments? Dry-clean them first, then slide them into mothproof garment bags, which are available for purchase from the dry cleaner, and at some discount stores.

Before storing a garment, clean it. Before you put a wedding dress or a prom dress into storage, dry-clean it. Even if the dress appears perfectly clean, you risk ruining the garment if it hasn't been dry-cleaned. You see, "invisible" stains—such as lemon-lime soda, white wine, even sweat—will turn into yellow or brown spots over time. Such spots, once they develop, are just about impossible to remove.There's another reason for making sure that any clothing is absolutely clean before you stash it away: Moths and carpet beetles are not only attracted to natural fibers such as wool and cotton, but they also salivate when you offer them clothing that is soiled, stained, or sweaty. ◀

10
SPACE-SAVING CLOTHING
storage
Tricks

Is the floor of your closet overrun with shoes? Are you strapped for belt storage? Are you up to your neck in loose scarves or extra ties? You are not alone—just about all of us have amassed so many clothes that we just don't have enough storage space for them. The ultimate solution, of course, is to take an honest look at your wardrobe and get rid of a lot of the items that you never wear. That—and learning to resist the temptation to buy that cute dress or sporty shirt that you don't need—will go a long way toward freeing up some clothing storage space. Still, there are very few among us who would not like to have more places to store our clothes. And manufacturers have been very adept at devising relatively inexpensive aids that will help you squeeze every conceivable bit of clothing storage space out of your homes. Try out these storage tricks, and you'll have that wild closet tamed in no time.

1 Closet them in canvas. When you consider construction costs, adding a closet to your home for a mere $70 is more than reasonable. Visit a storage-gear store in person or online and pick up a freestanding canvas closet, which you can set up in a spare room or basement. This will give your home an extra 3 feet (1 meter) of closet rod, plus storage for folded sweaters as well. The canvas will protect your stored clothes and let them breathe at the same time.

2 Sleep on it. If you'd like to find an extra 15 or 20 cubic feet (0.4 to 0.6 cubic meters) of extra clothing storage space, just take a look under your bed. Container manufacturers have devised a wide variety of clever gizmos for making maximum use of this space, including flat totes that will vacuum-pack bulky comforters, clear vinyl cases for shoes and accessories you want to peruse at a glance, and wide storage boxes with wheels, snap-on lids, or side drawer access.

3 Buy hard-working furniture. When you buy furniture, pick the kind that will perform more than one job—including storing clothing that you can't accommodate in your bedroom. Examples: A daybed with a hinge-up top and storage underneath, or a sofa with hidden drawers below the seat cushions.

4 Show them the door. Add shoe-bag-style organizers to the backs of closet doors and bedroom doors. The typical shoe bag has hooks that fit over the top of the door, draping a couple dozen pockets down the door surface. These are a splendid way of getting shoes off the floor of your closet, of course, but they also provide clever storage for rolled scarves, pantyhose, other accessories, and even kids' toys.

5 Get hooked. In the bathroom, install several hooks on the back of the door for hanging extra towels and robes.

6 Jacket? Rack it. Freestanding coat racks come in handsome designs, and they can turn a small bit of floor space into vertical clothing storage. Park one by the door, in the mudroom, or in the kids' bedrooms. With several hooks for jackets, scarves, and hats, coat racks go a long way toward freeing up space in crowded coat closets.

7 Send them packing. Pull out any suitcases that aren't in current use and fill them with the kind of clothing you don't need day-in and day-out. You'll gain some elbow room in your closet, and your luggage will take up no more space than it did before.

8 Spare the rod. To save closet-rod space, become a fan of the specialty hangers that are available at home stores, discount stores, and organizing stores. Such hangers take up very little rod space, but they can accommodate several skirts, a dozen neckties, a like number of scarves, or a score of belts, for instance.

9 Bin there, stored that. See-through, stacking bins are ideal for storing sweaters, other foldable clothing, and accessories such as handbags and shoes. When you stack such bins, they take up vertical space—but minimal floor space. Since they have transparent sides, you can quickly identify the items that you want. Drawer-type access makes this all the easier.

10 Hang 'em high. Install high shelves in your bedroom to accommodate hats, purses, or small storage bins. A shelf mounted 12 to 18 inches (30 to 46 cm) below the ceiling will be in no one's way, but it will provide a nice "relief valve" for an overstuffed bedroom closet.

Researching Purchases

6 Smart Strategies That'll Mean Less Hassle and Big Savings

Stay on top of fluctuating prices. Major retailers often make a big deal out of their 30-day price guarantees, proclaiming that if the price for a product, like a television or DVD player, drops within 30 days of your purchase, the store will refund the difference in price. But this is a calculated marketing decision. What these retailers don't mention is that they know that few shoppers watch the price *after* they've made their purchase. Not long ago, watching a price meant returning to the store. But thanks to the Internet, you can beat the major retailers at their own game by watching the price online. It should only take a couple of minutes a day. And if the price goes down because of a sale, you'll get some of your green back.

Ask salespeople if they work on commission. Salespeople are legally obligated to tell you the truth about this. And the truth, as they say, can set you free. It works two ways: If you're looking for an honest opinion about a computer or stereo—not just some spiel that will put quick dough in the salesman's pocket—do your research at a retailer whose employees do not work on commission. But sometimes that spiel can mean a deal, since salespeople working on commission usually have the flexibility to slash prices. If they work on commission, ask for a discount—just be wary of the advice that they're giving you.

Sniff out spiffs. Retailers often offer their salespeople "spiffs," or special

How I Do It A Kitchen and Bath Designer's Way of Checking Product Reliability

"When it comes to choosing a brand, it's bewildering," says Jodi Fitzpatrick, a kitchen and bath designer for Home Depot and an associate with the National Kitchen and Bath Association.

"My suggestion? Get the real dirt from a guy with the dirt under his nails: the repairman. Go to an independent, local appliance dealer. First, talk to the salespeople. Next, talk to one of the repairpeople. Then try to figure out who to believe on which brand. Once, when I was shopping for tankless water heaters for one of my clients, I checked with my local bath products distributor, who recommended a certain brand. Then I talked to my favorite plumber, who installs tankless water heaters. He also liked this brand, but he did not like a competing brand because he had had numerous calls about problems with them. Why talk to the installer? Because he or she knows the problems and performance of the product in real-life, local situations. Salespeople, even from a local independent dealer, may be pushing a particular product for a weird reason—like, if they sell 50, the company will send them to Hawaii."

incentives, to sell products that are not selling quickly enough. While commissions might already make salespeople biased toward the more expensive products, spiffs encourage them to sell an unpopular or brand-new (read: no customer feedback) product. If you've done your homework online or by talking to others, you'll figure out in a hurry which ones are being pushed.

You may have more warranty than you think. Salespeople have been known to downplay a manufacturer's warranty if they think they can sell you their own warranty. You're much better off with a warranty that comes from the company, not the store. Ask to see a copy of the manufacturer's warranty, and read over it carefully. You may find that it covers problems for quite a bit longer than the salesperson would have you believe. Refrigerator compressors, the most expensive replacement part on any fridge, often come with a manufacturer's warranty for up to five years.

Skip the extended warranties. Salespeople are good at making two- to five-year warranties sound worth the extra money, but some of these plans can cost you hundreds of dollars! Here's what they don't tell you: Proft margins on electronics are only about 10 percent. Extended warranties are one way that retailers and manufacturers pick up the slack. The repair rate for the first three years of ownership for camcorders, digital cameras, and standard televisions is less than 10 percent. That means 90 percent of the time, all the warranty money goes to the store or makers.

One extended warranty that you might actually go for is one for a laptop computer—laptops have a three-year repair rate of 33 percent. Consider a one- to three-year extension of the standard one-year warranty. Buy the extended warranty from the computer manufacturer, however—this will give you tech support too. Warranties from retailers tend to cover just the hardware, not the tech support.

Have your dealer do the installation. There's always a lot of finger-pointing when something goes wrong with a new appliance. Say the new dishwasher you just spent $500 on doesn't work. The appliance dealer might say it's the installer's fault, while the installer might say it's the retailer's responsibility. You can prevent this kind of hassle by having your retailer also do the installation—most do offer this service. When the same business is both selling and installing your appliances, it's pretty much on the hook for any problems that crop up. ◄

Appliance Care
4 Pro Secrets for Keeping Your Machinery in Tip-Top Shape

Lubricate your icemaker. Finicky automatic icemakers keep many an appliance repairperson in business. If your freezer's icemaker has ground to a halt, try this simple cure before you spend a bundle on a repair call: Remove the ice cube tray and dump out any ice. Buff the tray with a dishtowel until it's perfectly dry. Then give the inside of the tray a light squirt of cooking oil spray. A common reason that icemakers quit producing is that the tray clings to the new ice cubes and can't dump them out. The cooking spray will prevent this bond and will lend no taste whatsoever to your ice.

Unclog your dishwasher. Repairpeople get a good chuckle when you tell them that your dishwasher isn't cleaning as well as it used to. That's because homeowners have a good shot at fixing this problem themselves with this easy, three-minute procedure: Look at the top of the spray arms inside your dishwasher (there are usually two, one at the bottom and one under the upper rack). If mineral deposit or other debris is closing off the holes along the top of the spray arms, they won't clean anymore. Unfasten the clips or screws holding the spray arms in place and put the spray arms in your sink. Unbend a paper clip, insert the end of this stiff wire into each spray hole, and move it around to dislodge the blockage. Rinse the spray arms out under the faucet and return them to duty in your dishwasher. Your dishwasher will now work properly again!

Think *inside* the box. There's hope for cash-strapped appliance owners. Easier access to replacement parts means that if you can get to that broken dryer belt or busted dishwasher spring, you can save on repair bills. Instead of having to drive to the nearest appliance parts dealer, flip through dog-eared manuals and catalogs, and try the patience of a behind-the-counter type who's used to selling to trained technicians who don't ask so many questions, today you can turn to the Internet for parts and advice.

But there's one hitch. Appliance manufacturers have made machines tougher for do-it-yourselfers to get into. "I was out there servicing appliances in the 1970s and '80s," says Wanda Martens, former field technician and major appliance instructor at Dunwoody College of Technology in Minneapolis, Minnesota. "Access has gotten trickier, but appliances are easier to work on once you get in there. Replacing parts is usually a matter of removing a few screws or brackets. The manufacturers build them so that highly paid technicians can fix parts and get out of there."

Many repairs, of course, are too complicated (or potentially dangerous) for homeowners to attempt on their own. The DIY-er has to make that call. You can usually use the Internet to diagnose your problem, find repair manuals (sometimes manuals for similar models give you all you need to know about accessing a machine), and buy parts through mail order. A great place for appliance DIYers to start online is www.repairclinic.com.

Clear a clogged drain tube. It's one of the most common things that go wrong with a fridge. In a typical two-door unit with the freezer at the top, there is a drain tube running from the freezer compartment to an evaporation tray underneath the fridge. You'll find the drain hole on the floor of the freezer compartment, near the back. Its purpose is to drain the runoff that develops when your unit periodically melts its frost to keep itself, as advertised, frost-free. The problem is that algae spores often develop in the tube, blocking it. This causes water to back up on the floor of the freezer, usually forming ice. The solution is simple: Use a turkey baster to force fresh water through it to flush it out. You may have to turn off the fridge to let the ice melt first. The water will run into the tray under the fridge, so empty it. Then pour a teaspoon of ammonia or chlorine bleach into the tube to prevent a recurrence of the algae spores. See—you just saved the cost of a hefty repair bill! ◁

How to Ruin Your Appliances

Appliances eventually wear out. Certain parts simply fail with time. It's inevitable. But appliance abuse and neglect can speed up the breakdown rate of washers, dryers, refrigerators, ranges, and dishwashers, helping keep appliance repairmen busy. Here are some of the most common ways homeowners contribute to appliance demise, along with advice for avoiding these errors.

Washing machine

Repairman's tip:

Never wash anything with heavy metal fasteners.

Some washer parts are easy to replace, but a chipped or cracked inner tub can sound the death knell for your machine. The exposed metal will rust—and keep rusting—and the rust will spot your clothes and linens. The cost of the new tub plus labor to install it makes this repair prohibitively expensive.

Bonus tip: Overloading your washer may not ruin it, but it will create wear and tear on certain parts that glide and spin, making these parts fail prematurely and forcing you to call the repairman or fix it yourself. Be sure to always follow the manufacturer's suggestions for load size.

Clothes dryer

Repairman's tip:

Follow your dryer manual's instructions for proper venting. Replace plastic or vinyl exhaust hoses with rigid or flexible metal venting, making the pathway from the dryer to the outside vent as straight as possible. Clean the lint filter before or after each load. Clean the places in the dryer where lint collects—the back, around the mouth of the lint filter, around the door. Once a year, have a professional clean the interior of your machine.

When the typical 12-pound (5.5-kg) load of laundry comes out of the washer, it contains a half-gallon (2 liters) of water. The dryer's job, of course, is to remove the water. It heats the clothes, converting water to water vapor and forcing it out of the dryer (and the house) through the exhaust vent, along with lint. Dryers are designed to push this lint-laden wet air only so far—between about 40 and 90 feet (12 and 27 meters) when rigid metal pipe is used, but only half that when flexible tubing is used. Every elbow in the pipe (around a corner, up a wall) dramatically cuts down on the maximum distance. Some newer homes have exhaust pipe runs of up to 200 feet (60 meters), making it impossible to adequately vent. So what happens? Your dryer has to work harder to dry your clothes (leading to potential part burnout), moisture problems arise in your home, and lint builds up in the machine and vent pipe. This last consequence is the most serious, because lint is flammable. The U.S. Consumer Product Safety Commission estimates that dryers are the cause of 15,500 fires each year. Lint buildup is a major cause of dryer fires.

Glass-top electric range

Because ranges don't have many moving parts (no motors, no belts), they tend to last a good long while—with one major exception. Damage done to a glass top, which can cost $300 to $400 to replace, makes the repair not worth the money. The most obvious way to break the glass is to bang a heavy pot on it—an impact break. But did you know that improper heating can also crack the glass? Using concave-bottomed pans can trap heat and cause the glass to crack. Using over-sized pots and pans can do the same.

Repairman's tip:

Use flat-bottomed pots and pans and make sure they are not larger than each burner.

Refrigerator

By far the most expensive part on your refrigerator is the compressor, part of the sealed cooling system. The sealed system is often protected under a special five-year warranty, and it should last at least twice that long. But you've got to clean the dust that builds up on the refrigerator's condenser coils, usually located behind a grille on the bottom of the fridge. If not, the compressor will be forced to work harder, and it may eventually overheat. If it fails prematurely—but after the warranty is void—you'll likely have to replace the fridge, since a repair will be too costly.

Bonus tip: A full freezer is more efficient than an empty freezer, which has nothing to hold the cold. An efficient freez-er not only prolongs the life of the compressor—and the fridge itself—but also saves energy. Fill your empty freezer shelves with bag ice, frozen veggies, or even plastic milk jugs filled with water.

Repairman's tip:

Once a year (twice if you have furry pets), snap off the grille and clean the dust from the condens-er coils using a vacuum cleaner and a condenser coil cleaning brush (an under-$10 accessory)—a tapered bottle brush on a plunger-length handle. Gently brush the bottom surface and in between the coils, then vacuum. Repeat until the coils are dust-free. Do not poke at the coils with a vacuum cleaner's hard-plastic crevice tool. That could damage the coils.

Dishwasher

Thanks to rust, dishwashers, like clothes washers, can be ruined by one small nick in the vinyl-coated rack. Once the metal inside begins to rust, you can't stop it. The rust will stain your dishes until you replace either the rack or the machine. Replacing a dish rack can set you back one-quarter the price of a brand-new machine.

Repairman's tip:

Hand-wash skillets, colanders, and other kitchenware with sharp edges. Never force a pan into a too-small space.

Computer Care
6 Slick Tips for Saving Money and Fixing 'Em Yourself

Shave time off the computer repair guy's clock. Here's a little-known secret among techies: The first thing a computer repairperson does when he arrives onsite is to make sure your operating system is updated. If you're like most people, you use Microsoft Windows. You can (and should) update Windows yourself, before the $95-an-hour IT expert arrives. And if you're lucky, updating Windows might even solve the problem you called about. (If a plug-in, such as a digital camera, MP3 player, or printer isn't working, it could be because your drivers are out of date. A Windows update will take care of this.) Think how great you'll feel calling and canceling that appointment!

To update Windows, here's what you do: Once you're logged on to the Internet, open up your computer's Web browser, go to the Tools menu at the top of the page, then click on "Windows Update." You'll immediately be taken to the Microsoft website, which will check to see if your computer needs any upgrades. If so, follow the prompts to download the upgrades. If you have Windows XP, you can have your computer download the upgrades automatically. To do so, click on the "Start" menu in the lower left corner of your screen, click on "Control Panel," click on "Security Center," then turn on "Automatic Upgrades."

For better computer health, get an Apple. Apple computers can be a little more expensive than most PCs. But since only about 2 percent of the population uses Apple's Macintosh computers, very few spyware and virus programs are written to affect them. Virus writers would rather affect 98 percent of the population than Apple's small population. So, if you're having a lot of problems with spyware and viruses, consider buying a Mac next. The peace of mind might be worth the slightly higher cost.

Kick-start a failed Internet connection. If your high-speed Internet service fails to work after a power loss or computer crash, it could be that some of your devices powered up in the wrong order. Instead of calling a computer consultant, save yourself some time and hassle by first trying the following: Shut down the computer. Turn off or unplug your modem, the device that connects you to your cable or phone line. If you have one, turn off or unplug your router, the device that connects the modem and your home network. Wait at least 30 seconds. Now turn everything back on in the following order:

1. Modem—it will send a message to your Internet service provider (ISP) saying you need a new connection.
2. Router—it tells your modem to connect.
3. Computer.

Nine out of ten times, this will fix your connection problem. If it does not, the problem probably has something to do with your Internet service provider, not your computer. At that point, it's time to make a phone call.

Boost your computer's speed without calling a pro. All those software programs that come bundled on your computer take up valuable real estate. They also fight for your computer's resources by constantly searching for updates of themselves, even when you don't have the program open. What the computer companies don't tell you is that when you buy one of their machines, it's already running slower than it should because of all the extra programs. You can free up space and resources by removing all the programs you don't use.

Just deleting the icon on your desktop will not remove the programs—you've got to uninstall them. If you use a Windows XP-based PC, you do this by clicking on the "Start" menu in the lower left corner of your computer screen. Next, click "Control Panel," then "Add or Remove Programs." Scroll down the list of programs and remove the ones you're certain you don't need. The rule of thumb computer technicians use

with clients who want faster machines: If you haven't used a program in a year, you can delete it without worry.

Drain, then recharge, your laptop batteries. Sure, the computer salesman makes it sound like the world will stop turning if you don't buy a second laptop battery. But you can do just fine without an extra, unless you travel frequently. A second battery is bulky and is almost never worth the money. Since batteries drain as they get older—after only a few years, a battery may only reach 95 percent of its original charge—it's best to stick with one battery and keep it healthy. The best way to keep it healthy is to only charge it after it has been fully drained. Leaving your laptop plugged into the wall all the time will actually make it weaker. Before a big trip, when you'll need as much battery power as possible, drain the laptop battery completely (running a CD or DVD is a good way to quickly sap the power), and then recharge it completely.

WHAT **SOFTWARE MAKERS** DON'T WANT YOU TO KNOW ABOUT Free Spyware

Makers of spyware, that insidious software that secretly gathers information about your Web surfing habits while also slowing down your surfing speed, have become very clever at fooling consumers into downloading their software onto your computer. They've even been

known to advertise spyware as "free spyware blockers." You should only download free spyware blockers from download.com, one of the most trustworthy sites for downloads on the Internet, according to computer technicians. Two of the best free spyware blockers?

Spybot Search and Destroy, and Ad-Aware from Lavasoft.

BUYING APPLIANCES AT
big-box
Home Stores

When you're out to buy a new appliance or power tool, it's only natural to make your local home superstore your first stop. But purchasing a complex mechanical device is not the same as picking up a new faucet or some paint or wallpaper—and you may not be getting quite the same good deal. Here are some things that you should consider before buying that washer or router at a big-box outlet.

These stores don't always have the lowest prices

After entering the appliance-selling game relatively late, retailers like Home Depot and Lowe's don't command the same volume discounts that they do on commodities like lumber and drywall. Nor do appliance manufacturers want to alienate the thousands of mom-and-pop appliance stores across the continent, stores that still offer competitive prices. Consider the potential benefits from buying from a small, local dealer—dependable service, accountability, and supporting the local economy. And if for some reason you buy an appliance from a big-box retailer (maybe you want to purchase everything for your kitchen remodeling in one place), bring the top competitor's lowest price quote with you. Most will match (or beat) that price.

Quality service is not their game

When it comes to large appliances, good service is important. Here's what the big-box stores don't want you to know about how their business models work:

1. They are typically too short-staffed to be able to handle service well (they have to keep those margins up for Wall Street, as well as Bay Street, every quarter!).

2. They provide you with a "customer-service department" rather than simply the "guy in charge."

3. Their organizational structure makes it very difficult to communicate with either your original salesperson or a single customer-service representative. Typically, there's no receptionist. You call in and must navigate your way through a huge phone tree, with no individual employee e-mail or voice-mail boxes for storing messages. Besides, the employees are too busy playing customer pinball to really give you their undivided attention. Think of big-box stores as retailers, period.

Think of big-box stores as retailers, period. If you call in for service, you must negotiate a huge phone tree.

Big-box stores do not have their own installers

When you purchase a large appliance that needs professional installation, it's not store employees coming into your home—they're employees of an installation company that the store has hired on contract. The big-box store acts as the middleman, charging you the installation fee, plus a markup that's usually in the neighborhood of 25 percent. Sometimes these installation companies are start-up outfits that can't generate enough business on their own and need the extra work. The whole setup creates a gap in accountability that can make it hard to solve any problems that crop up.

Power tools that use one kind of battery are a great idea

The battery is typically the priciest part of a new cordless drill, saw, or other power tool. And it's always nice to have a backup battery. Buying multiple tools that use the same battery basically gives you free backup batteries. It also cuts down on the number of battery chargers you have around the house, which reduces clutter and saves you money.

Buying tools that are exclusive to one retailer is risky

Some brands of power tools are sold at just one retail chain. Rigid power tools, for example, are only available at Home Depot. This can spell trouble for contractors working long distances from their hometowns, and for others who move to an area where there's no branch of that particular store. Without easy access to the store that sells your brand, you might not be able to buy nails or other accessories for your tools. Before you choose a brand, find out where accessories and parts for that brand are available, where repairs are made, and then consider if it's convenient for you.

Renting tools can be as expensive as buying them

Renting a power or garden tool can cost nearly as much as buying the same tool new. If you're going to use the tool more than once or twice, it makes sense to buy it. Even if it only takes you an hour to aerate your lawn, you may have to rent the tool for a minimum time period, for instance 24 hours. Instead, if you need expensive lawn tools like lawn mowers or tillers, ask your neighbors if they'd like to go in on buying one.

Upgrade your desktop PC. Computer companies thrive on a marketing strategy known as planned obsolescence—the idea that today's brand-new machine will be out of date in just a few years, thanks to ever-faster processors, bigger hard drives, and more memory. They figure most of their customers would never dream of tinkering with electronics the way they might replace a belt in their vacuum cleaner. But despite the ethereal nature of computer software, many desktop computer hardware parts fit together like high-tech Legos. Instead of buying a brand-new computer for $600 to $1,200, upgrade a few parts. Need more memory? Snap in a random-access memory (RAM) upgrade, which usually costs less than $100. Want to burn DVDs? Buy a DVD burner (another $100 purchase), and add it to one of the empty slots on the computer. This way, you can keep your old keyboard, monitor, and speakers, all of which work perfectly well. ◁

Computer Security
5 Ways to Keep Your Personal Information out of Strangers' Hands

Remember that nothing is free on the Internet. "When you see a pop-up ad for free screen savers, you might think they're cute as a button," explains Ontario-based computer guru Brian Muntz. "They seem innocent enough. But you pay a price: They contaminate your system with spyware. When spyware builds up on your computer, every time you start it up, you have a line of people at your Internet door waiting to collect information about you. It slows down your computer tremendously."

Read that license agreement. To download those "free" screen savers, you must first click a button that says "I accept." Most people click without reading the end-user license agreement (EULA) accompanying it, which is like signing a contract without reading it. Read the EULA, and it will explain (in legalese, of course) that in exchange for the free screen savers, the company will plant spyware on your computer.

Arm your PC with security programs. This is essential: If you're going to have a computer that is hooked up to the Internet, you should have reputable security programs installed on your computer. Spend the extra 25 bucks to get a quality security package. Norton and McAfee are two of the biggest names in computer security software. They each sell bundles that include an antivirus program, a firewall to stop hackers, a spyware blocker, and an e-mail checker (it scans incoming mail for contaminants). You need all these.

Get a router if you have broadband.
"When you use DSL or cable to link directly to the Internet, you're entering what I call the DMZ, the demilitarized zone," says Muntz. "You're a wide-open target," meaning any hacker out there can use scanning software to locate your open Internet protocol (IP) ports and remotely access your computer, accessing personal data or using it to distribute viruses or spam. "That's because you were visible," says Muntz.

Here's the trick. Buy yourself a router, a small modem-looking box that routes data between the cable or phone and a small network of computers. Even if you only have one computer at home—and no plans for creating a network—a $50 router can slam the door on all potential hackers. "If you add a broadband router, and then the router to your modem, you're now invisible. Now when the hacker scans, all he can see is your router, and he can hack that all day long and he's not getting through it, because there are no ports open."

Secure your wireless network.
Many people with more than one computer at home are discovering the benefits of wireless networks (which use routers to link those computers). But there's a big potential problem. "Like anything computer-related, wireless networks are all designed to work right out of the box. So you plug it in, and the next thing you know, you're online and surfing. A lot of users stop right there. They say, 'Beautiful! And I didn't even have to fish any wires through the walls.' But if you can surf, so can anybody else. Any passerby can get onto your network and spread viruses or traffic in child pornography." Some lawyers have even

suggested that homeowners are legally liable for the lack of security on their networks.

Securing the network is simple. You'll find instructions inside the box. Typically, they'll ask you to open your Internet browser and type in a series of numbers (your IP address, which in most cases is 192.168.1.1). This takes you not to a website but to your router settings. Click on the "Wireless" tab, and then click on "Security." Follow the instructions for creating a password, sometimes called a WEP (wired equivalent privacy) key. Choose a password, and voilà, your network is safe. ◁

Cell Phone Service
3 Tips for Outsmarting Cell Phone Companies' Sneaky Tactics

Time your cell-shopping trip carefully. An employee of a major wireless phone service provider let us in on some serious dirt about what goes on in that industry. In exchange for a promise to protect his identity, he revealed some of his company's trade secrets. Here is the first:

The best time to buy a cell phone is at the end of the month. Most phone sales teams have a specific "discount budget" or allotment of money they are allowed to discount in order to close deals. At the end of the month, when sales quotas must be met, salespeople tend to dip more deeply into their discount budgets. Sometimes the budgets themselves shoot up. So bargain for that phone at the end of the month—and don't let them tell you they "can't do any better on the price." What do you say? How about, "I'll sign for two years if you sell this phone to me at this price."

Skip the accessories. Cell phone salespeople typically only make commission off the accessories they sell you, not the phone itself. That's why they seem so insistent that you buy extra chargers and cases. Be a savvy shopper, and only buy accessories that you'll really use (if you don't travel a lot, for instance, a car charger might not be necessary).

Skimp on "replacement" insurance and save your old phone. Cell phone salespeople leap at the opportunity to sign you up for a phone replacement policy at anywhere from $3.99 to $6.99 per month. It doesn't sound like much at the time, especially when compared to the $200 or so they'll quote you for a full-retail replacement phone—but at the end of the year, you've already spent $50 or $100 and have nothing to show for it! Here's a trick for saving money by creating your own insurance policy against loss, breakage, or theft: Save your old phone. Most phone companies will switch your service to the old phone for free, or maybe $50—which is a lot less than $200. ◁

You Can Get Cheaper Cable Service

Cable companies compete fiercely for your dollars. Here are some insider tips for gaining your own competitive edge when it comes to getting the best cable TV and Internet service.

You are probably paying for a lot of channels you don't watch. Try a package with fewer channels.

Use your loyalty as leverage

Because of marketing costs, it can cost the cable companies 10 times more to recruit a new customer than to retain an old customer. You can use this bit of advice to your advantage the next time you find yourself dissatisfied with your service. Simply say that you'll take your business elsewhere. Chances are they'll address your problem, and they may even give you a deal on your cable rate.

Start over—with a signing bonus

Since most cable companies don't make you sign a contract, you can cancel your service, often without penalty, and then sign up again the next day to take advantage of sign-up incentives such as reduced fees or six months of free premium channels. Better yet, just call the provider and say you're going elsewhere unless they offer you the new-customer rates.

Shop around

If there are multiple cable service providers in your area, call around for the lowest price. If your current provider's price is relatively high, quote the lowest competitor's price (including incentives). Chances are they'll match or beat that price to keep your business.

Ask for the credit you deserve

Every now and again you have trouble with your cable TV or cable-based Internet service, don't you? The next time your cable goes out, don't just settle for restored service. Ask for credit. If you don't have luck with the first customer-service representative, keep asking for a supervisor.

Don't buy services you don't need

All cable companies offer a range of packages with names like basic, standard, and premium, each step up adding more channels and more cost. Take a very close look at the channels offered at each level and compare them to the channels you actually watch. What you are likely to discover is that you are paying for a lot of channels that you never watch. Most people only have at most ten or so channels that they watch regularly.

PRIVATE

part Three

EVERYDAY LIVING

Did you know that the best time to shop at a retail store is two in the afternoon? That you can get the best deal on a car at the end of the month? That the time to lowball a bid on eBay is over a holiday weekend? And if you want to find real bargains at a thrift shop, go in late December or early January? Timing is not the only thing that we've gotten normally tight-lipped insiders to open up about. They've shared a lot of other hush-hush secrets that can save you a ton of money. Discover why you should never, ever write or attach a note when paying a bill. Why mixing business with pleasure will get you ahead at work. Just turn the page to start discovering many, many more rarely disclosed tricks and secrets.

Auto Maintenance

10 Surprising Car-Care Shortcuts That Will Save You Money

Peel off that oil-change reminder sticker. Those quick-oil-change emporiums want you to think that the world will end if you don't change your car's oil every 3,000 miles (4,828 km). They even put stickers in your windshield reminding you to have it serviced. However, most cars do fine driving 7,500 miles (12,000 km) without a change—and some can go twice that. Check your car owner's manual—the manufacturer will give you the real story.

Pump the minimum. Despite what service-station ads want you to believe, very few cars really need expensive, high-octane gasoline. Most conventional automobiles are designed to run perfectly well on the cheapest (87-octane) gas.

Look for a detailer certificate. Detailing a car is just like any other professional service—some people are good at it, some aren't. How do you find a car detailer that's going to get into every crack and crevice and get your auto looking like new? Look for a detailer that has been licensed from a car detailing training facility. While there's no "official" master detailer designation (in other words, it's an unregulated industry) detailers who take the time to go through a certification program are probably better equipped to do a top-notch detail job.

Ignore that tire "dent" warning. If a tire salesman points out dents in the sidewalls of your tires, don't worry—he is just looking to make a quick buck. An unscrupulous tire dealer will tell you these dents are a problem and you need new tires, but in fact, these little concave depressions are more than normal. And they're not really dents—they're where the tire's poly cords are joined together. On the other hand, if you have a tire bulge—a convex lump that's a sign of an impending blowout—that's when it's time to consider forking over the dough for some new tires.

Keep tabs on tire pressure. What's the easiest way *not* to spend a ton of money on your mechanic's bill? Check your tire pressure every month. Reason number one: It's unsafe to have over- or underinflated tires, because the tires can blow out. Other big reasons to watch the pressure, says Lauren J. Fix, owner of Automotive Aspects in Clarence, New York, are that lousy tire pressure will lower your gas mileage, and add wear and tear to your car's brakes and handling systems, and it will also lower your gas mileage. The maximum tire pressure is marked on the sidewall of the tire; many cars also have a more important figure—the suggested tire pressure—marked on the inside of the driver's-side door.

Skip the spray-on wax at the car wash. A few more bucks for a hot wax job (or maybe they call it triple foam, or a sealant, or whatever) at the local car wash seems like such a deal. Does it make your car look better? Absolutely. Problem is, the shine (and additional protection) diminishes after about a week. A better idea would be to save the extra few bucks that the wax costs, and spring for one of those "express" wax jobs most car washes offer. They cost about $30, but they will give you longer-lasting protection.

Catch the wax on the rebound. Car wash owners certainly aren't going to tell you this, but you'll get the hot wax treatment for free at most car washes. How? Prentice St. Clair, president of Detail in Progress, an automotive detailing company in San Diego, says that if your car wash recycles its water—just ask, and you'll find most do—then the spray-on wax that gets applied during other people's car washes will stay in the water supply, and will get transferred onto your car. Just another reason to find an environmentally friendly car wash!

Put your mechanic behind the wheel. Something in the front of your car is squeaking. So you take it to an auto repair shop, you tell them about the squeak, and they throw the car up on the lift. Twenty minutes later, they're telling you that you need pricey new brakes and brake pads. How do they know this if they haven't taken the car for a test drive? One auto service manager we asked says you should get that car off the lift and take it to a different repair shop. A mechanic typically needs to take a car for a spin to diagnose big problems; those that don't are just selling you the most expensive fix to what could be a much smaller problem.

Beware shock absorber shenanigans. Many an unscrupulous mechanic has sprayed oil on a customer's shock absorbers, causing them to appear to be leaking oil. So if your mechanic delivers that kind of grim news to you, take your car to another mechanic for a second—and even third—opinion.

Look for the MAP on the wall. Never heard of the Motorist Assurance Program? Unscrupulous repair shops hope you haven't. The Motorist Assurance Program (MAP) is the first and only agency that accredits car repair shops, ensuring that these shops maintain a standard set of guidelines when diagnosing what is wrong with your car. The MAP guidelines cover exhaust, brakes, ABS, steering and suspension, engine maintenance and performance, HVAC, electrical systems, drivetrain, and transmission. The guidelines are not intended as a diagnostic tool (they won't help the technician locate the problem). However, the program offers peace of mind to the consumer—the knowledge that the repair shop is accredited. It's as close as you're going to get to finding a repair shop that's not out to pick your pocket. ◂

WHAT YOUR **CAR DEALERSHIP** DOESN'T WANT YOU TO KNOW ABOUT Maintenance

When you drive your new car off the lot, chances are your dealer will have given you a service schedule for your car. The manager of a New York-area auto-maintenance shop confesses that that schedule is the biggest "hose job" in the business. The dealer is trying to scare you into believing that your car needs all sorts of preventive maintenance work, and that it all has to be done at the dealership.

The only service maintenance schedule worth following is the one that comes from the car manufacturer; you'll find it in the vehicle's manual. This service schedule is a heck of a lot more conservative than the one your dealer has prescribed. We know of one woman whose dealer's service schedule said that she needed—all within the first year—an oil and filter change, a tire rotation, a brake system check, an air system check, and a transaxle service. In addition, the dealer said that an engine oil flush, fuel system service, four-wheel alignment, tire balance, and wiper blade replacement were all required. The total cost for this dealer service schedule? More than $600. What, exactly, did the manufacturer recommend after a year? Changing the oil filter, rotating the tires, and just checking everything else. Total cost? About $70.

Road Safety
6 Tips to Surviving the Most Dangerous Driving Situations

Stop your car from hydroplaning. Hydroplaning occurs when your car tires are driving on water, rather than directly on the pavement—usually when you're driving quickly and you suddenly drive through a deep puddle. If it's raining hard enough, you don't even need to drive through a puddle to hydroplane—it can happen anywhere on the road. This is a pretty dangerous condition; it's very easy to lose control of the vehicle. If it happens to you, *don't brake*—just let the car coast until the hydroplaning subsides (and if you're driving a manual transmission car, you'll want to engage the clutch).

Survive skids on ice and snow. Don't have a panic attack. Don't hit the brakes. Take your foot off the gas, and steer in the direction that you are skidding. If you must hit the brakes, apply steady but gentle pressure, but do not pump them or allow them to lock. The brakes will likely make some noise, but you should be back in control in no time.

Sit back to sidestep air-bag injury. Who's at highest risk for being injured by the air bags that are supposed to protect us? According to the Michigan State Police, it's drivers who sit too close to the steering wheel. Sit back in your seat, rather than hunched over, put at least 10 inches (25 cm) between yourself and the steering wheel—and, of course, always wear your seat belt.

Minimize the impact if the worst is inevitable. So a vehicle is coming toward you; maybe the driver is distracted (or even worse, asleep at the wheel). What should you do? Make sure your headlights are on—bright oncoming lights will get the driver's attention—and that you're driving as close to the right side of your lane (away from the oncoming lane) as you can. If the car is in your lane and it's not moving, don't play chicken with it. Slow down so that you minimize the force of an inevitable crash, then veer off the road to the right (not left, into the

Car Emergency Kit Checklist

Here are 15 things that'll get you out of most car-related jams. Keep them in your trunk or glove compartment so that they are always handy.

- ☐ Maps
- ☐ First-aid kit
- ☐ Flares or emergency lights
- ☐ Jumper cables
- ☐ Paper towels
- ☐ Flashlight, portable flashing light, and extra batteries
- ☐ Energy bars (or other nonperishable food)
- ☐ Drinking water
- ☐ Matches and emergency candles
- ☐ Brightly colored flag, banner, or "help" sign

In the winter, add these, if appropriate for your climate:

- ☐ Cat litter, sand, or salt (provides good traction in the snow)
- ☐ Snow shovel
- ☐ Ice scraper/windshield brush
- ☐ Extra clothing and shoes, particularly warm jackets, hats, and gloves
- ☐ Windshield wiper fluid and/or deicing fluid
- ☐ Gas-line antifreeze

oncoming lane). If it looks like you'll hit a street sign or another obstacle, so be it—at least it's not another moving vehicle traveling at top speed. Just try not to hit that obstacle head-on; see if you can maneuver your vehicle so that you hit it at an angle instead.

Don't swerve with deer. Most deer-car collisions happen in the fall, between the hours of 6 p.m. and midnight, say the Michigan State Police troopers. If it's dark out, the easiest way to spot deer is to drive with your high-beam lights on—they illuminate the animals' eyes. If you see a deer in your path, it's rarely prudent to swerve: It's better to strike a deer than another car, or a telephone pole or something else that can cause even more damage to you and your vehicle.

Stay calm if you get stranded in the snow. Avoid overexertion and overexposure to the cold. If you can't shovel your vehicle out of the snow—or if there are blizzard conditions—stay inside the car. Don't leave the car unless help is visible within about 100 yards (90 meters). Turn on flashing lights or set up flares. In daylight, tie a brightly colored cloth to the antenna to make your car more visible. Run the engine for about 10 minutes every hour to provide heat without burning too much fuel. For safety, make sure the tailpipe is free of snow and crack a window on the side away from the wind. Bundle up in a blanket; sharing it with another person gives extra warmth. Don't fall asleep; take turns sleeping if there is more than one person in the car. These tips come from the Canadian Centre for Occupational Health and Safety. ◂

Driving Violations
5 Tricks to Avoiding (and Getting Out of) Traffic Tickets for Speeding

Understand that your car says a lot about you. Most officers decide whether you're getting a ticket or a warning before they even approach your vehicle. A good rule of thumb is to keep your car maintained in such a way that you wouldn't be embarrassed to drive it to a job interview. Keep it clean, decluttered, and free of bumper stickers that are anti-police or pro-violence. Forgo aftermarket add-ons like spoilers, tinted windows, and neon undercarriage lights. You want to say "I'm responsible and law-abiding," not "I hate the police, I speed all the time, and I'm trying to hide something from you."

Wave at the hidden police cruiser. So you were driving down the road a little faster than you should have been, and you spot a police cruiser lurking behind some shrubbery. One former police officer says that the smartest thing that you can do right then is to wave at the officer. Why? He will either think that you know each other and wave back, or will think that you're acknowledging that you were driving too fast, and are letting him know that you're slowing down. Either way, you drastically reduce your chance of getting a ticket.

Never admit that you were speeding. If you do get pulled over, says one former police officer, never acknowledge that you were, in fact, speeding. You don't want to give the police any ammunition to use against you, should you contest your ticket in traffic court. When the officer tells you that you are speeding, giving a brief, noncommittal response like, "I see" or "I was not aware of my speed" is the way to go. (Asking sarcastic questions like, "What's the problem, Officer?" won't help your case!) Secret sources who have dodged more than one speeding ticket in their lives also advise that you just get through the meeting with the police as quickly and politely as you possibly can. You don't want them to remember anything about you, except that you were nice and did what you were told. Why? Read on.

Plead not guilty, and defer your court date as often as you can. The more time you put between your speeding encounter and your court date, the better, advise some ticket dodgers we know. Imagine how many people an officer pulls over in a month. How many of them do you think he'll remember two or even six months from now, especially if you take your ticket quietly and move on? The more continuances you can reasonably request, the more time you have to collect your evidence and prepare your defense—and the less specific that officer's recollection of you will be. Getting a continuance also increases the probability that the ticketing officer retires, transfers to another department, or just doesn't show up for your court date. In almost all of these extenuating situations, the case against you will be dropped.

Know the tactics that can get your ticket dismissed. There are dozens of ways to have your traffic violations reduced or dismissed—opportunities vary from region to region, so check to see if these apply in your state or province. Here is just a sampling:

POI Software

For those who have GPS navigation systems in their cars, here's an added bonus: You can download additional Points-of-Interest (POI) software onto your gizmo that will tell you when you're approaching stoplights that are hooked up to traffic cameras. You'll find links to this software on the GPS manufacturers' home pages.

- The issuing officer does not show for your court date.
- Two officers were in the patrol car when you received your ticket, and only one shows for the court date. In many jurisdictions, both need to be present to recount their testimony firsthand.
- A factual error on the ticket itself (your license plate number, name, date, or other inarguable fact is incorrect) may get you off the hook.
- There is no correct speed limit sign posted within a reasonable distance of where you were pulled over (in the U.S. this distance varies by state, but is usually about 1/4 mile). ◄

Buying a Car

6 Tricks for Beating Car Salespeople at Their Own Game When Purchasing a Vehicle

Realize that "certified" doesn't mean squat. You'll never get a used-car dealer to admit this, but the term "certified pre-owned" is virtually meaningless—it's nothing more than a marketing come-on. In fact, one auto expert said he's seen "certified" cars with bald tires and bad brakes. He said the "certified" tag just means someone went through a checklist in the garage before putting the car back out on the lot. Many times, a dealer selling a certified used car offers a long-term guarantee, which is good, but unless that guarantee covers everything—and we mean everything—chances are you're just buying a regular old used car with some problems. Before you buy that car, take it to your own mechanic for a careful going-over and let him certify it for you.

Know your extended-warranty options. After jacked-up financing rates, car dealers' biggest profit generators are extended warranties. Before you sign on the dotted line, know that there are other warranty options out there: The Internet can be a saving grace for consumers, with plenty of websites (such as www.warrantydirect.com) offering policies that beat or exceed the ones being offered by the dealer. Again, you may not buy your warranty over the Internet, but just knowing what your pricing options are will give you leverage with the dealer.

Don't fall for dealer sealer. Don't let a car salesman sell you on the protection programs that promise to keep your car looking shiny and new for years to come. Why? It's nothing but a big scam. "They charge anywhere from $300 to $1,500 to throw some stuff on the car, and they'll dazzle you with phrases like 'polymer paint sealant,'" says detailer Prentice St. Clair. "This adds very little value to your car." St. Clair says many of these treatments are guaranteed for five years, when in fact even the best sealants will only last 6 to 12 months. The dealerships are simply banking on the fact you'll never come back in to touch up any mischievous markings that appear on your car.

Specificity Saves You Money

EXPERT INSTANT ADVICE

Ever wonder just what happens when the car salesman tells you he has to "go speak to the manager"? One car dealer who asked us not to reveal his name explained exactly what happens: They spend their time formulating a strategy to sell you a car for maximum profit.

This same expert disclosed the very best way to buy a new car for the lowest price. It's almost too obvious, but he swears virtually no one does it: Know exactly which car you want to buy, including model, options, and color. Then go to five different dealers and tell them what you want. Tell each dealer that you're going to four competitors, and that you'll be back the next day and you want to hear his best price—no nonsense, no sales games, just the price. Our source promises that this is the shortest, quickest way to find a good deal.

How I Do It A Travel Pro Tells Why He Always Rents the Smallest Car Possible

At many popular vacation destinations, they don't stock enough compact and economy cars to fill the needs of everyone who wants to save a few bucks by renting a smaller automobile. This can work out to your advantage.

Let's say you're headed to a big-time tourist mecca, like Las Vegas or Disney World. According to Peter Wu, a frequent traveler (and former chief purser of a major airline), your best bet is to book the smallest car possible. Chances are you're not the only one looking to save a buck; therefore, the smallest cars will likely be the first ones off the lot. If all of the smaller cars are gone by the time you arrive at the rental office, the company will give you a free upgrade.

What if your ploy doesn't work and the car rental agency hasn't run out of the tiny cars? Don't feel bad, says Wu. If you really want a larger car, just tell the counter representative that you have changed your mind and will pay the higher rate. Upgrading to a larger car is much easier than switching from a midsize rental car to an economy model.

Carefully study the fine print of such protection agreements too. "For instance, some dealerships will tell you that bird droppings won't cut through the polymers," St. Clair says. "And then you read the fine print about exclusions, and it says, 'Bird droppings not covered.' "

Pass on rust-proofing. When your car salesman offers to sell you rust protection for your new car, take a pass. Cars are made so well nowadays that this protection is an out-and-out waste of your money. Stick to your guns—don't let his warnings and worries about road salt rattle you.

Check out the tire specs. The salespeople won't mention it, but some new cars are being sold these days with "performance" tires that are designed to give the car better handling on dry roads at super-high speeds—speeds the car can't even reach. Such tires can cost twice as much as conventional tires, and often come with no warranties whatsoever. Because the cost of these tires is rolled into the sticker price of your new car, you might not realize what you've ended up with until a few years later, when you have to replace those pricey tires. So research what the options really are for tires on the model you want to buy.

Buy your car in September. This is the time of year when the next model year cars are being rolled out. Dealers are anxious to liquidate the older new cars, and you can get a real deal. Visit the dealership on a weekday, preferably toward the end of the month (see next page). ◁

Bargaining Car Price
8 Ploys for Buying the Car You Want (Almost) Hassle-Free for the Best Price

Ignore the multiple-rebate ploy. Those car ads in your newspaper are there for one reason and one reason only—to get you into the showroom. And while there are many laws concerning truth in advertising, car dealers get around them by not telling the *whole* truth in advertising. For instance, one car dealer confesses that many of its ads list *all* the rebates you're eligible for—but what the ads don't tell you is that you're only going to be allowed to cash in on one of them. Misleading? Certainly. Illegal? Hardly.

Arrive armed with the car's invoice price. Edmunds.com is the last website that your car salesperson would ever want you to visit. It's a buyer's best Internet source for finding the invoice price (the price the dealer pays) on a new car. At www.edmunds.com, you choose the make, year, and model, and basically build your car with the option package that you're looking for. A few minutes later, you'll have the invoice price and the manufacturer's suggested retail price. Another cool feature on Edmunds.com is the True Market Value, "what others are paying," price, which clues you in on the amount (typically somewhere between retail and invoice) that customers in your area are paying for the same automobile. In Canada, you can try www.carcost canada.com for similar advice, but you'll have to pay a $40 membership.

Go car shopping at the end of the month. It sounds like one of those urban legends, but it's not—car dealers will be more aggressive on the last day

of the month, and this can work in your favor. Virtually all car dealerships have monthly quotas, and if quotas aren't being met, the last business day of the month—and the few days preceding—are the days when the car salesmen are really looking to move their cars off the lot.

So how do you know if the salesmen are scrambling for those sales quotas? Glance around the showroom. If they're nervously scrambling around the room, chances are they are scrambling for sales. While you're not going to get a car for free, just knowing there's a little pressure on the sales force should allow you more room to negotiate.

Order up a discount. Car dealers will never tell you this, but they'd much prefer to sell you a car off their lots (thus clearing out inventory) rather than special-ordering one for you. You can use this fact to your benefit. Tell salespeople that you want to order a base-model car that doesn't have all of the expensive options of the showroom vehicles. They'll likely be more willing to roll back the price of a luxury-packaged car if you agree to take current stock off their hands.

Don't mention your trade-in. New-car dealers love hearing that you want to trade your old car in when you purchase the new model. Why? Because the more variables that they can work into the equation, the easier it is for them to play the smoke-and-mirrors game with the price of that new car. It's a much better idea to negotiate the price on the new car and then, at the last moment, tell them you're interested in trading in your old car. Make it two separate transactions so they can't use "fuzzy math" to confuse you. Of course, no dealer is going to give you more than wholesale value for your trade-in, so unless you've got a real junker, it's almost always better to sell your old car yourself.

Pick apart that trade-in deal.
Sometimes a car dealer will promise you a generous trade-in allowance on your old car, and then neglect to mention that he is jacking up the cost of the new one. The cost of your new car should be the same whether or not you're trading in an old one; to be as prepared as possible, find out how much other dealers are asking for the new car. You should also ask the dealer whether his advertised generous trade-in offer applies to all used cars, no matter how much wear and tear they have. Also, ask whether his special offers apply exclusively to in-stock vehicles, or to those with the most expensive options packages.

Never pay more than $500 over invoice.
You've done your research on the car's invoice price—now use this knowledge to your advantage. If a car isn't the hottest new thing (meaning, the demand outweighs the supply), you should never have to pay any more than $500 over the invoice price. It's just that simple. The salesman won't be happy, and the sales manager won't be happy, but know this—they'd rather sell you the car and make $500 than not sell you

WHAT CAR DEALERS DON'T WANT YOU TO KNOW ABOUT Loans

Car dealers who lure you into the showroom with the promise of a low-interest car loan hope that you won't take a second look at their paperwork. However, there are a number of factors that could mean the "deal of the century" is not so generous after all. Here are some questions to ask that will expose car-dealer double-talk:

- Does the loan require an enormous down payment or a "balloon payment" at the end?
- Is the price of the car higher for people who accept low-interest financing?

- Are you given an unusually short period of time to pay the loan off—say, just a couple of years?
- Will you be required to buy extras that you don't want, such as an extended warranty?
- Will you have to give up the rebate offered by the automaker?

Before you go anywhere near that finance officer's desk, though, know your credit score, and be armed with the interest rates that you qualify for. You can order a free copy of your credit report in the U.S. at www.freecreditreport.com and in Canada at www.equifax.com. At www.bankrate.com, you can research the going rates for auto financing in your area.

the car, especially if that car has been sitting on the lot for a month or two. So go armed with the invoice price, and get the best price possible on the car.

Make them an offer they can't refuse. The second-to-last thing any car dealer wants to do is lose money on a sale. So what's the last thing he wants to do? Leave inventory sitting on the lot, says an anonymous New Jersey car dealer. This has a direct correlation to the amount of "holdback" money that the dealership gets from the automaker. "Holdback" is money meant to offset the costs of keeping the car on the lot, usually distributed in the form of interest payments. The more quickly a dealership moves cars, the more of the holdback money it gets to keep. But as months wear on and cars sit on the lot, the holdback money disappears and the dealership is left holding the bag. Oftentimes, just to move inventory, the dealer will sell cars for less than he paid for them. While there's no surefire way to know how long the dealer has had your preferred car in inventory, it's safe to bet that as the new model year's cars are coming in, last year's models are primed for sale. So make an offer that's a little below invoice, and see what happens. You may end up pleasantly surprised. ◂

Auto Insurance
4 Tips for Getting Good Coverage and Low Premiums on Your Car Insurance

Keep your credit score healthy. Clean up that credit score before shopping for auto insurance. Why? According to Loretta Worters, vice president of the Insurance Information Institute, drivers with long, stable credit histories are less likely to be involved in accidents. People who are lax with their financial affairs, according to the folks who study insurance data, are statistically more likely to file an insurance claim, so the insurance companies consider them to be a higher risk. It may sound like comparing apples to oranges, but the fact remains, this is one method insurance companies employ when determining your auto insurance rate.

Don't let your insurance lapse. Don't fall into the trap those car insurance companies have set up for you—namely, the trap of "I'm not driving my car right now so I don't need insurance." Even if you won't be driving your car for an extended period of time—say, you're traveling overseas for several months or health issues prevent you from getting behind the wheel—it's always better to strip down your insurance to the bare minimum than to cancel it outright. Why? Because car insurers like to see someone insured for 36 consecutive months. So if you let it lapse, you'll be starting from scratch, which means higher premiums and a tougher time landing a policy. That's why you're better off calling your insurance agent and whittling down the coverage to just the bare minimum. This way, you'll maintain your 36-month standing and find it a piece of cake to bring your insurance back up to its previous levels when you finally do get back behind the wheel.

Set up your own car insurance. Your insurance agent chuckles every time you renew collision and comprehensive insurance for a car that's more than five years old. If your car is only worth a couple thousand dollars, it makes better economic sense to lower your insurance premiums and put the cash you save into an account. If you have an accident or your car is vandalized, use your own cash to repair or replace it. Ask your insurance agent how much your premiums will drop if you raise your deductibles or eliminate collision and comprehensive altogether. (Collision covers damage from accidents, and comprehensive covers theft and other damage.) Coverage that once made sense for a brand-new car isn't advisable for an old clunker.

Caught cardless? Call your agent. A phone call to your insurance agent might just get you out of a pickle, under certain circumstances. Consider this scenario: You get pulled over by a police officer, and for the life of you, you can't find your insurance card. With a little luck, however, you won't get stuck with a $200 ticket for failing to produce your documents, says Lloyd Bezar, an Allstate agent in Pennington, New Jersey. Simply ask the officer if you can call your insurance agent and have her vouch for you. In most cases, assuming you actually do have the insurance, the officer will let you go without writing you a ticket. (That said, you're on your own if you were speeding too.) ◄

Getting a Break on Insurance Costs

Everyone knows that you have to do a lot of comparison shopping in order to find a good car insurance rate. The problem is, you may be eligible for some discounts that the agent giving you a quote isn't telling you about. Here are some of the things that can qualify you for a discount on your auto insurance:

- Insuring more than one car
- Having no accidents or moving violations over the last three years
- Being over 55 years of age
- Taking a driver training course or a defensive driving course
- Having an antitheft device
- Driving few miles each year
- Having antilock brakes, air bags, or daytime running lights
- Being a student with good grades
- Being a long-term customer

Recreational Vehicles
4 Travel Strategies That Every RVer Should Know

Land on free parking. Don't be gouged every night for RV campsite parking fees—you really only need to stop at a campsite when you need to dump your waste or pick up water. On the nights when you don't need a hookup, stop by a Wal-Mart or a Sam's Club; both will let you stay in their parking lots after hours for free. Churches, too, usually don't mind RVs in their parking lots, as long as you're gone by the time services start in the morning.

Get a tax break on your RV. Still on the fence about making the leap and buying an RV? Well, maybe this will swing you: If you pay taxes in the U.S. and you finance your purchase, you can write off the interest payments much in the same way you'd write off the mortgage interest on a second home. As long as you use the RV as security for the loan and as long as the RV has sleeping, toilet, and kitchen quarters, you're all set.

Make sure your RV isn't a heavyweight. Plenty of RV makers are building motor homes that are dangerously close to maximum capacity. In other words, each RV comes with a maximum weight the entire rig should carry, and if it's already close to that weight and you haven't even added your family of four or filled the water tank—watch out! Way too many buyers and renters overlook this crucial fact.

Watch out for water damage. Bruce Powell of Pappy's Motorhome Rentals in Salt Lake City, Utah, offers his professional advice on how to avoid buying an RV with water damage: Even if the RV looks pristine, bring it over to another RV dealer and have him check it out. The main thing to look out for is water damage that came in through the roof and settled back behind the walls. Water behind the walls will lead to wood rot, which leads to big bucks and big headaches. ◂

Keeping Pesky Pests Away

Give mice the rough treatment. Rodents can gain entry to your RV through the access slots where you hook up a cable or hose. To keep these critters on the outside, wrap the cable or hose in a bit of steel wool before you connect it, making sure the material fills the surrounding gap. Any mousie trying to enter your vehicle will scrub that plan.

Hate those love bugs? RV drivers who visit the southeastern United States know about the love bug problem. These creatures seem to make a beeline for the highways, only to plaster themselves across the forward-facing surfaces of your vehicle. To make matters worse, the acid in those crushed bug bodies will eat through the finish. The solution: Apply a light coating of baby oil to the vulnerable surfaces of your RV. When you stop for the night, your love bug "collection" will be easy to hose right off.

Secure the perimeter. Buy a gallon jug of pump-up bug spray at a discount store and keep it in your RV. When you set up camp, spray around any spots where the local bugs might gain access to your vehicle—the stabilizer jacks and the tires, for instance.

Motorcycles
6 Tricks to Make Two-Wheelin' a Breeze

Make yourself easy to see. If you ride a motorcycle, you have to put extra effort into being seen—your life depends on it. During the day, ride your motorcycle with the high-beam headlight on. Check the alignment of your headlight and running lights to make sure motorists can easily see them. Many headlights are pointed too far down. Replace weak brake lights with bold halogen lights that will command attention. Adding side lights and reflective devices to your cycle and clothing will reduce the odds of getting smacked by another vehicle in an intersection at night. Also, if your cycle is dark-colored, customize it with a touch of contrasting light color to increase your visibility.

Beware of oil slicks at tollbooths. When you're riding long-distance on your motorcycle, remember that tollbooths are one of the most treacherous locations you will encounter. There are fewer spots on the road that are more likely to be slimy with oil—a tricky obstacle for two-wheeled vehicles. So enter and leave a tollbooth very slowly, and stick to the left tire track to get clean pavement as you pay your "dues." Warn your passenger that tollbooths are a lousy place to make sudden weight-shifts.

Let the postman carry your luggage. If you take your motorcycle on long trips, you know how important it is to pack sparingly, no matter how commodious your saddlebags seem to be. Well, shipping and mailing companies can be your best friend in this respect. Learn the locations of the shipping stores and post offices along your route. Mail ahead to yourself bulky items such as fresh laundry and gifts for people you're going to visit. Mail home your dirty clothes, purchases, and gear you don't need anymore.

Prevent your visor from fogging up. Try this trick from veteran cyclists: Put a drop of dishwashing liquid on the inside of the visor, rub it all around until you can't see it, and wipe off any excess. No more misty visor!

Cleaning marked-up chrome. How do you get those "indelible" boot marks off your chrome exhaust pipe? Pull on rubber gloves and dampen a cleaning rag with oven cleaner. Mask off nearby parts of your motorcycle, then smear the oven cleaner onto the marked-up exhaust pipe; let it sit for 10 minutes. Scrape most of the oven cleaner off with a flat piece of wood or similar non-scratching device. Rinse with a clean, wet rag, and add wax for protection.

Fast, easy spoke cleaning. Cleaning spoked wheels is one of the more annoying motorcycle maintenance chores. Here's how to keep the hassle to a minimum. Buy three bottle brushes and use a separate brush for each of these tasks:

- Clean the spokes with a car-washing solution.
- Apply a car wax according to the package directions.
- Polish the wax.

Hang the brushes side by side in your garage. Put a masking-tape label on each so you can tell them apart at a glance. ◁

General Savings

8 Ways You Can Always Be at the Top of Your Game When It Comes to Finding Bargains

Watch the economic news. Toward the end of the year, pay special attention to the financial section of your newspaper or stories on the evening news about the economy. The retail industry will never tell you when business is slow—store managers *hate* for you to have this information. But the media will certainly let you know. If media forecasts are saying that holiday sales will be sluggish, you can bet that stores will start discounting their merchandise during the fall shopping season. Head to the store and take advantage of discounted merchandise. If you learn on the news the day after Christmas that the shopping season indeed turned out to be disappointing for retailers, plan to head to the store and stock up on bargains, since prices will *really* be slashed.

Check your junk mail. Day in and day out, your mail brings into your home all sorts of offers for cheaper versions of services you purchase each month, such as your cable television and cell phone. Don't just drop these solicitations into the recycling bin—use them to your advantage, urges Jeffrey Strain, a frugality guru and the founder of savingsadvice.com. When a great offer shows up in your mail, call up your current service provider and explain that you're considering switching to the competitor. Read the competitor's offer over the phone and ask whether your existing provider can match this deal. Most of the time, you'll be able to save money with one quick call. When Strain made one of these calls to his mother's cable television provider, the discount he grabbed saved his mom $230 over the next six months!

Become a pro at shopping. An ancient lost art will put thousands of dollars into your pocket every year. Here's what to do: Establish a specific price in your mind—let's say $20—and anytime you're going to buy an item that costs more than this amount, first thoroughly educate yourself about the product, urges Alan Zell, a retail expert in Portland, Oregon, who calls himself "the ambassador of selling." Long ago, shoppers researched the difference between quality brands and poorly made brands. They learned to recognize high prices and bargains. They thought long and hard over their purchases before they put their money on the counter. Shopping carefully like this has become a lost art nowadays, and that's how businesses like it! Stores are more than happy for you to simply grab whichever item is convenient, since you often give them more of your money than you would if you took a little time to make a well-informed purchase. Remember: Stores are professionals at selling you stuff. Level the playing field by becoming a pro at shopping. Once the price passes $20, give all purchases your full attention.

Use credit to your advantage. If your credit card doesn't offer rebates or other incentives, take out a pair of scissors and cut it up, then sign up for one that does. Credit card companies have so thoroughly blanketed the country with their cards—and pleas in the mail for even more people to get them—that they're desperate for your business. Use this inside information to your advantage. Many credit card companies are offering incentives for you to use their cards nowadays. One card may offer you a small discount or rebate when you use it to buy gasoline or groceries. Others may let you earn money toward a new vehicle, discounts on air travel, or discounts for tickets to major amusement parks. If you see an offer for a credit card that provides discounts on items you plan on buying anyway, sign up for it. Then every time you make a purchase, put it on the credit card so you can rack up the benefits. However, remember that these incentives are bait—the credit card companies are trying to lure you into giving them more money than you'll save. Avoid these sneaky traps by paying off your balance every month so that you aren't hit with finance charges and late fees. And avoid cards with a high annual fee, because they eat into your benefits.

Pay some bills in big chunks. Are you still paying bills every month? Put your checkbook away so you can save your time—and money. Many of the service companies you pay regularly, such as your insurance or lawn maintenance, may charge you a lower fee if you pay every six months or annually rather than monthly. Always ask the service provider if you can lower your charge by paying in big chunks once or twice a year. If you can get a discount this way, take it! Not only will you save money on the service, but you'll save time and money on filling out checks and buying postage stamps.

Plan ahead and buy off-season. When it's hot, people want to buy window air conditioners and barbecue grills. When it's cold, they want sweaters and winter coats. And businesses charge a lot of money for these items because demand is so high. Instead of shopping with the herd, make your purchases at times when demand is low so *you* hold the upper hand. The shopkeepers will be happy to offer you a bargain just so you'll take the merchandise off their shelves. This will require you to look a little farther down the road when planning your purchases, and also know when stores are eager to reduce their inventory. If your air conditioner or grill is on its last legs, buy a replacement during the early fall. New models of big appliances such as stoves tend to arrive in stores in early fall too. Store managers will give you a great deal on *last* year's model, since they just want it out of the showroom.

Learn the skill of negotiation. In plenty of locales around the world, the price tag on an item is merely the starting point—you then discuss a more reasonable price with the store owner. Make haggling a regular part of your shopping

experience, urge Toronto-based Anna Wallner and Kristina Matisic, bargain-hunting hosts of the TV show *The Shopping Bags* and authors of *The Shopping Bags: Tips, Tricks, and Inside Information to Make You a Savvy Shopper.* You'll be astounded how often retailers will give a discount in order to make a sale, they say. Look for a small imperfection in the item—perhaps a bouquet of flowers looks less than fresh—and ask for a discount. However, never name the discount you'd like. Just ask for a better price and let the salesperson toss out a figure. When *you* name the price, you may be offering a figure that's higher than the salesperson would suggest.

Stock up on gifts. A steady stream of coworkers, acquaintances, and distant relatives will always be having birthdays. That's just a fact of life. And when you suddenly remember that a birthday is coming up in a few days, you'll probably buy a knickknack or gewgaw that's too expensive just because it's convenient. That's often a fact of life too—but it doesn't have to be. Instead, always be on the lookout for bargains on items that would make a neat gift when you want to give someone *something* but it doesn't have to be perfect. Try a candle in a nice candleholder, or a funny gift book from the rack at the front of the bookstore, or a silicone spatula or other new-fangled kitchen implement. Tuck these into the back of your closet. When a birthday pops up, pull an item from your stash, wrap it up, and pat yourself on the back for your thrifty thoughtfulness. ◂

Special Savings Tricks
8 Secret Ways a Little Ingenuity Can Help You Cut Your Money Outflow

Form a "hand-me-down" club.
Children's clothing stores have a great racket going: Since kids grow so fast, their clothes quickly become unwearable even though they still look nice. So parents have to buy a constant stream of new apparel just to keep up with their growing kids. Instead of enriching the coffers of your local kids' clothing store, organize a club of parents from your child's school or day care to exchange hand-me-down clothing. Twice a year, in the fall and spring, everyone can bring in the clothing that's still in good condition but no longer fits, and you can quickly assemble a new wardrobe for your child while getting rid of items you no longer need. Just make sure a wide range of ages is represented at the gathering, rather than only kids in one grade. That way you'll always have bigger clothes working their way into your trading system.

Get socks of one color. Always buy the same color and style of socks for your child—preferably white, since you can bleach them when they're stained. Since socks invariably vanish, when you lose one of a pair, you can simply pair it up with another, because they're all identical. You'll never be stuck with an "orphaned" sock that has no match. Just imagine how the clothing manufacturers will grit their teeth as you stroll right by that display stand of socks in every imaginable color and texture.

Get the most at the gas pump.
When gas prices soar, every extra block you drive to find bargains puts more money into the pockets of big oil com-

panies. But you can do your bit to get back at these giant corporations with one simple step: Fill up your car during the morning or late evening. Gasoline becomes denser when the temperature is cool. Since the gas pump only measures the *volume* of the gas you put into your car, when the gas is denser, you get a greater quantity for each gallon (or liter) that the gas pump measures. You'll get more distance for your buck than you would if you filled up at noon, when the temperature is higher.

Take a job for a discount. If you're looking for a part-time job, fill out applications at stores where you frequently make purchases, such as clothing stores or sporting-goods shops, which give their employees a discount. If you have teenagers in your home who are ready for a job, encourage them to work at your family's favorite stores with employee discounts too. Not only will you benefit from the discount, you'll also gain access to a new world of inside information on upcoming sales!

Skip the premium channel. If you pay for a premium movie channel just to watch a particular original series, you can bet that some cable bigwigs are getting a laugh over how much they're charging you for a few hours of entertainment. Call your cable company today to cancel your subscription to the channel. These series typically only contain 12 or so episodes per season, and you then have to wait for many months—or even years—before the next season begins. All the while, you're paying those bloated fees to the cable company. Instead, ask a friend who pays for the cable channel to tape the show for you (this is really a small favor to ask of a friend, don't you think?) or just wait a few months and rent the whole season for about $20 when it comes out on DVD. Or, even better, go the to library, take it out, and view it for free.

Turn your back on the vending machines. Want to get a $250 raise for the coming year? Stop buying your sodas and snacks from the vending machine at work. If every day you only brought in one soda and a resealable plastic bag of chips (refilled from a big store-bought bag), you could save $1 each day. If your worksite has a refrigerator, store your sodas and cold snacks there. If not, just bring them in a tiny cooler. Quit being a sucker for vending machines that are more about convenience than they are about product.

Help your friend move. Always help friends pack their belongings and load the truck when they're moving—this simple favor can save you big money. When people are loading their households into boxes, they usually find items that they no longer need or don't want to bother packing and unpacking. As a result, you can bring home hundreds of dollars' worth of spices, frozen food, videos and DVDs, books, toys, furniture, and other handy household items. Best of all, at the end of the day your friends will still think you've done *them* a favor!

Get a reporter's help. Companies live in absolute dread of looking like "the bad guys" in newspaper or TV news stories. If you have tapped out all of the possible ways to air a consumer complaint within the offending company, contact the consumer reporter at your local newspaper or television station. Reporters love "little guy vs. unscrupulous company" stories. Once they make an inquiry, your consumer problem will probably be solved very quickly. ◁

WHAT RETAIL STORES DON'T WANT YOU TO KNOW ABOUT Gift Cards

If a salesclerk tells you that your gift card has expired, don't take it lying down. Retail stores don't exactly advertise this fact, but many gift cards have an "expiration" date on them. They're hoping that the $30 gift card you got for your birthday will languish in your dresser drawer for a year and then they'll get to keep the money. Check your state's or province's consumer laws. In some places, such expiration policies aren't allowed (California, for instance), and in others a generous time frame is mandated (in Massachusetts, it's seven years). Act quickly and complain up the chain of command at the store. If your gift card just expired recently, you're more likely to get your money back.

Grocery Savings

9 Tricks for Getting the Best Quantity and Quality When You Go Shopping for Food

Food-shop just once a week. If you're hooked on impromptu food shopping, break that expensive habit right now. Attach a magnet-backed notepad and pen to your refrigerator, and the moment a food container runs empty and you need to replace it, add it to your list. This simple discipline will have a major impact on your family budget. When you don't keep a list, you're likely to drop into the store for one item here, and two items there. Instead, establish a time each week that you can go to the store when you have time to focus on your shopping and you aren't in a rush. Be sure to take your list with you on your way out the door. Supermarket managers love it when you don't keep a list, for several reasons. First, the more times you go into the store, the more chances you'll have of picking up unnecessary items on impulse. Also, when you buy goods on the spur of the moment, you're more likely to pay full price for them, since you didn't have time to look for a sale or wait for one to arrive. In addition, the more trips you make to the store, the more gas you burn, which adds an invisible cost to your groceries.

Get the smallest carrier possible. If you're going to the supermarket to buy only one item, refrain from getting a basket. If you're only buying three items, get a basket, not a cart. Only get a cart if you're picking up a bunch of items. When you venture into the store knowing you're going to have to carry your purchases up to the counter, you probably won't make impulse buys. Since you've already scouted out the bargains in the sales ads and made a list of the items you need, you shouldn't be buying more stuff anyway, right?

Look for "limited purchase" signs. When you see a sign in the supermarket or clothing store that advertises a low price—but only lets you buy a few items at this price—take advantage of the deal. You may never see this product at a price this low again. When a store sets these limits, it's a sign that it's selling the products at, or even below, the price that it paid for them, says Eugene Fram, Ph.D., a professor of marketing at the Rochester Institute of Technology. Stores don't set limits because they're worried that customers will pile their carts high with the discounted items—they're fearful that owners of smaller mom-and-pop stores will buy out the inventory and resell it at a higher price in their own stores. So mom and pop may be out of luck when these limited offers come around—but it'll be your lucky day.

Know prices of one dozen products. Buy a small spiral-bound notebook, and look through your refrigerator, freezer, and pantry for the 12 products you buy most often. For many people, this list will include sodas, milk, juice, and bread. Give each item its own page and write its name at the top of the page. Take your notebook to the store whenever you shop, and each time you buy the item, jot down the price. And each time you see the item listed in a supermarket sale circular, note the price in your notebook too. It won't take long for you to become aware of when you should stock up on bargains and when you should wait for a sale. As savvy shoppers have learned through their adventures in bargain-finding, you *have* to know the difference between great prices and expensive markups in order to save money. Although a large supermarket may contain 30,000 items, just being able to find your top 12 items at a discount will save you big money. One frugality expert shared this information with us: By simply stocking up on chicken breasts *only* when they're on sale—rather than paying the going price every week—she saves $325 every year.

Watch the register. The checker at the supermarket will want to discuss the weather or make other small talk with you as she rings up your purchases. She may or may not have been trained to do that to help the store

make more money from you, but either way, this distraction can certainly do it. Politely respond that you need to pay attention to something else instead— and keep your eyes trained like a hawk on the register readout. Cash registers aren't always updated with the latest sales prices on items, and some stores pledge to give customers an item free if the register rings up the wrong price. Since you've done your homework and know *exactly* how much the items should cost, alert the clerk if any wrong prices come up. If the store has a generous mistake-finding policy, your moment of attention has earned you a free item. But even if you don't get the product free, at the very least you're ensured that you're getting the low price that you took the time to find.

Check your discount card carefully. Many supermarkets offer discount cards so you can save money on certain products. Often these cards come in the form of tiny plastic rectangles that go on your key chain, which the clerk passes over the register scanner. Be careful when you hand your key chain to the clerk if more than one store's discount card is attached to it. If the clerk scans the wrong card, the machine may still beep as if it's going to give you the discount— but it never does. Hold the right card between your fingertips as you hand your key chain over at the checkout counter,

How I Do It **A Bargain Hunter Tracks Sales Patterns**

You don't have to monitor the constant pricing activities at all the supermarkets in your town to save on groceries, says Stephanie Nelson, a bargain-finding author and founder of couponmom.com. All the sales will ultimately come to each store, she says, and running back and forth between stores eats up your precious time and expensive gasoline. However, develop a fundamental understanding of the store's sales programs. Choose a store that doubles or triples the value of the coupons you use. If the store offers a special member-ship card so you can save money, use it. Read the store's advertising section in your newspaper each week for upcoming sales. When you see a great sale on an item, buy a six-week supply so you'll have enough to last you until the item goes on sale again.

and watch the register to make sure that it's displaying your discounts.

Hit the farmers' market late in the day. Farmers' markets are great places to buy fruits and vegetables—the produce is fresher because it's grown close to your home. And when you show up at the right time, you can take home your favorite fruits and veggies at a steep discount. Late in the day, sellers are faced with the prospect of having to cart home or throw away unsold merchandise. They hate having to do that. So they're likely to sell you their remaining items at a reduced price so they won't have to figure out what to do with them. To find your nearest farmers' market, visit the U.S. Department of Agriculture's website at www.ams.usda.gov/farmersmarkets. In Canada, search for "farmers' markets" and your province's name.

Do it yourself to save money. Food companies like you to think they're doing you a favor by offering bags of prewashed salad and individual servings of soup. Actually, they're just looking for a way to charge you more money. Buy individual salad components instead of bagged salads, and soup, oatmeal, cereal, and other foods in regular-sized containers instead of tiny ones. Washing the salad or dividing the food into multiple bowls only takes a few seconds, and you won't be paying extra money for conveniences that you don't really need.

Keep your beer in the dark. If you're a big beer drinker, you can save a bundle by taking a tip from wine connoisseurs. Create a "beer cellar." Find a cool, dark spot where you can leave cases of beer without moving them—under these conditions, beer will stay fresh for six months. Watch for the summer sales, when you can buy in bulk and get the best discounts on your favorite brands. The convenience store manager—the one who has been charging you those outlandish markups on six-packs—will just weep when he sees his bottom line. ◁

Using Coupons
4 Special Ways to Get the Most from Your Coupons When You Go Grocery Shopping

Get more coupons. Coupons are a great way to gradually save big money on your grocery bills each year. So why stop with getting only one set of coupons from the Sunday newspaper or door-to-door packets when you can get two, three, or even more bundles of coupon circulars? Ask your friends and family if they receive the coupons but don't use them. If so, ask for them. In addition, swing by the supermarket late on Sunday evening. They may let you buy any leftover newspapers at a steep discount. If your main source of coupons is flyers in the supermarket itself or the website of the supermarket chain, you can pick up or print out as many coupons as you want.

Combine your savings. You'll never get your grocery store manager to volunteer this information, but when you use your coupons on items that are also on sale, you may get the merchandise for just a few cents—or even free. Most items in a supermarket will go on sale every six weeks or less, says Stephanie Nelson, known as the Savings Mom on ABC News' *Good Morning America*. Looking at the store's weekly advertisement in your local paper is a good way to find these sales. When you find an item that's on sale, review your coupon file to see if you have a coupon to lower the cost even further. If this is a store that doubles or even triples your coupons, you may have just found a free product. When you find a great bargain, stock up on it so you'll have enough to last until it's on sale again.

Watch for the bonus coupons. A lot goes on as you leave the checkout counter—you're paying, grabbing your receipt, and preparing to wheel your bargain-laden cart to your car. But don't forget one more slip of paper: Many checkout lines have a machine that spits out

---

WHAT **GROCERY STORES** DON'T WANT YOU TO KNOW ABOUT Product Placement

While you're wheeling your cart down the aisles, do plenty of stooping down low and reaching up high. Food makers may pay extra to stores to have their products stocked at eye level so consumers see them easily. And guess who pays the extra cost so these foods can have prime real estate in the supermarket? That's right—you. Supermarket managers cross their fingers and hope you'll drift through the store with your gaze firmly at eye level. So be sure to look up and down. The items stacked on the highest and lowest shelves will probably be better deals.

coupons for items you might be interested in on your next trip to the store, based on the products you've bought on this trip. It's easy to ignore these coupons in the hustle and bustle of the checkout stand. When the coupon emerges from the machine, tuck it into your purse or pocket rather than putting it into a bag of groceries, where it will likely get lost.

Organize your coupons with coupon mom.com. Stephanie Nelson hates the thought that grocery manufacturers offer consumers *$318 billion* in coupons each year, but we don't make use of 99 percent of these savings. So she's created a tool to help you grab thousands of dollars of this bounty each year.

Most people find coupons too hard to use, since hundreds of them are jammed in random order into circulars in your Sunday paper with no organization by name or product type. It's a chore to hunt through piles of coupons to find just the one you need. Her tool quickly and easily solves these problems for American bargain hunters. You'll find it on her website, www.couponmom.com. Founded in 2001, the site offers a feature she calls the Virtual Coupon Organizer. To use it, you must first start saving the coupon circulars from your Sunday paper or other source. Write the date on them—along with an S or a V, which stands for SmartSaver or Valassis, the two companies that produce these circulars—and stick them into their own section in an accordion file. Before you go grocery shopping the next time, call up the virtual coupon tool on the website and select your state from a menu (this feature works for 44 states). The site will then tell you *all* the products with coupons that have run in your

newspaper that are still valid. If you need kitty litter, simply search down the list of hundreds—or even thousands—of items to see if there's a coupon for kitty litter. If there is, you'll see the date that this coupon appeared in your newspaper, and which of the two circulars contained it. Go to that circular in your accordion file and pick out the coupon with ease.

Along with this ultra-cool money-saving tool, the site also has a feature that allows you to choose your state, then see a list of dozens of *other* great discounts at particular supermarket chains and drugstores in your area that don't even require a coupon.

In Canada, you can go to www.frugal shopper.ca, which partners with some of the country's largest retailers and has coupons featured in store flyers listed by province. Or visit www.save.ca to select coupons for your favorite brands. Just specify your province and click on the coupons you want to receive. They will be mailed to you free of charge the next business day. ◁

Retail Shopping
11 Secrets That Renegade Shoppers Use When Buying General Merchandise

Speak your mind. You needed to find out if the pair of jeans you admired on your friend were available in your size—but the 20-something store clerk was too engrossed in her cell-phone conversation to help you. Don't handle the situation by vowing never to go to the store again. If you're steamed over any issue in a store, from an encounter with a rude or unhelpful salesperson to shoddy merchandise—use the situation to your advantage. Store managers want their customers to return, and they have a lot of leeway to give you a special offer when you're disgruntled to make you happy with the store again. Ask for a refund or a discount, store credit, or some other type of incentive on your next purchase.

Don't be afraid to ask for a discount. Similarly, forget about feeling embarrassed or uncomfortable when you call a company and threaten to take your business elsewhere if it won't offer you a discount. This call might be the best conversation the customer-service representative has had all day! Many customer-service reps get bonuses for keeping customers who are thinking about leaving, says frugal-living advisor Jeffrey Strain. That's because it costs companies a lot of money to bring in new customers, and many are happy to offer a discount to keep you from canceling the service. So make that call—the company's representative should be happy to work with you to offer you a deal, and a few minutes on the phone can put hundreds of dollars back into your pocket.

Follow the return policy. Before you fork over $100 at the mega-electronics store for a portable DVD player for your kids to watch in the car, visit the customer service desk and read the fine print about the store's return policy. If you don't, you could get stuck with a bad purchase. Stores often require you to follow complicated directions in order to return a product. You may need to provide the receipt and all of the item's original packaging to get a refund or replacement item. So be sure to review the return policy before you leave the store to cut down on confusion later. When you get home from shopping, take your receipt out of the shopping bag and stash it in a special folder in your desk drawer. Then stow the item's box and other packaging in the original shopping bag in the back of your closet until the period of time in which you can return it has passed. If you become dissatisfied with the item, you can quickly reassemble all the elements you need to return it to the store.

Show up at the right time. The more information you have about a store and its products, the more chance you'll have of finding a great bargain. And when, exactly, is the best time of day to find the inside scoop on a store's merchandise? About 2 p.m., says Anne Obarski, a St. Charles, Missouri, consultant who advises businesses on how to provide good customer service. At this point in the day, the morning shift is still working and the evening staffers are just starting their shift. Avoid hitting stores during the first 45 minutes after they open—the few workers are still busy getting the store ready for the day. Late in the evening, they're often more interested in closing up the shop than helping you with your purchase.

Write a nice letter to get freebies. Wouldn't it be nice if manufacturers filled your mailbox with free cosmetics and other products? They're happy to do so; all you have to do is say something nice to them. Manufacturers get lots of letters from customers complaining about items, and it makes their day when they get a letter *complimenting* their products. If you use a product often and really enjoy it, write a letter to the manufacturer, recommends Donna Montaldo, the coupon and bargain expert at about.com. She's written letters to show her support for her favorite cosmetics, and by doing so, she says, "you can usually get a ton of coupons in the mail." Find the mailing address of the company on the product's package or on the company's website. Make sure you mention the exact name of the product you enjoy and how long you've been using it when you write the letter. Apply a stamp, cross your fingers, and wait for those coupons as a thank-you for your letter.

Act promptly on rebates. Many manufacturers offer rebates on their products, from toothpaste to televisions. These can put $20—or even more— back into your pocket. But companies don't always make the rebate process easy, and when you don't follow their rules, you probably won't get your money. After all, they count on a certain percentage of their customers failing to apply for the money. Since you often need to mail in a receipt to claim your rebate, ask for a duplicate of the receipt at the checkout counter. This way you'll have a backup copy in case the company loses the one you send in or you need to

WHAT **WAREHOUSE STORES** DON'T WANT YOU TO KNOW ABOUT Prices

Managers of warehouse stores—those no-frills stockrooms with bare concrete floors and pallets stacked high with bulk goods—want you to think these stores offer the best bargains you'll find. That's not really true. These stores *do* tend to offer better deals than you'd get if you simply filled your cart at the grocery store without comparison shopping and seeking out bargains, says Jonni McCoy, founder of miserlymoms.com. However, now that you have the inside scoop on finding bargains, you're not just an average shopper anymore. You can find better deals on many items than the prices that warehouses offer. When you use coupons and wait to buy items when they're on sale, you'll generally get your household goods more cheaply at the supermarket (she's made spreadsheets to prove this!) You can save 50 percent or more on cereal, meat, toilet paper, paper towels, and many other staples when they're discounted at the supermarket versus the warehouse store. Plus, at the supermarket you don't have to pay an annual membership fee, which takes away some of the value you gain at the warehouse store.

How I Do It A Penny Pincher One-Stop-Shops for Bargains

Annette Economides, a Phoenix-based bargain finder, publishes "The Home*Economiser* Newsletter." She knows virtually every trick in the book when it comes to saving money. But she doesn't always have time to use every trick. When she needs to go shopping but is in a time crunch, she'll run down her shopping list and look through the newspaper sales circulars from several stores to find the cheapest prices. Often these are the loss leaders, or absurdly low-priced items that stores set out solely to bring in customers. Once she finds the lowest prices for as many items as possible, she'll head off to one store that has a policy of matching its competitors' prices. When she pulls her cart up to the register, she pulls out her advertising flyers and shows the clerk the low price that the store needs to match on each item. This way, she reaps the benefits of sales all around town—but only has to expend time and gasoline shopping at one place.

return the item because it's defective. As soon as you get home from the store, immediately send off for the rebate. You often have to fill out a form and include the proof of purchase—which is often found on the package—along with the receipt. If you don't stuff all these bits of paper into an envelope right away and mail it to the manufacturer, odds are good that you'll lose one of these crucial elements, and your rebate will slip away.

Befriend the store's staff. You have your eye on a particular backpack that you're planning to buy before your hiking trip later in the summer, but it's not on sale now. Engage the salesperson—or even better, the store manager—in a little chitchat to establish a friendly atmosphere, then ask if the item will be on sale anytime soon. You're not just a run-of-the-mill customer anymore—you're a person about to reel in some inside scoop. Since you have a casual banter going, the staffer may share some inside info on upcoming sales that the other shoppers don't know about. Next weekend, or even a few months from now, you may be able to stroll back in and snag the backpack at a 20 percent discount.

Take advantage of loss leaders. Stores often advertise products at a super-low price just to bring you into the store. They may lose money on these loss leaders, but they'll make even more money because they're using the bargains to lure customers toward other items in the store that are marked up in price. When you head into the store to buy one of these great bargains, just buy the loss leader, turn right around, pay for it, and leave. When you buy other things, you're almost guaranteed to blow any money you've saved on the bargain.

Check out new apparel thoroughly. Clothing retailers are perfectly happy when you take home damaged goods and decide, later, that complaining is not worth the bother. But think about it: There's a good chance that some other customer has tried on the garment that you're thinking of buying. Sometimes a hurrying shopper will get a foot caught in a hem and rip it. Some unscrupulous shoppers will even snip off the extra buttons from a garment while they're in the fitting room. So before you head for the cash register, check that a new garment's hems, extra buttons, fasteners, and other details are intact and operating correctly.

Beware "sales" bins. When you're cruising through a department store, you find all of the display racks in impeccable order—until you come across a bin of items dumped in a disheveled heap. Your immediate reaction is, Oh boy, steeply discounted items! That's just what the store manager wants you to think. Hold on to your wallet and check the prices carefully. An unkempt display does not necessarily mean a good deal.

Use coupons for bargains. Coupons are not just for groceries. Department store ads in newspapers often have coupons for 10 to 20 percent off in certain departments or for certain kinds of clothing. Combine that with a sale, and you can snap up some dazzling duds at truly bargain basement prices. If you have a store credit card, check the inserts that come with your bill. You may find a coupon or two tucked in there to lure you back to the store. And stores often have special sales offering an extra 10 to 20 percent off for using their credit card. ◄

Shopping Alternatives

6 Tricks for Finding the Best Bargains at Yard Sales, Outlet Stores, and Thrifts

Plan your yard sale attack. One of the penny pinching-est people on the planet revealed to us her personal game plan for scooping up scores of cents-on-the-dollar yard sale bargains in a single weekend. Now you know too: Go to a nearby convenience store and pick up a street map that covers all the residential neighborhoods in your town or city. When your Friday newspaper arrives on your doorstep—with its classified section brimming with ads for garage sales—plan your attack. Circle the ones that fall within pricier neighborhoods, and use your map to list the order in which you'll hit each sale. Homes in more expensive areas of town tend to offer more upscale goods, says Shelley Kincaid, author of *The Garage Sale Decorator's Bible* and host of a home-décor-on-a-budget TV show in Colorado. She should know: She says she goes to dozens of yard sales *each weekend.* By carefully planning your route to all these sales, you'll cut down on wasted miles driving back and forth. When you spend $5 or $10 less on gasoline, the bargains you'll find become even better deals. To *really* cut down on driving time, look for community sales, in which dozens of households in a neighborhood or subdivision are selling their items at the same time.

Equip yourself for yard sales. Finding great deals at yard sales depends on speed—so you can find the good items before other shoppers get to them—and a discerning eye that lets

Break the Secret Yard Sale Code

The most experienced yard sale shoppers can hit sales early by understanding a subtle code embedded in the classified ads. By mastering this code-speak, you, too, will be able to zoom directly to all the sales that offer the particular items that you want.

- At a *moving sale,* you'll find household items that are useful, but that the soon-to-be-moving owner can't move or won't bother bringing–think plants, lawn mowers, and gallons of paint.

- An *estate sale* is likely to showcase items from an older person who has passed away, such as antiques and vintage collectibles.

- The contents at a *divorce sale* will vary according to which member of the split-up couple is hosting the sale. If the man is doing the selling, expect to find items such as appliances, dishes, and women's clothing. If the woman is hosting the sale, look for sports memorabilia and power tools. Divorce sales are particularly good places to find a bargain–sellers are inclined to sell stuff for a song, since they just want the merchandise out of their lives, says yard sale expert Shelley Kincaid.

you pick out the quality merchandise from the junk you don't want. Load up a fanny pack with the following weapons so you can move quickly from sale to sale and pounce when you find a great deal:

- *Small bills and coins.* Your debit and credit cards are no good in the yard sale world, and sellers may not want to take checks either. You don't want to lose that beautiful lamp because you ran out of cash.

- *A tape measure.* From curtains to couches and from mirrors to mini-blinds, you need to know if certain items will fit in your home before you buy them. Know what sizes you're looking for before you take off for the yard sales, and measure these sorts of objects at the sale before you purchase them. If you forget your tape measure, you can also use a dollar bill to check sizes—it's six inches long.

- *A magnifying glass.* Quickly check for dents, loose threads, and other imperfections before you shell out any cash.

- *A map.* When you finish at one sale, it's time to make a beeline for the next one.

To call it your own, take a piece home. It's nothing short of a tragedy: You find a beautiful chest of drawers late in the day after you've spent most of your money on garage-sale bargains, and you don't have enough cash left to buy this new treasure. Sure, you could give the owner a few dollars as a deposit, but who's to say he won't go ahead and sell the chest of drawers to some other buyer who happens to have cash on the barrelhead? Here's a crafty trick gleaned from one of the world's best bargain hunters: Give the owner as much money as you can for a deposit. Then, before leaving to get the rest of the money, take a drawer with you. No other shopper will be willing to buy the incomplete chest, so you're assured that it will be waiting for you when you return. Top-drawer advice!

Plug into irregulars at outlet malls. A salesperson at a regular retail store would *never* steer you away from a full-priced pair of jeans and suggest you buy a slightly damaged version for a 30 percent discount. But that's exactly the sort of offer you'll find at an outlet mall. On your next shopping trip, skip the retail mall and head for the nearest outlet mall. Many clothing chains operate stores in outlet malls that offer merchandise for a lower price than you'd find at a regular retail mall. Some of the best bargains you'll find in outlet stores are items with tiny irregularities. These imperfections may be so small that you can't even find them! Ask the store manager to show you the section containing irregular items. Once you pick the item you want, ask the manager for his or her opinion on whether the defect will significantly decrease the usefulness or life span of the item. Odds are good that it won't. At outlets, you do have to be careful of brand-name merchandise that is made specifically for outlets and is of a lower quality than the brands' department store merchandise. So inspect items carefully for workmanship, fabric quality, and such.

Buy slightly vintage bread. It probably takes your family a few days to finish a loaf of bread—so what's one more day? Steer your cart right past the bread aisle in the supermarket, and buy your bread and other baked goods from your nearest day-old-bread outlet. This is where bread, rolls, and other bakery items go when they don't sell quickly in the supermarket, and these bread thrift stores offer the products at a very steep discount. When you get them home, just pop them into the freezer and take out a few pieces as you need them. Bread freezes very well.

Shop at year's end at thrift shops. Secondhand outlets run by charities such as Goodwill Industries or the Salvation Army would like your business year-round—and shopping there frequently is a good idea, since you can get clothes and other household items for a fraction of what you'd pay in retail stores. But there's a special two-month period during the year when you'll find an extra-large variety of bargain merchandise: December and January. Crowds of people flock to these stores to drop off their donations at the end of the year for tax purposes, and you'll find that the extra assortment of goodies on the shelves lasts even into the new year. If you only go to these stores once during the year, this is the time to visit! ◁

WHAT **HOUSEHOLD PRODUCT MAKERS** DON'T WANT YOU TO KNOW ABOUT Amounts

Even though labels tell you to pour a cupful of detergent into your washing machine, squirt the cleaner into the reservoir in your dishwasher until it's full, or add a level scoop of coffee into your coffeemaker—you don't *have* to use this much. Manufacturers are in business to make money, and the more times you return to the store to replace their products, the more money they make. Experiment by using a little less—pour out a quarter-cup less laundry detergent. Keep your toothbrush an extra week beyond what the package recommends. Squirt only half as much cleaner into your toilet bowl. You'll find that you can cut back on many household products without seeing a difference in results—and all those bottles, jars, and tubes of product will last longer!

Buying Online
5 Little-Known Ways to Safely Get Those Great Savings Available in Cyberspace

Buy from auction sites on holiday weekends. When you bid on items on the eBay auction website, you will always see when the bidding will end. Watch for items for which the bidding will close at a time when most people are away from their computers, says Steve Economides. (The aptly named bargain guru is operator of americas cheapestfamily.com with his wife, Annette.) If bidding stops at 9 p.m. on July 4, or 8 a.m. Christmas morning, few people will be adding bids and running up the price at the last minute. You can sneak in at the closing seconds, place your bid, and claim the item for yourself.

Be creative with your spelling. If you're looking for a particular item on an auction site—say, an Armani suit—try searching for it under a few misspellings, say bargain hunters Anna Wallner and Kristina Matisic. Sellers who aren't good spellers may be offering the suits as Aramani or Armane, for example. Since most people searching through the site would only look for the suit under its proper spelling, you'd be competing with fewer shoppers when you cast your bid.

Look for a reputable rating. When considering whether to buy an item on eBay, consider the seller's rating. Unscrupulous folks hiding behind a pseudonym online may take your money and never send you the product. However, people who buy merchandise over the site can rate sellers based on criteria such as whether the item was described accurately, whether it arrived on time, and if it showed up undamaged. Steer clear of sellers with less than a 98 percent positive rating, Annette Economides warns. Your risk of having an unhappy transaction goes up as the seller's approval rating drops. If you're tempted to buy an item but the seller's reputation seems questionable, send the person an e-mail asking about the product. If you receive a thoughtful response in a timely manner, this is a good sign that you're dealing with an honest individual.

Let the Web shop for you. A number of websites have sprung up in recent years that will hunt down bargains for you. Before you start driving from store to store to compare prices on electronics, appliances, clothing, or other household goods, first visit several shopping comparison sites to get a sense of what a bargain price for the item looks like. In 2006, *Consumer Reports* magazine investigated six of these sites: froogle.com, nextag.com, pricegrabber.com, shopping.com, shopzilla.com, and shopping.yahoo.com. The magazine found that Yahoo and Froogle displayed the lowest prices. But search for your desired item at more than one of these sites to make sure you find plenty of options. Be sure to find out what the shipping and handling charges will be from each source so you're comparing the full cost from all the potential sellers.

Google those online vendors. Check the reputation of any company you buy from over the Internet. There are swarms of companies willing to sell you merchandise online, some of them reputable name brands and some of them fly-by-night shysters. Such companies would be embarrassed to have you do this, but go to your favorite Internet search engine and enter the company's name. You will probably be able to click your way to a forum where other customers air their opinions of the service they received. Another check to make: On the company's website, make sure there's a phone number and an address—signs of the company's stability. Make sure the address and phone number are accurate by checking them in the business listings of a standard directory search site such as 411.com, WhitePages.com, or superpages.com. You might also want to call the phone number. Be especially wary of doing business with websites that have offices that are based in other countries, since they are harder to check and you'll have fewer alternatives if your deal goes awry. ◄

Online auction sites are a great place to find bargains—but they're also cyber-hangouts for very sneaky crooks. Plenty of fraudulent folks will advertise cool merchandise at tantalizing prices, then take your money and run as soon as you pay them. These scams are especially painful when you're trying to buy big-ticket items that cost thousands of dollars. On smaller purchases, you may be protected from online fraud; for instance, when you use eBay, the site protects you up to $175, and when you use the PayPal method of paying, it may protect you up to $1,000.

To protect yourself on larger purchases, arrange to pay the seller through an escrow account. An escrow service will hold your payment until you verify that you've received the merchandise, then it will turn the money over to the seller. This way your money's in neutral hands until you're happy with your purchase.

But not every escrow service is safe. Plenty of services exist only to scam you. Here's how to protect yourself:

- Some of these scammers work hand-in-hand with fraudulent sellers to rip you off. As a result, eBay endorses escrow.com.

- If you choose to use a different service, be wary of any escrow providers that the seller suggests.

- Steer clear of escrow services that don't list their address and phone number on their websites, or services that have misspellings or odd language on their sites.

- Call the phone number to see if someone answers.

- Also, services should be licensed and bonded; verify this information with a state or provincial consumer-protection agency in the state or jurisdiction in which the company is located.

Auction Strategies

6 Best Bets for Getting the Best Bargains When Buying by Bidding

Check out storage-unit auctions. Check your newspaper classifieds for storage facility auctions, and visit your local storage companies to ask if they have any upcoming auctions scheduled. People keep all sorts of valuable items in storage facilities: seasonal sporting equipment, collectible comic books, china dishes, and other cool stuff. However, they don't always pay their monthly fees! When this happens, managers regularly sell off the contents of abandoned storage units to the highest bidder—which could allow you to bring home great bargains.

Know your auctioneer. At an auction, the auctioneer's obligation is to make money for the people selling the merchandise, says Gary Peterson, president of the Auctioneers Association of Canada and the auctioneer with Hudson Auctions in Hudson, Quebec. However, the auctioneer wants *you* to leave satisfied with your purchases too. Strike up a conversation with the auctioneer before the sale begins. Mention the items you're interested in buying and ask the auctioneer if he knows any helpful information about the items, such as their age, condition, and value. Once you get to know an auctioneer—particularly if you're a regular at auctions in your area—he can help you out in a number of ways, Peterson says. An auctioneer may choose to "ignore" your bid if he thinks you're trying to pay too much for the item. Or if he notices that you're not paying attention to an item that you'd probably be interested in, he may mention during his high-speed patter that you should consider bidding. By having a good rapport with the auctioneer, you'll notice these helpful little signals.

Bid reasonably. If you're going to toss out the first bid at an auction, start with a low price, but not a price that would be a "steal" for the item, says auctioneer Peterson. For example, if you think the item is worth $1,000, don't start your bidding at $5. Offer $100 or $200 instead. The auctioneer needs to make money for the seller hosting the auction, and if certain items aren't going to fetch a reasonable price, the auctioneer can halt the bidding. If few people were going to bid against you anyway, your excessive bargaining just lost you the prize!

Set your limit ahead of time. Before bidding begins on an item—whether it's an in-person or online auction—write down on a piece of paper how much you're willing to spend, then add an extra 10 percent. During a heated exchange of bids, most people lose their ability to stick to a reasonable price. Once you reach your limit, and then the added wiggle room you've allowed yourself, stop bidding. Don't go a dime higher. Let the winning bidder realize with dismay that she's just paid too much on an item, and save your money to win on an auction bid another day.

Avoid publications promising big savings at auctions. Government auctions that sell property such as seized vehicles and foreclosed homes can be places to find decent bargains. However, pay no heed to advertisements that want to sell you guides on finding auctions that sell this type of property for next to nothing. For starters, you may be charged for more guides than you really want, according to the Federal Trade Commission. At around $50 a pop, these get expensive quickly. Another reason to skip these is that they only provide information that you could easily find on your own. Finally, they tend to exaggerate the deals you'll encounter. Don't get your hopes up *too* much about the savings you'll find at these auctions. Plenty of people know about them and show up to bid on worthy sales. If indeed you find a car for a few hundred dollars, or a house for a few thousand, they're going to be very questionable in value. Instead of purchasing one of these guides, visit your local city hall, which may have information about upcoming auctions. Or find auctions on the Internet by searching for the words "government auctions" and looking at sites ending with ".gov" in the search results in the U.S. In Canada, the Public Works and Government Services Canada website is a good one to access at www.pwgsc .gc.ca. It provides a list of Crown Assets that are on the auction block; to view featured items go to crownassets.pwgsc .gc.ca.

Seek out auctioned furniture deals. When home interiors retailers receive a truckload of products, if one box inside the truck is damaged or open, they will typically refuse the entire truckload, not just the one box. Instead of having the shipping company return all the products, the manufacturer of the products often sells the truckload of refused goods to the shipping company. The shipping company then auctions it off for pennies on the dollar. Most of the material is perfectly fine, and the auctions are open to the public. Contact the major shipping company in your area and ask about these auctions. You can save a lot of money. ◁

When Shopping for Anything, Free Is the Best Price

EXPERT INSTANT ADVICE

Whenever you need to buy anything, always work your way up the "shopping hierarchy" from the cheapest to most expensive to find the best deal, urge Steve and Annette Economides, authors of the book *America's Cheapest Family Gets You Right on the Money.* Here's how the hierarchy works:

- First, try to borrow the item from a friend or neighbor. If you only need to cut down a few trees, *borrowing* a chain saw makes a lot more sense than buying one.

- Can't borrow it? Try to get it *free*. Websites such as craigslist.org or freecycle.org will identify all sorts of useful items that people in your area are giving away free. Steve is well on his way to collecting thousands of free bricks he wants for building a walkway—instead of paying hundreds of dollars for new bricks.

- If you can't get things free, buy a *slightly damaged* version. A new washing machine may have a small scratch on the side but will still work perfectly fine.

- If a dinged version isn't available, then shop around for a store offering the item at a *discount*.

- Finally, if you can't get the item free or cheap, only then should you pay full price. But odds are very good that you'll find what you're looking for long before you have to settle for the most expensive option.

Budget and Savings
6 Easy Ways to Keep More Cash in Your Pocket

Keep a slush fund handy.
Something—be it a car repair, an emergency root canal, or a job layoff—always comes up to throw you off your monthly budget. To keep these incidents from running you into debt, you need to have an emergency stash in an easily accessible account, preferably a money market account (they earn a little more interest than regular savings accounts).

But how much is enough to get you out of a bind? Easy. Track all of your spending for a month (including everything from your mortgage payment to lunch at the deli), and multiply that monthly total by three. That three-month operating budget is a scary number, eh? Well, this is the minimum you should have on hand in case the roof caves in (literally or figuratively) and you need some dough to get you through the rough spots. And don't worry if this money isn't accruing the big interest; it's there for emergencies.

Ditch the ATM card. We're always making impulse purchases, from a pack of gum at the supermarket checkout line to that new Van Halen-meets-bluegrass CD. How can you stop your bank account from hemorrhaging? Take a page from the old-timers and shred your ATM card. It's just too easy to take out $100 at the local 7-Eleven when you're jonesing for a Snickers bar at 2 a.m. Instead, figure out how much cash you'll need each week for your regular, cash-based purchases (things like lunch at the cafeteria and your daily cup of coffee), head on over to the bank teller's window, and get your walking-around money for the week. With a finite amount of cash, you'll start to think twice before those spur-of-the-moment spending sprees.

Unionize your money. There's a better place than a bank to park your dough for your checking account needs, and if you want to take out a home equity loan, there's a better place to get that as well. It's called a credit union, and it acts much the same as a bank, but it has better loan and savings rates. Here's how they work: A credit union is a cooperative venture that doesn't have to make profits for clamoring stockholders. The people who do business with the credit union—you, with your checking accounts and loans—more or less "own" the credit union. Many credit unions now offer the same services as banks, including debit cards and online banking. You can find a credit union at the Credit Union National Association's website, www.cuna.org. It has a searchable list of credit unions broken down by state, and eligibility criteria. In Canada, try the site cucentral.ca, run by the Credit Union Central of Canada.

Put yourself on your payroll. There comes a time every month when the bills start piling up and you force yourself to sit down and write out all the checks. Well, there's one more check you should be writing—one to yourself. Jay Fine, a longtime financial planner based in Monroe, New Jersey, offers this easy way to put your retirement planning into high gear. "Put yourself on the payroll," he says. "Every month—or even better, every paycheck—make sure you set an amount aside for investment. A good number would be about 6 percent. Anything more would be great. If you have to, you can even write yourself a check to deposit or send to another account. But just as you pay your mortgage and your electric bill without fail, now you'll be making sure to pay yourself as well."

SECRET WEAPON

Budget Formula

So you diligently track your income and every expense that you have. But how do you know if you're spending reasonable amounts of money on things like housing, debt, and groceries? Follow these parameters offered by E. Kim Dignum, a financial planner in Fort Worth, Texas, courtesy of CNNmoney.com (all figures are percentages of your gross household income):

30 percent: Housing and debt (mortgage/rent, credit cards, auto loans, student loans, etc.)

26 percent: Living expenses (food, clothing, utilities, transportation, medical, entertainment)

25 percent: Taxes (federal, state, local, and property; FICA and Medicare or CPP in Canada)

15 percent: Savings and retirement (401(k), stocks, mutual funds, college savings, RRSP in Canada, etc.)

4 percent: Insurance (life, health, disability, auto, homeowners, etc.)

Make, and stick to, a budget. Budgets are the first steps to gaining some financial order in your home. Stanley Kershman, an author, lawyer, and creator of the website www.debtonadiet.com, has a six-step plan to accomplishing just that:

1. Don't attempt to do your entire budget in one sitting. Take a few days, breaking the work down into manageable pieces.
2. Gather up all of your income information, including salaries, interest, and gifts.

Easy Financial Rules of Thumb

Concerned about how much you're spending, how much you should be saving, and how much house you can afford? Use these easy equations to determine how financially healthy you are:

- The **price of your home** should not be more than 2.5 times your annual gross household income.

- Your **total monthly debt payments** (including mortgage, student loans, car, and credit card payments) should not be more than 35 percent of your monthly gross income. Some mortgage brokers will stretch this ratio up to 40 percent, but that leaves you very little budgetary wiggle room.

- To **retire comfortably**, your nest egg should be about 20 times what you want your annual income to be. If you anticipate needing about $75,000 a year to live on when you retire, you'll need to save a nest egg of about $1.5 million. Of course, this will vary if you retire early or continue to work longer than usual.

3. Next, gather up all of your expense information. Do this thoroughly, even if it takes three days, a week, or a month. Make sure you're not missing anything.

4. Using a budget worksheet—the free one on debtonadiet.com or one you mock up on your own—add up all of the totals for the income and outflow.

5. Figure out where you can do some fine-tuning, either to pay down your debt or increase your savings goals. However, above all, make sure you're making as much money as you're spending. Stay out of the red.

6. Redo the budget with the new totals, and post it around your house, lest you forget you are now living within the cozy confines of a household budget.

Divvy up any unexpected income. When you have a windfall—a bonus, gift, or extra cash for extra work—use the rule of thirds to determine how to use it:

- *One third for the past.* Use one third to pay down debt you owe.

- *One third for the future.* Put a second third immediately into some sort of savings or investment.

- *One third for the present.* Use the final third to make a home or personal improvement or purchase you want.

If you follow this rule, you'll see your debt shrink and your savings grow, and you won't feel deprived. ◀

Credit Cards

8 Little-Known Tidbits That Will Help Get You Out of Debt Fast

Pay down the expensive debt first. Let's say you have $5,000 of debt built up on a high-interest-rate credit card (perhaps 18 percent) and you also have a $50,000 home equity loan at 8 percent interest. You only have so much money to devote to paying down loans each month, so which of these debts should get priority? First pay down the high-interest-rate debt, even if it's the least amount of money you owe, say financial planners. If you must, just pay the minimum on the home equity loan while you aggressively eliminate the credit card debt. You'll save a lot of interest in the long run.

Drowning in debt? Ask for a life raft. Here's something that you'll never hear from a Visa or AmEx customer service rep: If you owe so much money on your credit cards that you're seriously considering bankruptcy, chances are the credit card companies will strike a deal with you. In most cases, a very good deal. Here's what you have to do, according to Howard Dvorkin of Consolidated Credit Counseling Services in Fort Lauderdale, Florida, and author of *Credit Hell: How to Dig Out of Debt.*

Start calling the phone numbers on the backs of your credit cards. When you explain your situation to a credit supervisor, you do nothing but tell the truth: You are considering filing bankruptcy. The B-word is one that the credit card companies hate to hear. If you did declare bankruptcy, credit card companies would usually be left holding the bag. (While bankruptcy may sound like an attractive way to get out of your financial predicament, keep in mind that it seriously blemishes your personal financial record.) Tell them that if they want to see any money, they should make you an offer you can't refuse. In many cases, according to Dvorkin, the credit card company will make a deal with you then and there—it may slash what you owe by as much as 50 percent. Other options it may give you include rejiggering the monthly payment plan or eliminating future interest on your account. From the credit card company's point of view, it's better to get something instead of nothing.

Pay credit card bills twice a month. Credit card companies will never offer you this brilliant idea, but it's yours

SECRET WEAPON

Prosper.com

Tired of paying 20 percent interest on your credit cards? Get a "prosperous" personal loan. In the U.S., a new website, Prosper.com, allows you to borrow money from regular folks, at interest rates that *you* determine. How does it work? Simple. Go to www.prosper.com, sign up, and type in the loan amount you need, along with the interest rate that you are willing to pay. Prosper will review your financial situation, and then lenders will bid on your proposal, and a match is eventually made. Prosper.com acts as the mediator and takes a small percentage of the deal—a one-time 1 percent charge from the borrower, as well as a 0.5 percent annual service fee from the lender. Backed by Accel Partners, Benchmark Capital, Fidelity Ventures, and Omidyar Network, Prosper had already done more than $20 million of business as of late 2006. Loans for first-time users range from $100 to $25,000.

right now. If you owe a lot on high-interest-rate credit cards, make a payment every two weeks instead of once a month, even if you're just paying the minimum amount due. Why? Because this will cut into the interest as it accrues. It may not seem like much, but over time, you'll save a bundle.

Pay credit card bills immediately. While it's wonderful that credit card companies give you a grace period before interest accrues on your balance, keep in mind that the longer you wait to make your payment, the more interest accrues on your previous debt. So don't file that bill away for later—pay it at your first opportunity.

Resist pre-approved credit card offers. Credit card companies know how to ensnare new customers: Keep up that barrage of offers. Once you take the bait on a card and they have you, chances are you're going to run up some debt. Here's a way to resist temptation: Stop receiving them. That's right—you can opt out of receiving credit card offers. There are two ways to do it:

- The first one you can do on the Internet, at www.optoutprescreen .com. When you get to the site, which is the only official site that credit rating companies will use for this service, you'll find three choices. You can stop receiving offers forever, for five years, or if you had previously "opted out," you can opt back in. Your information and preferences go directly to all of the major credit rating companies.
- If sending this information over the Internet still spooks you, you can call 888-567-8688 and accomplish the same thing.

Canada does not have one central service like this, but if you receive a lot of solicitations from one or two companies, you can call them and ask them to remove your name from their mailing list.

Use good penmanship. Here's another easy way to avoid credit card late fees: Write legibly, because it's perfectly legal for credit card companies to hold, reroute, and otherwise stall payments that they say they can't read. They can do this for five days without having to contact you. If your payment due date passes in the meantime, tough luck.

Stop writing notes. Don't write notes to your credit card company and enclose them with your payment. Why? Those companies are allowed to take the notes, along with the bills and checks to which you attached the note, and reroute them back and forth to different departments for up to five days. As a result, you may miss your payment deadline. It will also give the credit card companies another few days to suck some interest charges out of you. Even a small notation on your bill means your bill is being redirected and, quite possibly, late.

Can those yearly credit card fees. Want that annual credit card fee waived? As with many things in life, you may just get your way if you ask. Simply dial up the number on the back of the card, and tell the representative that you don't want to pay the fee any longer, and you'll switch to a different credit card if you have to. One credit counselor says that most of the time, the first customer service rep on the line will have the authority to waive or discount the fee. If you routinely carry a balance, it's likely that you'll get your way. ◂

Lower Your Bills

11 Ways to Pay Less for Cable, Groceries, and Phone Service

Get 4-1-1 for F-R-E-E. Here's a way to sidestep the directory assistance charge on your phone bill, which can cost 75 cents to a dollar per request: Call 800-FREE-411. It's completely free, though you may sometimes hear a brief commercial. You can access this service from both your landline and cell phone. This does not apply in Canada—although you can use websites to get phone numbers, including whitepages.ca, canada411.ca, and 411.ca. In the U.S., you can get phone numbers online at anywho.com, switchboard.com, superpages.com, and many other sites.

Cut those cable bills. Cable and satellite TV companies won't yell from the treetops, "You're paying too much for your service!" but almost all of them are open to negotiating your service rates Here's how you do it. Call the "billing inquiries" number on your bill. When you get a human on the phone, tell him or her that you've been receiving offers from satellite or cable (whichever one you don't have) and that you're being offered a significantly better deal. It helps if you actually have a real offer in hand. Chances are, this operator will pass you along to a different department. Tell this

WHAT YOUR BANK DOESN'T WANT YOU TO KNOW ABOUT Fees

You can negotiate the fees that banks and credit card companies charge you for their services. Try these:

- ☐ Overdrafted on your account? "Insufficient funds" fees on checks start at around $25, and go up from there. If you've been an otherwise good customer and ask, this fee can usually be waived. All you have to do is call the number on your statement or credit card—no crying or pleading necessary.

- ☐ If you're going through a major bank to secure a mortgage, virtually all the fees are subject to discussion, most notably the notion of "points," which is an extra percentage or two you pay up front to secure the loan. Appraisal fees of the property you're purchasing are also often waived. Just ask the bank manager for a face-to-face meeting, point out the fees, and politely ask if they can be waived. The fees are negotiable, and there's a lot of competition for your business—so there's a good chance the bank manager will comply. Just because a host of other people blindly pay them, that doesn't mean you have to.

- ☐ Credit card issuers love sticking you with late fees, even for your first offense. But a phone call to the customer service number listed on the back of your card will more often than not result in the fee being waived without any red tape, provided you've been a good customer up to that point.

next person that you're happy with your service, but the price differential has you thinking about switching. Ask if he can offer a similar price. You will almost be certainly offered a price break.

Keep your eye on the cash register. Don't "check out" mentally at the checkout counter—it may cost you! You might think that modern scanner systems don't make mistakes. However, studies show that discrepancies between the sticker price and the scanned price happen in about 5 percent of all cash register transactions. Speak up if you see an error—many stores will even credit you the full value of the item if you point out price mistakes.

Study your grocery store's sales patterns. They might not admit to this, but many supermarket chains put foods on sale at regular intervals—for example, a certain ice cream might go half-price once every four weeks. Other foods that regularly go on sale include breads, orange juice, soda, spaghetti sauce, apples, lettuce, shrimp, chicken breasts, yogurt, and cereal. Once you become aware of the patterns, you should never have to buy these products at full price again!

Seek out savings "triple plays." While most retailers limit you to one discount at a time on a product, grocery stores allow you to apply multiple discounts at the same time on a product. It's rare, but every now and then a store will have a sale on a food product that you love, that you happen to have a coupon for, at a time in which the store is offering double- or triple-coupon discounts. At moments like these, stock up—you'll be getting a favorite food nearly for free! This strategy works well for yogurt, bread, ice cream, and frozen prepared foods (items for which discount coupons are often available).

Go directly to the source for coupons. Pretty much every national brand has a website, and many of them provide printable coupons, rebates, and

WHAT **MANUFACTURERS** DON'T WANT YOU TO KNOW ABOUT Refunds

The dirty secret of companies that offer refunds is that many if not most of the people who buy an item with a refund offer don't actually bother to claim it—or they make some mistake that disqualifies their claim. Claiming a refund takes time and patience, but if you're buying something that you would buy anyway, applying for a refund puts money back in your pocket—and in the case of big-ticket items, it can be significant amount. To make the most of refunds, keep these points keep in mind:

☐ Apply for the refund as soon as you get home. The longer you wait, the less likely you are to do it. The expiration dates can be very short.

☐ Remove the product code or other part of the package designated as the proof of purchase. Fill out the refund form, photocopy it, and mail it. Be sure to include the proof of purchase, a copy of the receipt, and anything else that is required. Send exactly what is specified or you'll be disqualified.

☐ Keep a log of refunds that you have requested, listing the item, the company, the amount due, and the date you mailed it.

other special offers (sometimes including free samples). Our best strategy: Look at your local grocery store's current sales flyer, and find what products are on sale and that you need. Next, go to the website of the product and see if there is a coupon available! The result: huge savings (as a test, we just did this, and discovered we could buy cans of tuna for 25 cents each!).

If you cook, plant herbs—not vegetables—in your garden. Fresh herbs bought at a grocery store are incredibly expensive, no matter what time of year. Serious cooks can save a small fortune if they can harvest basil, oregano, thyme, mint, and rosemary from their own gardens. However, you won't see the same cost benefit with vegetables. The week your zucchini harvest comes in is usually the same week that it comes in at local farms—meaning the grocery store will be selling them at a deep discount.

Don't double-buy long-distance service. For people with both home and cell phone services, it's highly wasteful to pay for expensive national calling plans for both. Choose the most cost-efficient or convenient service for your long-distance calls, and use the other service for local calls only. Or skip long distance on both if you use an Internet phone service.

Upgrade to a digital cable box. Even if you don't have a new television, this can pay. Most televisions sold today are high-definition sets that require an upgraded, digital cable signal to deliver a great picture. To keep customers loyal, many cable companies will let you exchange your old cable box for a digital box, for free. The benefit? Many more channels at no extra charge.

Get free telephone service over the Internet. Phone companies don't want you to know this, but if you have broadband Internet service, then you can use your computer as a telephone at no charge! All you need is a headset with a microphone or an inexpensive telephone that connects to a USB port on your computer and some free software that you can download in minutes. Skype (www.skype.com) is the best-known Internet phone service—it allows you to call any other similarly equipped computer around the world for free. And if you want to use Skype to call regular phones in the U.S. and Canada, it's just a modest annual fee, far less than the cost of one month of typical phone service. Calls to most countries overseas cost only pennies a minute.

Cash in on store courtesy cards. Sometimes called club or thank-you cards, store courtesy cards have proliferated in recent years. There's not a major drugstore or supermarket chain that doesn't offer one now. And even some big-box electronics stores have their own version. The stores offer the cards because they want to make you a regular shopper, and some consumers are suspicious about the cards—especially if there is a fee associated with them. But today most of the cards are free, and the savings can be significant, and there is no limit to how many stores you can have a card from. Some cards work by giving you a coupon rebate, say $5 off future purchases once you buy $100's worth of goods. Others give you a reduced price on certain items when you flash the card. Either way, you win, provided you regularly comparison-shop and make sure that you are not paying any more than you would at another store. So fill your key chain up with these little money-saving tags. ◁

Stocks and Investments
3 Questions to Ask Yourself to Determine If You Have the Right Broker

Have you researched him? Here's a secret tip to determining if your stockbroker is legit: All of the complaints filed against him, and all the settlements he's been involved in, are public knowledge and easy to find. In the U.S., all you have to do is look your broker up on the National Association of Securities Dealers' website, www.nasdbrokercheck.com. The site will list your prospective broker's employment history, plus either the nasty details of the broker's professional career or a clean bill of financial health. (You can also call 800-289-9999 to get the same information.) In Canada, find your provincial securities commission through the Canadian Securities Administrators site, csa-acvs.ca, and contact them to check a broker's references or to see if complaints have been filed.

Is he pushy? One broker who asked not to be named said that you should start worrying if your broker is pushing a particular stock, especially one that has been in the dumps recently. Unscrupulous brokerage houses sometimes engage in what's known as a pump-and-dump scheme: They highly recommend a stock to their customers, the price rises as those customers buy it up, and the brokers quickly sell their own shares of the stock behind the scenes, pocketing bucketloads of cash. It's ugly, and it's illegal, but it happens.

Does he crow about his "hot tips"? Keep this in mind next time your broker tells you about some "undiscovered gem" of a stock: It's almost certainly not "undiscovered." The odds of any one Wall Streeter knowing something the rest of them don't know are between slim and none. By the time the "secret" reaches you, chances are that the Wall Street highfliers have already made their move on the stock, leaving latecomers little chance of making a profit. ◁

SECRET WEAPON

Free Cash Flow Multiple

Want to know the secret to picking successful stocks? The "free cash flow multiple" is a measure that top Wall Street analysts use when trying to determine the health of any one particular stock. The number measures how much cash a company generates after it's finished paying its bills, including reinvesting capital back into its business.

To figure out what a stock's free cash flow multiple is, do this: Subtract a company's capital expenditures from its cash flow from operations. This information can easily be found on the face of a cash flow statement (which can be found at Yahoo!, Google, or tons of other Internet financial sites). That's free cash flow. Next, divide that free cash flow figure by how many diluted shares the company has outstanding (also found on any number of financial websites). This will give you the free cash flow multiple. You can feel pretty good about buying stock in a company at 12 times the current year's free cash flow, and very good at 10 times. The lower the multiple, the more attractive the company is. Don't like to do math? Your broker should be able to get you the free cash flow number very easily.

Investment Cautions
2 Traps to Avoid in the Pursuit of Quick Wealth

Be aware of investment scams. The moment you get a few extra dollars in your pocket, investment advice starts leaping at you from every corner of your life—from a favorite uncle, from coworkers, from strangers on the telephone, from unsolicited e-mails, and from magazine ads. Greet all unsolicited investment suggestions with an enormous amount of skepticism. Here are seven signs of a possible investment scam trying to pluck dollars out of your wallet.

- A promise that there's no risk
- A promise that you'll make lots of money quickly
- A promise of tax sheltering in an "offshore" investment
- An offer of offbeat investment "opportunities" such as oil leases, artwork, coins, or jewels
- A woeful story from a stranger who wants your help in accessing a large bank account or other funds
- An investment based on information that, supposedly, no one else has access to
- An investment plan that asks you to recruit other investors

Think twice before becoming a day trader. It sounds like the ideal life. Rather than reporting to an office or waiting on tables every day, you're going to sit at a computer at home in your pajamas, making quick buy-and-sell stock decisions and racking up bucketloads of cash. Well, hold on to your wallet, hotshot. Here's a reality check.

- *Don't bet the farm.* The harsh reality: Most day traders lose money big-time. So never, never, never day-trade with money you need for routine living—tuition money, retirement funds, money you need to cover household bills, and the like.

- *Understand the expenses.* Many day traders have to pay the company they're affiliated with enormous commissions in exchange for training and equipment. They work with borrowed ("on margin") money and can quickly ring up mountains of debt. Given the hefty expenses, have a clear idea of what it takes to turn a profit in this scenario.

- *"Easy" is a myth.* Day trading requires that you be glued to a computer all day, every moment, monitoring prices and trends. Done right, this is hard and gut-wrenching work. Anyone who tells you otherwise is scamming you.

- *Consider the source.* Once you become known as a day trader, you will be barraged with hot "insider" advice, primarily from people who are trying to drive up their own investments. Don't act on advice if you aren't sure of the source.

- *Check out that class.* You may have been invited to find out about day trading at a special class or seminar. Find out whether the instructor will benefit if you decide to become a day trader. If so, the information provided in the class might be seriously skewed. ◁|

6

SECRETS TO
boosting
Your Credit Score

In our modern society, where most people pay for all their major purchases—from houses to appliances and cars—with loans, your credit rating is extremely important. The better it is, the more likely you are to get a good loan rate, and a few points' difference in your rate can add up to a substantial amount of money over the life of a car loan or a house mortgage. Here are some inside tips on keeping your credit rating in tip-top shape.

1 Ask for leniency

The quickest path to a low credit score is making late payments on obligations such as your credit card, mortgage, or car payment. But if you're coming up short this month and have been a good loan customer up to this point, there's an easy solution: Call the lender and ask for an extension. Or ask if you may make a smaller payment this month. If you have a good track record, chances are you'll get a free pass and be able to keep your credit rating high. But keep in mind that this is a one-time maneuver designed to give you a little breathing room. You can't call up month after month and expect to receive an extension from your lender.

2 Limit the number of credit cards you apply for

Want to watch your credit score go into a downward spiral? Never apply for more than two credit cards at any one time, says Stanley Kershman, a lawyer, author, and financial whiz based in Ottawa, Ontario. If a credit bureau sees that you have applied for three or more cards in a short period of time, the company will probably assume you're in desperate need of cash—and desperate people do not make good credit risks. An even worse scenario, says Kershman: The credit bureaus think your identity has been stolen, which would also send your credit rating down the tubes.

3 Shred your financial statements

The one surefire way to see your credit rating head south is to get your identity stolen. Not only will it ruin your credit rating, but it's going to take a lot of time, effort, and aspirin to restore your previously sterling credit rating.

So how do you avoid this mess in the first place? Don't throw your mail away—shred it. This includes bank statements, credit card bills, and anything with financial information on it. Shredders range in price from about $30, for the most basic model, to more than $1,000 for one that turns your important financial documents into dust. In truth, a simple shredder is all you need. That's because crooks—the bums that they are—always take the easiest route. It's a lot easier to read a bank statement that was ripped in half as opposed to one that was shredded into 50 pieces.

4 Don't be ruined by late payments

Did you know that if you miss a deadline on your car or credit card payment, your *other* lenders can jack your rate up to the default rate? This clause is called "universal default," and you want to avoid it at all costs. If you read the fine print on your credit card agreement, you'll read all about it. In a nutshell: If you are more than 30 days late on any payment, all of your credit card lenders earn the right to treat you like a financial pariah. Your low 0 percent or 3 percent credit card deal can skyrocket to a default of 20 percent or 30 percent. Remember, the credit ratings and reports will be seen by anyone who's holding your credit, and if you're making late payments for one credit card, you can be sure your other credit card companies are going to find out. Be sure to make your payments like clockwork.

5 Watch your credit account online

Identity theft is a multibillion-dollar business now, and hordes of thieves are hoping you won't do this. But if you check your account on the Internet religiously, you'll spot any criminal spending quickly and you'll be able to take action. Check your hard-copy statement or go to your credit card company's website for information on how to get online access to your account.

6 Never use a P.O. box

Oddly enough, using a post office box can harm your credit rating. When credit rating companies see that your bills are headed for a P.O. box, they worry that you have either lost your home or that someone has stolen your identity. Both scenarios raise a red flag.

Insurance

6 Secrets to Buying the Right Policies for You and Your Family

Don't buy worthless disability insurance. Some disability insurance is what's known as gainful occupation coverage. This kind of coverage means that if it's possible for you to work at *any* job you're qualified for—for example, as a fry cook at Burger King—no insurance dough for you. Don't buy this kind of coverage. Instead, ask your insurance agent for either an "own occupation" policy or an "income replacement" policy. The former will pay out if you're prevented from doing the job you have—for instance, if a writer loses his ability to type, the insurance will pay the claim. He'll continue to get paid even if he changes careers and goes back to work. An "income replacement" policy will continue to pay benefits to that writer, but will cut his benefits should he decide to go back into the workforce and pursue another career. These two kinds of policies make a lot of sense considering that, according to the U.S. Social Security Administration, 30 percent of Americans between the ages of 18 and 35 will one day be forced out of the workforce for a long-term disability.

Don't get canceled; get renewed. Disability insurance doesn't come cheap, so don't let the insurance companies talk you into making it even more expensive down the road. It's better to put a little more money into the policy up front and get what's known as a noncancelable and guaranteed renewable policy. This covers you in virtually any situation. Changing your profession from accountant to javelin catcher? They still can't cancel you, and must renew you. The other two types of disability insurance—plain old "guaranteed renewable" and "conditionally renewable"—have major disadvantages. The "guaranteed renewable" policy may be just that, but it allows the insurance company the flexibility to make changes to the policy, and "conditionally renewable" means, well, don't expect to get renewed once the company finds out you're catching javelins for a living.

Get your long-term-care insurance now. Even if you're only 35, signing up for this fast-growing segment of the insurance industry is a smart move. Why? Because your premiums will be very low, and as a result, you'll save money over time. Long-term-care insurance covers you in the event of disability or prolonged illness. The insurance can grant you all sorts of protection, such as covering nursing home costs and in-home health care. The trick here, though, is that very few young people think that far enough in advance. By the time they are senior citizens, the monthly premiums can be too much to bear.

Factor inflation into your long-term plans. So you're smart and got your long-term-care insurance now—great. But don't let the insurance companies snooker you down the road. Make sure inflation, and your own advancing age, don't get you in the end. Today's $5,000-a-month coverage might just be pocket change in 50 years. So when you buy your policy, you'll be faced with two choices for combating inflation—you can either choose to buy more coverage at a later date, or choose to have the insurance company automatically increase your coverage each year in step with inflation. Bet on the latter, because if you have to buy added insurance down the road to keep up with inflation, you're going to be charged a price in relation to your current age.

If it's not excluded, it's included. Here's something you need to know when it comes to your insurance, especially homeowners' policies: Unless the policy specifically excludes something from coverage, the insurance company has to cover it. Let's use a wildly hypothetical example to explore this. Say aliens from planet Xenon land in your living room and demand your self-cleaning oven. They claim they need it to get back to their homeland. Because they have their laser guns pointed at your dog, you allow them to take the oven. Now you need a new oven, so you call your insurance company to file a claim. "Aliens stole my oven," you'll say. "Sorry," the insurance agent will then say, "but you're not covered for alien thievery." Well, guess what? You are. And you can tell that drone on the other end that if it isn't excluded, then it's included.

Become a loyal customer. Here's something not all home insurance agents are telling you up front: If you give your insurance company your business over an extended period of time, you may be eligible for a loyalty discount. In fact, the Insurance Information Institute claims many home insurers will reduce your premiums by 5 percent if you've been with the company for three to five years, and up to 10 percent after you've been a customer for six years. The only way to find out about these loyalty programs is by asking. ◁

WHAT YOUR **INSURANCE AGENT** DOESN'T WANT YOU TO KNOW ABOUT Riders

You really don't need all of those life insurance riders (extra benefits for more money) that you have attached to your policy. For most people, a typical, basic life insurance policy—be it term or whole life—is all you really need. Here are some that you may have that you can get rid of:

☐ Accidental death and dismemberment, better known to Billy Wilder fans as "double indemnity," is not necessary. Should you die in any "accidental" manner, this rider doubles the payout. For a $100,000 policy, expect to pay an extra $10 to $12 per month. That's not much now, but it adds up over time. And the chances of your dying in an accident are—knock on wood—slim.

☐ You can also forget about the "waiver of premium" rider. This rider, for about 8 to 10 percent of your yearly insurance payment, would have the insurance company continue to pay your premiums should you become disabled. If you're concerned about this, just buy disability insurance.

☐ A spousal rider allows your spouse (and children) to get term life insurance after you die if you had whole life insurance. This is useless, because kids generally don't need life insurance and your spouse could probably do better shopping for a new policy.

Taxes and Estate Planning
8 Tips to Surviving Tax Returns, Audits, Wills, and Probate

Don't do your own taxes. It may sound like we're advertising for H&R Block, but it's really worth it to pay someone a couple hundred dollars to prepare your taxes for you. Why? "What people don't understand is that nearly 80 percent of the IRS hit list—returns that are audited—are self-prepared," advises Dan Friebis, EA, ATA, ATP, a tax professional in Port Orange, Florida, with 28 years of experience. This number is staggeringly large because "people don't really know how to use [tax-preparation] software," he says, and get overly eager to pad their returns as they watch the amount in the "refund" box grow. In the process, they make trouble for themselves because the IRS has its own averages for what people of certain professions, in certain areas of the country, should reasonably claim as deductions. (To give you an idea of how low audit rates are for those who use professional tax services: Over the past seven years, Friebis has prepared over 13,000 returns, only two of which were audited. In the end, neither of those two audited parties ended up having to pay the IRS any extra money.)

Don't donate your car. As you've probably heard on the radio and from your tax professional, donating a car is tax-deductible—but that doesn't mean that it's a smart idea You'll probably be able to pocket a lot more money by selling it to a used-car dealer. Let's say you're in the 25-percent tax bracket, and you have an old junker that the Kelley Blue Book—the bible of used-car pricing—says is worth $2,000. You can deduct 25 percent off your taxes—$500—if you donate the car. If you're keen to have the car benefit those less fortunate, donate a chunk of the cash you got from selling the car.

Don't file a Schedule C, if possible. The "single-highest audit risk, bar none, is a person who's self-employed and files a Schedule C/sole proprietor form," says Friebis. By filing as a sole proprietor, you have about a one-in-three chance of getting an audit letter from the IRS, because the IRS has something similar to a points system about how your return should measure up regionally and nationally, and if you're even a little bit out of these parameters, watch out. You're much better off making your sole proprietorship an S corporation or a limited liability company, if you qualify and if you will earn enough to make the paperwork worthwhile. Changing your business to one of these lowers your risk of being audited to about 1 in 1,000, depending on region (and if you file as an S corporation, your personal assets are also protected if your business is ever sued). If you're starting your own business, Friebis advises, your first visit should be to an accountant, not a lawyer.

If you *do* get audited, seek professional help. Even if you prepare your tax returns yourself, don't face the IRS without a professional in your corner. The IRS "is hoping that you pay just out of fear" of being audited in the first place without even fighting the audit, confesses an anonymous tax professional. And don't just pick a random pro out of the phone book—get a recommendation from someone you know who has had success with that preparer. Another thing: Look for someone with the letters "EA," which stands for "enrolled agent," after her name. EAs have licenses to practice before the IRS and their specialty is strictly tax law; CPAs may be good number crunchers, but relatively few are well versed in tax codes, or in dealing with government auditors.

Eat, drink … and deduct? A tax pro we talked to was more than happy to dish, no pun intended, on little-known deductions. Our favorite? If a husband and wife own their own business together, any meals that they eat together at which they discuss business are *100 percent deductible*, not limited to the entertainment deduction, which is only 50 percent allowable. (Who *doesn't* discuss work with his spouse over dinner, even if he doesn't work with her?) By the same token, if you work for someone else and have lunch

SECRET WEAPON

Public Records

There's a good reason why you better behave yourself during divorce or other court proceedings. A tax pro who didn't want us to use his name offered this shocking revelation: IRS auditors are literally hunting for tax dodgers on a regular basis, and it's very easy for them to find you. Auditors first check the newspapers for recent court cases, especially granted divorces, and then they go straight to the depositions. Divorce cases are fertile grounds for finding folks who have been cheating the government. Why? Think about all the he-said, she-said accusations that go on when warring spouses are trying to divide their assets and battle for custody. Everything you say during these proceedings is part of public record. Accusing your ex of declaring less income than she made, or hiding a million dollars in blackjack winnings under the mattress, will get you *both* audited faster than you can say "ex-wife." For your sake, if not for hers, keep your mouth shut about your financial status in court and make an attempt to be reasonable with each other.

with a coworker or your boss, and you buy yours and he buys his, your meal is deductible. It's called a "corporate meeting meal" deduction. Finally, say you're on a deadline at work and can't get out for lunch. If you order in and eat that meal at your desk while you're working, this "meal on premises" is also 100 percent deductible. The key to taking these deductions is to document carefully, and save your receipts.

Put your trust in trusts. Everyone needs a will, but most folks need much more than that. In the U.S., options you should consider:

- A revocable living trust keeps all of your assets (except, in most cases, your principal residence) under one umbrella. You put your name on the trust and name a beneficiary; when you die, the assets all transfer to the beneficiary, bypassing probate altogether. If you don't have this trust, a probate lawyer can take up to 3 percent in fees off the top "just because he can," says one estate pro, and your assets could be tied up in the courts for up to a year and be subject to estate tax. If your assets are in the trust, the lawyer (and the government, if your estate is under the maximum net assets allowable) would get zilch.

- A pour-over will is a part of the revocable living trust that takes precedence over any prior wills and directs where and how your assets will be distributed. You should retitle all of your assets, with the possible exception of your principal residence, into the trust; any assets that you forgot to mention or retitle (or didn't know about) would be automatically assumed part of the trust and would avoid probate.

- An AB trust protects your assets in the event that your estate is valued at more than the estate taxable maximum. Let's say that your family fortune is valued at $4 million, and the maximum estate tax exclusion allowed before taxing it is $2 million. An AB trust is one in which you can divide the money equally among spouses. Say you and your husband adopt an AB trust, which separates $2 million of your $4 million estate into the surviving spouse and a trust in the name of the other spouse, which the surviving spouse has the use of for health and welfare. When a surviving spouse dies, the trust of the spouse who predeceased goes directly to the ultimate beneficiary. The last surviving spouse has use of his or her deceased spouse's money, but these assets do not have to be included in the surviving spouse's estate. When managed properly, you can eliminate most of your estate tax this way. Consult your tax professional for specific advice.

Change personal debt to a home equity loan. A distressing number of people pay high interest rates for the personal debt they carry (credit card balances are a prime example), and sadly those fees are not deductible on your taxes. If you must have personal debt, cover it all with a home equity loan. Home equity loans, which are based on the value you have already accumulated in your house, generally come with lower interest rates. The bonus: For home equity loans up to $100,000, you can deduct the interest. Be disciplined with your home equity loan, however. If you're going to use it to wipe out your other personal debt, make sure the term of the loan lasts no longer than the original debt would have. If you prolong the payments, a home equity loan might not save you money after all.

Deduct your charity mileage. Log the miles that you drive while helping a charitable organization. For instance, when the Boy Scouts hold a holiday food drive and you drive all of those goods to a homeless shelter for them, you can deduct that mileage on your taxes. Go to the IRS website (www.irs.gov) to find the current cents-per-mile rate it allows for charitable driving—it's lower than the business mileage deduction, but a savings nevertheless. ◁

Retirement

3 Clever Moves for Your Career Endgame

Play catch-up. Maybe during your first few decades of work, you failed to see the wisdom of socking away cash for retirement when there were so many more fun things to do with it. If you're now age 50-plus, retirement is just around the corner and some age-old bits if investing advice apply to you in spades:

- It's never too late to save.
- Contribute the maximum allowable to your IRA or 401(k).

The good news is that U.S. taxpayers who are age 50 and up are allowed to contribute more into these tax-deferred accounts than other folks. For the year 2007, for instance, most workers were allowed to put as much as $15,500 into their 401(k) accounts. The 50-and-older crowd was allowed an extra $5,000. So start playing catch-up—it's time to mend those wanton ways.

Roll over, play smart. Many people in the first couple of decades of their careers change jobs every few years. If they have a 401(k) with the former employer, they often take the cash out of the account and pay the early withdrawal penalty. Big, big mistake. There's no wiser savings plan available to you than funds that are allowed to grow tax-free. So when you leave an employer, roll your 401(k) savings into an IRA, where your cash will grow with similar protection. You'll be so glad you make it a career-long habit—just ask anyone nearing retirement age.

Delays pay—up to a point. Everyone's retirement needs are different, but if you qualify for Social Security in the United States, waiting to file will put more money into your pocket—up to a certain point, anyway. For one thing, for every year that you delay retirement, that's an extra year of earnings from the work you do—and higher lifetime earnings can translate into a larger Social Security payout. On top of that, for every year that you delay retirement, the Social Security folks will permanently increase the benefit that you receive when you do eventually retire. These benefits stop increasing when you hit age 70, however—so that becomes a magic number for you. Once you reach age 70, there's no longer a reason *not* to file for benefits. And if you want to, you can keep working without penalty.

Even if you've decided to delay retirement, sign up for Medicare—the U.S. health plan for older people—before your 65th birthday. Unless you are still covered by insurance at your or your spouse's employer, delaying will usually actually cost you more. ◁

Getting Hired

9 Inside Tips on What to Do and What Not to Do When You Are Looking for a Job

Sweep the Internet for your own name. They won't ask your permission, but you can bet that prospective employers will punch you up on Internet search engines to find out every juicy little detail of your life that's posted online. Googling applicants is standard practice now, human resources directors confide, but they don't exactly broadcast that fact to the general public.

Actually, getting googled is a positive sign, because it means a company is interested in you. But it also means that just about everything you've ever "shared" in cyberspace is available for them to see and judge you by. Fair? Probably not. But it's a job-hunting reality these days.

Your first countermove is to do a Net search on yourself to see if any surprises are lurking out there. Then run through all the sites you have posted to—chat groups, discussion forums, friends' blogs or home pages, your own blog or home page, and social networking sites like MySpace or Facebook. If you find something you'd rather not have come up at a job interview—beer-soaked beach party photos, say, or an angry tirade you once wrote about the very industry you're trying to land a job in—see what you can do to make them disappear. Ask your friends to take those party photos off their sites, and see if more formal sites offer a "private access" option for archived material.

You might be stuck with having some embarrassing material stay posted, but at least you'll be aware of what your prospective employer may have seen. That way, you'll be better able to deal with it if it comes up. And from now on, remember the 21st-century version of your grandmother's advice: Never post anything on the Internet that you would not want to discuss at a job interview.

Give your letter the stamp of character. Here's a secret straight out of the human resources office: You are being judged even before your résumé is opened. Did you use stationery from your current employer to try to find your next job? Did you run your letter through the company mail meter? If so, the HR person receiving your letter is going to make some instant judgments about your character—and drop your résumé in the "round file."

Instead, make sure the first correspondence you send to your future employer screams, "This is special!" Choose an attractive envelope, and interesting stamps. Always—without fail!—address it to a specific person, such as the head of human resources, the personnel director, or the person in charge of the area you're applying to. Use that person's name on the envelope, not just a title. Spell it right. And don't just scribble your return address any old way. If you don't have a personal address sticker you're proud of, print your name and address in lettering that says, "I am somebody!" Yes, you want your communication to be businesslike, but you also want to make an impression. The best résumé in the world won't do you any good if it doesn't get opened.

Use e-mail like a professional. Applying by e-mail? Keep in mind that the person reading it will notice things that you don't.

- Rule #1 is to show some professionalism. Will an e-mail address like yugogirrrl@yahoo.whatever be the first thing your prospective employer sees? That's pretty far down the professionalism scale. So are jokey instant messenger screen names. So are sign-offs without enough contact information because you're assuming they'll just hit "Reply" to get back to you. Solution: Set up a separate e-mail account just for job searching.

- Another thing they're looking at right away is your spelling and grammar. Forget about the quick-typing culture that's connected with casual e-mail. Proof your cover letter and your attached résumé. HR types are unanimous on this: If they see typos and sloppy grammar, you won't be considered even if your résumé is CEO caliber. Their thinking is that if you don't care enough to check for errors, you won't be much of an employee.

- Also, remember that sending your correspondence to a specific person, by name, is even more important when you're applying by e-mail than by regular mail. You can usually find out the name of a human resources person, as well as his or her e-mail address, by checking the company's website. If you can't find that information online, there are reference volumes at your local library that provide data on companies, such as the Harris directory.

Surprise: HR's on the phone! There's a trend among human resources hirers you should be aware of: They're likely to hit applicants with an unexpected phone call as the first step in the interview process. It's nothing to get panicky about. It's just that they've read your cover letter and résumé, checked your references, and looked you up on the Internet, and now they want to learn more about you before committing to an in-person interview. So be prepared for that phone call, and keep any notes or talking points you think you may need by the telephone, or otherwise handy.

One extra piece of advice: If they've caught you at a bad time, it's okay to say so. It's much better to arrange a call back in an hour than try to make a good impression while the kids are screaming, dinner is boiling over on the stove, and dogs are barking. And a little extra time to collect your thoughts won't hurt, either.

Tout skills and strengths, not hopes and dreams. One of the most common résumé formats calls for placing an "objective" at the top of the first page. Something like,

"Experienced widget designer seeks new challenges within an innovative organization," blah, blah, blah. Your potential employer would never be this blunt, but in truth he doesn't care what your hopes and ambitions are. He wants to know what skills, talents, and traits you have that will benefit his company. So craft a concise, one- or two-sentence "positioning statement" at the top of your résumé instead. This feature in particular should be tailor-made for every prospective employer you write to.

Leap on job prospects immediately. Have every element of your personal presentation ready to spring into action on a moment's notice—particularly a polished résumé, work samples, and a list of references. If you see a classified ad for the ideal job in the weekend newspaper, you want your materials on a hiring manager's desk on Monday morning. Why? The inside secret is that companies typically pluck the best prospects out of the first batch of applicants and give them the most consideration. This may not be scientifically wise on their part, but it's human nature. If you respond immediately, you could be getting called in for a job interview while other applicants are still dusting off their out-of-date résumés.

Respect your friendly recruiter. Many a job opportunity is lost because the applicant doesn't realize what the hiring team in the company knows only too well. Which is: The human resources staff "recruiter" has as much say about whether you get hired as the department head with the vacancy. Often your first interview is with this personnel department staffer. Treat it as the real thing, not a preliminary formality, or you may never get that second interview.

"If I'm the HR recruiter and I sense you're talking down to me or dismissing me in your mind, you're not going to get past me," says Dale Kurow, a New York career coach and former human resources director, who is author of the e-book *Surefire Networking Tips*. "I'm reading your personality and looking for a cultural fit with the company, so an arrogant attitude is not what you want to have coming across."

True, the HR gatekeeper usually doesn't have the expertise to grade your technical capacity, but you need to see this as a communications challenge. "I always made sure that I knew enough about things like systems and applications programming, for example, to ask intelligent questions," Kurow says. "Applicants who really know their stuff are able to frame their knowledge in a way that even a six-year-old can understand."

Take The Lunch seriously. So, the hiring manager and two other company Ms. or Mr. Bigs invited you to lunch? What a nice, friendly gesture. And they'll do everything in their power to encourage you to think that's all it is. Don't believe it for a minute. Their motive is to evaluate you in a social setting. For some jobs—especially higher-level ones—The Lunch is the part of the interviewing process where you need to show that you have good casual communication skills, that you fit into the corporate culture, and that you can represent the company to outsiders gracefully and confidently.

How to Ace That Job Interview

There's so much advice floating around on how to handle job interviews that you'd probably make a fool of yourself if you tried to follow it all. Stick to the following simple tips and you'll do fine:

- **Rehearse the interview.** Have a friend play the role of interviewer and practice answering questions. It may seem silly at first, but you'll learn a lot. Some career coaches even suggest interviewing for jobs you don't really want just to get used to it.

- **Do a dry run to the interview site.** The surest way to get to your interview on time is to make the same trip the day before. See how long it takes to get there, notice the traffic, figure out where to park, and time the walk from the parking lot (or public transportation stop) to the building.

- **Dress like you care about the position.** Err on the side of conservatism. For most professional or office jobs, that means suits for men or women—even if a suit isn't "you." You're not making a fashion statement; you're showing them that the job is important to you.

- **Impress the receptionist.** He or she might be asked their opinion of you. "I know people who didn't get the job because they were rude to the receptionist," says Alison Doyle, a veteran human resources professional.

- **Stride confidently as you enter.** The biggest impression you make is visual, not verbal, and it comes in the first 10 seconds. So don't walk in chewing gum or finishing off your Diet Coke. Smile, walk into the room purposefully, and shake hands firmly.

- **Refuse the coffee.** Or the soft drink. Or the glass of water. You don't want to be worrying about spilling, or wondering where to put an empty cup.

- **Bring only what you need.** Some notes or work samples might help your cause. Shuffling through piles of folders definitely won't.

- **Turn off the cell phone.** Better yet, leave it in the car.

Are you up to it? Of course you are. You wouldn't have made it this far if you didn't have plenty on the ball. But get the details down. Arrive on time (yes, they're watching for that). It's okay to order a pre-meal drink if they do; it's also okay not to. They invited you, so let them pay. Turn off your cell phone, your BlackBerry, and anything else that can be turned off. You're not impressing anybody about how busy you are by taking calls or messages during lunch. Don't order the most expensive thing on the menu, but don't be a killjoy by saying something like, "I think I'll just have a small salad today." Order something you know and like. Show them you can enjoy yourself and be a pro at the same time.

Finally, feel free to cheat by scoping out the restaurant in advance. Check out the menu, the wine list, the service staff, the bathroom location, and the dominant attire among the clientele—anything that will help you feel more at ease is a definite plus.

Check your personal life at the door. In a job interview, focus on professional issues and avoid personal matters altogether. If you blather on about your childhood or your marriage, the interviewer will assume that personal issues will intrude upon your work life as well. This will leave you with plenty of "personal time," all right—and no job. ◁

Maximizing Compensation
5 Important Things to Keep in Mind When You Are Negotiating Salary or Benefit Matters

Pin down the benefits before saying yes. Don't accept a job offer without being clear about the benefits package you'll be getting, even if you're happy with the salary offer. Sometimes a company can meet your salary requirement only because they are seriously skimping on the benefits package, though of course they won't tell you that unless you ask. Remember that your compensation is a package, not just a salary. Employee benefits can make up as much as 40 percent of that package. If you have to pay all of your medical insurance premiums and shell out $300 a month for parking, that so-called acceptable salary is in effect reduced considerably.

Never lowball yourself. When you offer to work at a low salary or inadequate benefits, you're probably assuming that the hiring manager thinks you're eager to work and a good team player. And you hope you'll be rewarded down the road. Forget it. What he or she is actually thinking is, We can get away with paying this sucker less than others. And chances are they'll keep thinking that for years to come no matter how good a job you do. Greed is not an issue in a salary negotiation. You are expected to ask for the salary (or raise, or benefits package) you think you deserve. Then you negotiate from there. You are not scoring points by lowballing yourself. You're only undermining your position.

Sympathy is not a factor. The man or woman on the other side of the desk will probably nod with sympathy when you say you need a better medical plan or more money because your child is sick. But that doesn't mean you're going to get it. The only thing on his or her mind is negotiating in the best interests of the company. Push for what you deserve (based on your qualifications), not what you "need" (based on your family situation). Convincing the company that it needs you and that you've earned what you're asking for will get you much further than any personal plea.

Money isn't everything. If your raise request is turned down, you may be able to get the equivalent of what you were asking for in better benefits. That could be some combination of a pension hike, more vacation time, broader medical coverage, or a more flexible schedule. But even though your boss may be willing to boost your benefits, he or she probably won't bring it up. That's your job. In fact, you should go into your raise negotiation with a backup benefits request ready.

Getting a raise takes time. Getting a salary increase, especially a merit raise, is rarely something you can just ask for and expect to receive. You have to build up to it. You not only have to do your own basic job well, but you need to take on more responsibilities and get a reputation as a person who can get things done. When you do ask for an increase, have a list of your accomplishments—and documentation to back them up—and know how they connect to the bottom line (sales increased, costs reduced, problems solved, processes speeded up). And another thing: Never give an ultimatum, threat-

Understanding a Company's Benefits Package

EXPERT INSTANT ADVICE

The benefits package confuses most employees, and the companies like it that way because it leaves you at their mercy. Here's a checklist that will clear the fog:

- **Start date.** Do you get the benefits right away or after a trial period?

- **Medical plan.** Does it cover pre-existing conditions? If not, what qualifies as a pre-existing condition? Is there a waiting period? Is your family covered? Is your unmarried partner covered? Will you have to pay some of the premium? How much?

- **Retirement/pension.** What program does it fall under? Does the company contribute all, some, or none? Are you required to contribute? How much? How much will you get upon retirement?

- **Vacation.** How many days? At what rate does vacation time increase with tenure? Are your vacations paid? Do you lose vacation time if you don't take it? When are you eligible for vacation time? Can you split it up?

- **Holidays.** What are they? Do you get your birthday off? Will you be asked to work on some holidays?

- **Life insurance.** Is it provided? How much? Do you have to pay?

- **Disability coverage.** Does the company offer coverage if you can't work? Is it long-term or just short-term?

- **Education/vocational training.** Does the company pay for work-related classes?

- **Day care.** Is it offered? Is it on-site? Is it free?

- **Parking.** Does it exist? Is it free?

ening to leave if you don't get the raise. Your boss may surprise you and accept. If you're that dissatisfied, start quietly looking for another job while you still have the current one to support you. ◄

Getting Ahead

9 Secrets for Honing That Competitive Edge and Advancing Your Career

Recruit yourself a mentor. You learned your work skills with the help of at least one experienced teacher. Learn your career advancement skills the same way, and you'll leave the lone rangers behind. "I can't stress enough the value of having a mentor in your job, especially when you're new and trying to get the lay of the land," says career coach Kurow. "A mentor will offer advice, act as a sounding board, give you professional support, and provide that objective feedback which is so crucial."

There's nothing formal about a mentor-mentored relationship. Once you've done some people-watching in the workplace and found somebody you might want to enlist as your mentor, simply ingratiate yourself with that person. First offer help. For example, you might mention that you're interested in a project she or he is working on, and you'd like to assist if possible to gain experience. Then offer friendliness.

If you're graceful about it and the person turns out to be a good choice, things will work out better than you may have thought. "It's not like you're being manipulative and going in with a hidden agenda," Kurow says. "If the person is sharp enough to have become a success in the company, they'll know what you're up to. They'll usually appreciate it that you chose them as a mentor."

A secret source of power. The pipeline to valuable information in a typical workplace runs through the administrative support staff. Administrative assistants and receptionists know this, but most of your coworkers are too busy feeling superior to give them the time of day. So get a leg up on the competition by making sure you're friendly, helpful, and respectful to all different kinds of people, up and down the ladder. To get ahead, you need informal as well as formal sources of information. And trust us, good administrative assistants know what's going on. The best ones know what's happening before it happens. So make it a habit to always say good morning, and occasionally ask, "What's new?" You might get an answer.

Another reason for respecting the clerical help: self-defense. "Law offices and accounting firms are full of people who won't even look at receptionists or secretaries," says Susan RoAne, a California personal communications consultant and author of *The Secrets of Savvy Networking*. "What a foolish mistake. Who's in a better position to botch up your stuff intentionally than they are?"

Solve future problems now. Figure out what your company's future problems will be within your area of responsibility, and create innovative solutions that will nip them in the bud. Missy Cohen-Fyffe has an example. She is president of Babe Ease in Pelham, New Hampshire, which creates and distributes baby products. The company requires a complex system for storing and shipping its goods. One day one of her workers asked her, "Do you mind if I come up with a different organizational system?" Without being asked to, the worker devised an amazing system for keeping the back office more organized in respect to reordering supplies and goods. Need we say she got a hefty merit increase?

Stop fixating on the time clock.

Managers don't expect you to be a slave for the company. In fact, most respect people who value and guard their private time. But if you consistently put in the bare minimum time required at work, or fixate on getting every last half-day of time off possible, or take every single minute of each day's lunch time no matter what deadlines are looming, you send a clear statement to your managers that what comes first is you, not your work. The better approach: Show passion for your work, and as it ebbs and flows, adjust your schedule to get things done. More than anything, managers love a worker they can depend on. Show you can be trusted and are flexible, and the free time will take care of itself.

Stay up on popular technology.

An estimated 80 percent of jobs in modern cultures involve daily use of a computer. In fact, for many people, computer proficiency is vital to workplace success. So go out of your way to learn and practice the computer skills you need to thrive at work. Then go the

---

WHAT YOUR **WORKPLACE COMPETITORS** DON'T WANT YOU TO KNOW ABOUT Promotions

- **Your work skills are not enough.** If you don't communicate well, promote yourself, establish alliances, fit in with the company culture, and stay informed about what's going outside your workstation or cubicle, somebody with less talent is going to pass you by on her way up the ladder.

- **It's a small world after all.** While you stick to your own kind, your rivals are connecting with every conceivable kind of human being. They're taking advantage of today's workplace diversity to expand their cultural horizons—and their contacts. Who's better positioned for advancement in a globalized market?

- **The action's outside too.** You may focus on the in-house environment, but your workplace competitors have joined professional associations, established links to colleagues in other companies, and befriended vendors and suppliers who flit from company to company like pollinating bees. Your competitors know that sometimes the best information about the company where you work comes from the outside.

- **Red tape is for cutting.** Your rivals are delighted that you work hard to be a regulation-respecting "loyal" employee who sees that those around him toe the line. Because while you're creating red tape, they're cutting it. And guess what? The can-do person gets promoted before the can't-do person.

next step and monitor what's hot in terms of electronic gear, software, and websites. No work manual will tell you this, but people who are savvy about technology often move ahead faster than people who don't care much about it.

Learn how to write power-packed e-mails. For such a common mode of workplace communication, intra-office e-mails as a rule are terribly written. What easier way to stand out from the crowd than to consistently send sharp, welcome electronic messages? Just do the following:

- *Hone your subject line.* The key is to be specific, not necessarily short. Instead of giving your e-mail the name "Byrne project," call it "Byrne project: new deadline for phase 2." Your e-mail is already more interesting than most.

- *Don't bury the lead.* If you want to annoy people, make them read three paragraphs before you get to the point. If you want to rise in the company, state your purpose in the first sentence or two and then get to the why and how of it.

- *End with an action request.* Example: "I will call you on Monday at 10 a.m. to follow up on this." Or: "When can we get this done?" Otherwise, nothing is likely to happen.

- *Be human.* Decent people who would never dream of being cold and abrupt in person often come off that way in their e-mails. Being businesslike doesn't have to mean being impersonal. Remember that the sender and receiver are both human beings.

- *Proof your e-mail.* It's worth repeating. Just one misspelling, grammatical error, or typo makes you look foolish. It also makes you look disrespectful to the recipient. Sending clean e-mails automatically lifts you above the sloppy crowd.

- *Behave yourself.* Irony doesn't work in e-mails. Neither do sensitive subjects, such as sex, race, religion, and politics. Stay away from them, because every message you send is being judged.

- *Stop cc-ing everybody.* All you're doing is making all involved feel less important.

- *Pick up the phone.* If you have to spend more than five minutes on an e-mail message, call instead. It's easier to explain things on the phone, and you can always follow up with a shorter e-mail.

How I Do It **A Human Resource Director's Self-Promotion Strategy**

Before career coach Dale Kurow starting helping others get hired and promoted, she was doing the hiring and promoting herself as a human resources staffer at a major company. It was there she learned a key trick:

"I once had a boss who was trying to get me fired, but it had more to do with his problems with his own boss than my performance. I knew I was doing a good job, so I asked other directors and people I worked with to let him know that. They did, and everything turned out fine."

The moral of the story: Don't wait until there's trouble. Have others toot your horn for you when the occasion arises.

"If somebody tells you that you're doing a fine job, ask them if they wouldn't mind passing that word along to the boss," Kurow says. "It's a way to shine your light, but more effective because somebody else is doing the shining for you. And most of the time they're very happy to pick up the phone or send a memo or e-mail on your behalf. All you have to do is ask."

Read the trades. Every industry has newsletters, magazines, and websites that are devoted to it. Subscribe to the ones relevant to your work. You'll learn about trends, the competition, key vendors, government actions, even your own company. There are two benefits: First, you'll be smarter about your job. Second, you'll impress and help your managers and coworkers with your expertise.

Managers, learn to manage "sideways" and "up." Most managers focus their time and energy on the people they oversee. But there are two other constituencies you need to manage as well: your peers (that is, managers at the same level as you), and your bosses. Often, these two groups are harder to win over than your employees! But work hard at it anyway. When your peers respect you, and bosses appreciate the way you communicate and assist them, you greatly increase your value to the company.

Never let your manager be surprised. It's one of the unstated rules of workplace survival: Don't let your boss learn about bad news, angry customers, accidents, or even positive developments from anyone but you. There is nothing worse for a boss than not knowing about something significant in her area of responsibility—and then finding out about it from an angry superior or a cutthroat peer. Make it a policy to let your boss know quickly about everything noteworthy that is going on—good *or* bad. She will be grateful for the candor. ◁

Office Politics

4 Tricks for Dealing with the Wide Variety of Human Interactions You Encounter in the Workplace

Learn to love office politics. Hard workers may hate to hear this, but "keeping your nose to the grindstone"—that is, concentrating on nothing but the job at hand—is a strategy for failure. You may think it's admirable to stay away from office politics, but all that really means is you're limiting your potential. "Office politics" is just a term for the range of human interactions that go on in any workplace.

"Being involved in office politics doesn't have to be something cold and calculating," says communications skills counselor Susan RoAne. "It's just being savvy, alert, aware of what's going on around you, and it's ultimately a means for doing a better job and having a more successful career."

So the most important tip concerning office politics is this: Embrace it. Get good at it. How? By doing what real politicians do—form strategic alliances. Establish relationships with some peers, some superiors, and some below you in the hierarchy. Go out of your way to help a person you like or respect, or somebody who has something to offer. Then ask her to help you. That may lead to a second link with somebody else as well. If not, create a second on your own, then a third.

Cultivate these work relationships. No matter how dedicated an employee you are, at some point you are going to need people to back you up. And no matter how well you do your job, you're going to need allies to help you up the ladder.

That's why you need to be involved in office politics.

Mix business with pleasure. The advice you usually get is to keep your social life separate from your work life. Balderdash! Make sure that you *do* have a social life at work. Not only are office friendships natural, they're also essential if you want to shine. Friends make for loyal allies, honest advisers, information sources, and links to other allies, advisers, and sources. So by all means, cultivate friendships at work.

But don't limit your socializing to individual relationships. Never miss the company picnic or Christmas party. Even if you'd rather stay home and watch the paint dry, lighten up and attend anyway. Such events are priceless opportunities for making the connections you seek in the comfort of a social context. Remember, RoAne says, it's as much about who knows you as it is about who you know.

"You need to have a presence in your job, a visibility," she says. "Socializing lets people get to know who you are and what you do."

Keep an eye on fellow workers. You'll never find this in the employees' manual, but the most useful habit you can develop at work is to carefully observe your coworkers' actions and behavior. And the best time to do it is when they don't know you're watching. Start looking from the first day on the job and don't stop until you get your

- **You're involved in office politics whether you realize it or not.** As knowledgeable personnel staffers like to put it, anytime more than two people are present in a work environment, office politics rage. If you're not an active participant, then you're a passive victim. That's why your rivals love it when you insist on "staying out of it." They know they can eat you for lunch.

- **Staying aloof gives you a bad rep, not a good one.** By refusing to play the office politics game, you do not come across as morally superior. And you are not impressing higher-ups. You are perceived instead as lacking in social skills, short on savvy, and not the kind of "people person" deserving of promotion.

- **Management actually approves of office politics.** Management likes engaged, action-oriented workers—in other words, office politics' primary participants. Management likes the creative ideas that arise from employee interaction, even if the motive is self-interest. Management likes the stability that results from in-house social relationships, since studies show that employees who socialize at the office are less likely to leave. In fact, management likes office politics so much that it watches to see who swims best in the office politics pool.

- **"Negative campaigning" is for losers.** There's certainly no shortage of would-be career climbers who turn to backstabbing and bad-mouthing because they think that's what office politics consists of. Smart office politicians love it when rivals do things like that, because they know it will backfire. Sure, a well-timed backstabbing of a fellow worker pays off on occasion, but in the long run that kind of negative behavior is a career killer. A good office politician makes alliances, not enemies.

gold watch. Watch everybody—colleagues, subordinates, and superiors. Watch them at meetings, at parties, at lunch, and during the workaday routine. Eavesdrop when you can (without being sneaky, of course). Observe body language. Use small talk to probe.

Here are some of the things you're looking for when you're new: Who takes lunch together? Who does what at lunch (cafeteria, brown bag, catering truck, restaurants, a gym or a jog)? Who commutes together? Who laughs at whose jokes? Who supports whom at meetings? Who comes early? Who stays late? Learn your fellow employees' individual interests, their status in the office, their family situations, and their hobbies. Notice how they talk and the tone of voice they use. Discern their values and their lifestyle.

You care about all this information because it constitutes the workplace culture in which you are performing. It is the raw material of your success. You will be able to make better decisions.

You will see opportunities you otherwise may have missed, and you will be able to act on those opportunities more efficiently.

Example: Your surveillance reveals that Mary in IT is an avid collector of dolls. A month later you run across an article on a famous person who is a doll collector, so you pass it along to her, saying you thought she might be interested. Another month later you need some quick help from IT on a project. You have a casual contact there, don't you?

That's just a little thing, maybe, but if you make a true effort to observe constantly, you'll multiply it by a factor of thousands.

Are you practicing office politics by doing this? Of course. Are you spying? Not really, because you're not seeking information to use against them. You're seeking information in order to work with them—albeit for your own benefit. Besides, a lot of them are watching you too.

Hear it through the grapevine.

As a source of factual information, the company grapevine is by definition unreliable, since rumors aren't facts. But as a barometer of workplace mood, it's essential. And as an indicator of what the future may hold, it's priceless. There's a reason for the grapevine's value that you're not supposed to know about: Management uses the grapevine to float ideas, to test employee reactions to possible new policies, or to slowly break the news of upcoming layoffs. You can't afford to ignore the grapevine.

Find out who the grapevine perpetrators are. Instead of shunning them as hopeless gossips, cultivate them as sources. Don't take their word at face value, of course, but register it and follow up. Remember that informal information is as valuable as formal information in the world of office politics. And in many cases, knowing that the top brass is monitoring your reactions to the rumors, you can make sure you respond in ways that make you look good. ◁

Legal Problems

3 Secrets for Handling Difficulties Arising from Harassment and Discrimination on the Job

After complaining, stick it out. Once you complain in writing that you've been a victim of harassment on the job, management and their attorneys are secretly afraid of one thing above all else—that you will also sue them for "retaliation." That's because they are not allowed to punish you for filing a claim against them. In fact, if you can prove that they disciplined you unfairly, you're more likely to win an award on those grounds than on the original harassment suit. So look for and document post-complaint actions that smack of retaliation. Your lawyer would love to file such a suit, and their lawyer shudders at the thought.

But that doesn't mean they won't go after you in more subtle ways. You may find yourself getting assignments you despise, loaded down with paperwork, or otherwise made uncomfortable. Their secret goal is to get you to quit. Don't. Because once the company can claim you "abandoned" your job—which you technically have if you quit—your harassment case immediately becomes so weak that lawyers are unlikely to take it.

You have little to lose. Employers have spread the word that trying to win harassment or discrimination cases against them is a losing proposition. They've been pretty successful at making employees think that there's little chance of winning, and less chance of collecting a worthwhile amount. What they don't want getting out is the truth, which is that you really can't lose in most cases. "If you win the suit, they have to pay your attorneys' fees," says Charles Joseph, a labor lawyer with Joseph & Herzfeld. "But if you lose the suit, there is a slim-to-none chance that you have to pay theirs."

How to Document Discrimination on the Job

- **Keep a record.** Start a diary at the first hint of discriminatory behavior or harassment. Write down the date, time, and place, along with who did what and who witnessed it. Example: "On June 30, 2007, in the coffee room Jack Pigg, my supervisor, called me an old fogy and said he resented having to work with geezers. My coworkers Jane Doe and Tom Katt were in the room and heard him."

- **Collect evidence.** Make sure you keep the evidence, even if it doesn't amount to much on its own. A note or memo with an ethnic slur, for example, that possibly refers to you goes into your discrimination case file. If the offense is public, such as a racist or sexist cartoon posted in the rest room, you have the legal right to take it down and copy it, or even keep it in your file. Remember that you're amassing evidence, not necessarily finding a smoking gun.

- **Skip the tape recorder.** Don't tape conversations with the discriminator or harasser unless you know for sure that it will produce a smoking gun otherwise not available. Even if you live in a state or province where it's legal to tape without the other's consent, don't do it. Labor lawyers say it hurts you with jurors, who tend to see "tapers" as unethical.

And if your case is solid, the judgment in your favor could involve a considerable amount of money. After all, discrimination and harassment are odious practices. "They do not want you to know that punitive damages are not as uncommon as people are led to believe," Joseph says.

It is true, of course, that it's pointless to pursue legal action when you have little chance of winning. But the strength of your case is for your lawyer to decide, not theirs.

Get counseling. There's a little-known fact of legal life that company lawyers hope like heck will never come up. It's not uncommon for victims of discrimination, harassment, or other illegal on-the-job practices to suffer from depression or other harmful mental conditions. But it's also not uncommon for victims to shun counseling, or at least put it off until their cases are resolved. That's a mistake. Besides providing the help you need, seeking professional care can help your legal cause. "Seeking counseling from a mental health professional can increase your award at trial," Joseph says. ◀

Getting Fired

8 Things You Should Consider Doing If You Are Unexpectedly Booted Out of Your Job

Ask for a good letter of reference. How crazy is it to ask somebody who just fired you to provide a reference letter for your next job? Not crazy at all, really. In fact, you should bring up the subject before you empty out your desk or locker and head home, says Alison Doyle, a job search expert at about.com. It will go a long way toward diffusing your worries about how this stain on your résumé will go over with prospective employers.

What are your chances of getting a positive reference under the circumstances? Better than you think, Doyle says. "It's something you can negotiate," she says. "If they won't offer a letter, you can ask for a good verbal reference if they're contacted. Or they might agree to just verify your period of employment and salary, with no reference good or bad."

At the very worst, you'll find out if they're going to give you a negative reference when future prospective employers give them a call. At least you'll know what you'll be dealing with. But there's some inside information involved that helps your cause. Unless you've been fired for punching a coworker or something equally unforgivable, many if not most companies are loath to say anything negative about a former employee. "They don't want to raise possible legal issues that can result form giving somebody a bad reference," Doyle says.

Or get a reference from a friendly manager. Whoever fired you may not appreciate it if somebody else in the company agrees to put in a good word for you with a potential new employer. But there's nothing they can do about it. If the company itself won't give you a reference letter, seek out another high-ranking staffer—a supervisor, a manager in another department with whom you worked often and well, or a respected veteran. Even if that person cannot go on the record with a formal letter on your behalf, he or she may agree to be listed as a reference and speak well of you when called. That will certainly water down the negativity when you're dealing with a prospective new employer.

Quit before you're fired. You remember the old cliché: "You can't fire me, because I quit!" In the movies, the characters say things like that to save their pride. But in real life, quitting before it comes down to an unpleasant firing makes sense if you're truly dissatisfied with your job situation.

Because your boss may know something you don't—that your job performance really has been suffering. The real forbidden knowledge in this case may be something you're keeping from yourself: Which is that deep inside, you know you're dragging because, frankly put, you hate your job. You may even unconsciously want to be fired.

If that's the case, the solution is to start looking for another job right now. Don't just up and quit; the best time to look for a new job is when you already have one. You have the security of a paycheck coming in, and you're out there in the workaday world with all its connections and energy instead of making phone calls from your kitchen table. Don't feel guilty about looking while you're working; you'll probably be doing your current job better with the new energy fueled by your decision. Just take advantage of your lunches and off hours to job-search. Use private e-mail, and check your home phone messages. And be up-front with prospective employers about your current situation.

Do tell your current boss about your plans, but not right away. First decide what it is that you're really looking for. Then get some résumés out there and wait until you've had some bites and prospects before breaking the news that you're "looking." The boss may be hurt or angry, but he or she may also be relieved that the situation is moving toward a solution that won't include a firing.

If you're leaving, ask for a promotion. Here's a variation on your pre-emptive dodge-the-axe strategy. After some soul-searching, you decide that you're so dissatisfied with your job that quitting is the best solution. Your next move is to march straight into the boss's office—not to tell him or her that you're leaving but to air your grievances. "Don't show your cards by revealing your plans to quit," says Karen Schaffer, a Halifax, Nova Scotia, career coach and author of *The Job of Your Life: Four Groundbreaking Steps for Getting the Work You Want.* "Instead, roll the dice, tell them how you feel, tell them what you want, and ask them what their plans really are for you."

Why bother if you're quitting anyway? Because that's the best time to do it. "You go in feeling liberated, with nothing to lose," Schaffer says. "At least you're creating parameters about what you want." In other words, just voicing your desires provides a context when you do give notice, and will even help make things clear in your own mind as you look for a new job.

But beware: You may get what you want and end up not quitting after all. "Sometimes management has no idea that you have a problem with your job," Schaffer says. "If you're valued, they may try to accommodate your concerns." And if you're not valued enough for them to do that, then you know your decision to leave was the right one.

Turn getting fired into a positive future job asset. The moment of truth has come, when the hiring manager asks about your termination from your previous job. You can handle it if you know

what the interviewer is really thinking: He doesn't want to be judge and jury. Nor is he interested in rescuing your career. He just wants to know if there's a problem or not.

Don't plead your case. Don't try to defend yourself with detailed complaints about what "they" did to you. Don't act morose, angry, repentant, or bitter. Don't bad-mouth anybody. All you're accomplishing with defensive behavior is convincing your would-be next employer that this thing is still festering.

Do this instead, says Karen Schaffer, the Halifax career coach: Use a general, big-picture description of the situation, like "bad fit," "unfortunate situation," or "unresolved conflicts." Then, in two or

---

WHAT **COMPANY LAWYERS** DON'T WANT YOU TO KNOW ABOUT Overtime Pay

Some salaried employees classified by their employers as "exempt"—that is, not eligible for overtime pay because their work doesn't fit into a schedule—are not really exempt under U.S. federal labor laws (most provinces in Canada have similar laws; check on your provincial government's website under "Hours of Work and Overtime Pay" for specific details). They are entitled to time-and-a-half for every hour over 40 in a week, even if they don't know it.

It doesn't matter if you're the one who volunteered to work overtime. If they let you do it, they have to pay you extra.

If you work 35 hours one week and 45 the next, it doesn't average out. You're owed time-and-a-half for those extra five hours in the second week.

Automatic clocking-out doesn't deprive you of overtime pay. If you work extra hours during lunch or after your shift, you must be paid time-and-a-half for that time no matter what the time clock says.

If you're required to arrive early to "prepare" for work, you're owed for that time, and you get time-and-a-half for it if it brings your weekly hours past 40.

You can collect three years' worth of back pay if you weren't properly compensated for overtime work. Executives, professionals, and most white-collar staffers who work independently are exempt; if you are otherwise, check with a labor lawyer on your status. You may have money coming to you.

---

three sentences, show that you've dealt with it, understood it, put it behind you, and moved on. Say something like this: "It was one of those unfortunate situations that had to end in a separation, and they moved before I did. I realize now that I should have taken some action on my own instead of letting things fester, but I've learned from the experience."

"Put a positive but still realistic spin on it," says Schaffer. "If you convince them that you 'own' the situation, management will usually accept that."

Call the unemployment office immediately. You were fired, but you managed to walk away from your old job with several weeks' or months' worth of severance pay. So it will be quite a while before you need to bother with calling the unemployment office, right? Wrong. You may be shocked to learn that, in the U.S., many states ignore severance pay as just another benefit of your old job, and they're willing to send you an unemployment check even during the period that you are covered by the cash payout from your former employer. Call your state's unemployment office to get the particulars. When your unemployment checks start arriving might depend, for instance, on whether you took a lump-sum severance payment from your old job or if it's paid out over time like a continuing salary. In any case, register immediately with your unemployment office so you do not miss any funds that you are entitled to. Some states don't pay benefits for the first week in which you qualify for unemployment. Also, it typically takes a few weeks for your first unemployment check to arrive. So you want the clock on your case to start ticking right away.

Make your case anyway. Maybe something untoward happened at work, and the bosses told you that you were fired "for cause." So surely you could never qualify for unemployment funds, a benefit reserved for workers who lose their jobs through no fault of their own? No, don't make this assumption if you live in the U.S. The laws vary from state to state for deciding who qualifies for unemployment. You may be surprised to find a sympathetic ear at the unemployment office when you describe the circumstances of your firing. If you actually resigned from your job and weren't technically fired, you might be able to persuade the state that there were compelling reasons you felt pressured to quit. Even if you are turned down initially by the state unemployment office, you will probably be offered a chance to make your case in person at a hearing.

Ashamed? Get over it. As smart and talented as you are, you might never have imagined that you would be without work for an extended period of time. What's more, the idea of filing for unemployment benefits makes you feel uneasy—as if you're accepting handouts when you're not actually destitute. Get past that mental block. If your car or home got damaged, you would accept the insurance money. Unemployment benefits are just an insurance program that happens to be run by the government. You deserve the money, so take it. ◁

Home Security

7 Shockingly Simple Tips to Put Prowlers Out of Business

Secure your door. Locksmiths will probably quote you a hefty fee to "burglar-proof" your front door. You can accomplish the same thing by spending a few bucks on a good dead-bolt lock, a few pennies on the right screws, and a few minutes with a screwdriver. The secret is a strong strike plate, which is the metal square that the bolt fits into when you lock up. Make sure the dead-bolt kit that you buy has a strike plate with four screw holes rather than just two; it's twice as strong that way. If the screws that come with the set are tiny, replace them with four 3-inch (7.6-cm) screws, which will go deep into the hard wood of the door frame and hold fast. You want your strike plate attached to the hard wood on the door frame, not just to the decorative trim that surrounds the door. That way, anybody intent on breaking into your home cannot kick in your dead-bolted door—the strike plate won't give. Do this with all your doors (back, side, garage) and you've eliminated a burglar's favorite points of entry.

Secure a window the easy way. Security specialists want you to believe that barred windows are the only safe windows. True, putting bars on all your windows will keep intruders out, no question about it. What those installers won't mention is that burglars usually look for open—not bar-less—windows. (Drive around any residential area for a few minutes and you'll be amazed at how many windows are left open.) Just by closing and latching your windows, security experts say, you make your home significantly less likely to be burglarized.

But latches are not locks, and they can be forced. Solve that problem by driving a long, fat screw into each of the two tracks that the window slides along (either up or sideways) to open. That way, even if the latch is broken, the window will be blocked before it can slide totally open. Position the screw so that it allows the window to open no more than 4 inches (10 cm)—enough for ventilation, but not enough room for a probing hand to remove the screw.

If the window simply opens inward instead of sliding up or sideways, install extra mini-dead bolts or simply hammer in strong, 3-inch (7.6-cm) nails on both sides of the frame and bend them to block the window's inward path. Such simple "secondary blocking devices," as they're known among security folks, aren't exactly at the Fort Knox level of security, but they deter burglars, who hate struggling with stubborn windows.

Adopt a pooch. If you don't have young children in the house, adopt a *big* pooch—they're one of the best burglar deterrents around. Good watchdog choices include Doberman pinschers, huskies, Great Danes, German shepherds, and retrievers. If you're not able to care for a dog or if they're not allowed in your building, it still doesn't hurt to get a tape recording of a dog barking to play every now and again (and have it running on your answering machine's

WHAT **BURGLARS** DON'T WANT YOU TO KNOW ABOUT Break-Ins

- [ ] **They prefer to break in during the day.** While most people fret about night prowlers, competent burglars look for open windows in the morning or afternoon, when most folks are out of the house.

- [ ] **They hate barking dogs.** Even a small pooch will help protect your home, as long as he makes a lot of noise when strangers come by. Big, mean-looking dogs are even more effective. Don't forget the prominent, menacing "Beware of Dog" sign either.

- [ ] **They'll come right up to your front door and knock.** What better way to find out if anybody's home? As long as they look like they have some reason to be there, they don't attract suspicion. If there's no answer, they can look for your hidden key or an open window—or just kick in your front door if you don't use a strong dead-bolt lock.

- [ ] **They don't care if your income is modest.** Don't think you're safe because you're not swimming in jewelry or valuable art. Burglars are usually looking for quick cash, not the big score. Criminals break in because they want small, easy-to-grab and easy-to-sell items—like laptops, video players, watches, CDs, and small electronic devices.

outgoing message). Consider posting "Beware of Dog" signs.

Resist a pricey monitoring alarm system. If home security vendors can't scare you into signing up for an expensive monitoring system that you don't need, they may try an appeal to your pocketbook. After all, everybody knows you get an insurance discount when you buy the top-of-the-line home security package. What "everybody" may not know is that the insurance discount you get is peanuts compared to the yearly fees you'll be paying for the monitoring system. Stick with the basic package of alarms and signs. On the other hand, experts do recommend that you consider a monitoring service if fire is a big concern—for example, if you live in a high-fire-risk area such as brushy foothills. The police may not get there in time to catch a thief, but firefighters will certainly be welcome if your system is set up to trigger a call at the first sign of a fire.

Get this important alarm protection. An anonymous stalking victim offers this advice to people who fear for their safety: If you have a home alarm system, always opt for the "phone line cut" service, which can detect whether an intruder has cut your phone line. It automatically sends police to your house, even though you're not able to call them yourself.

Give your neighbor that spare key. You'll hear a thousand different ideas on the best hiding place for your spare home key, but you'll seldom hear the only one that counts: "Nowhere." You'll never find a spot that a burglar hasn't thought of. Instead, give that key to a neighbor. That solves a number of problems (besides getting in when you've locked yourself out). If you're expecting service people while you're away, a neighbor can let them in and see them out. A key exchange also establishes a mutual trust with your neighbor that is an important security strategy in and of itself. When you're away, have neighbors keep an eye on your home, gather mail and newspapers, watch for strangers, and even park their car in your driveway from time to time to simulate occupancy. You should have a pact of mutual protection that kicks in when one of you isn't home. Tell them what days you'll be gone, who will come by in your absence, who they can let in, and how they can reach you if they encounter anything suspicious.

Watch the foliage. Overgrown shrubbery and high hedges around the perimeter of your house provide as much privacy for burglars as they do for you. Trim foliage in your foundation plantings often so that it can't camouflage a burglar's activities from the view of neighbors and passersby. Think twice before installing a tall privacy fence or planting a tall hedge. You may just be inviting an intruder to take advantage of the cover they provide. Also check out large trees near your house and prune branches if they provide ready access to second-floor windows or a balcony. The same is true of trellises on the side of your house that make an inviting ladder for a burglar. Another thing to keep in mind is that basement windows are often obscured by shrubbery, making them a favorite access point for burglars, especially because they lead to an area of the house that is often not occupied. Keep these windows locked whenever possible. ◁

Personal Security
4 Little-Known Safety Tips That Can Save Your Life

Don't look like a target. You know the cliché: "It can happen to anybody." But criminologists know something else—that bad things are more likely to happen to those who make themselves more attractive to muggers. How? By walking along looking lost, distracted, or vulnerable. Don't be like them. Stay aware of your surroundings and adopt purposeful, assertive body language that projects confidence. That doesn't mean that you should try to come off as tough or threatening. Just don't act like a potential victim.

"There's really no such thing as 'random' street crime," says Jon French, a security consultant who works with U.S. companies doing business in Mexico. "The muggers go after who they perceive to be the easiest targets. If your body language says 'Don't mess with me,' you're less likely to get mugged."

Know your enemy. The politically correct message you hear is that you shouldn't stereotype criminals—they could be anyone. But if you could be a fly on the wall when cops and security pros are chatting it up, you'd know that there is one category of human beings responsible for the overwhelming majority of violent crimes: young men. "It's almost always young males who are the perpetrators," says personal security guru Chris McGoey. True, the proper public posture is to avoid stereotyping, and in most cases that's good advice. But not when it comes to protecting yourself from muggers, robbers, and thieves. It's not that all young men are criminals, it's that most criminals are young men. Just exercise caution when unknown males in their teens and 20s cross your path in vulnerable situations.

"You have to use common sense," McGoey says. "If you're getting gas at night or running into a convenience store and you see young guys loitering, don't go that way. If you're walking through a parking lot, be suspicious of young men hanging out in parked cars."

Don't bring your stalkers home with you. If somebody is following you, your natural instinct may be to get home as quickly as you can and lock the doors. After all, that's what they do in the movies, isn't it? In truth, though, heading for home is a bad idea—you don't want your stalker to know where you live.

"If you are being followed, never lead the person back to your home," the U.S. State Department instructs its overseas diplomats. "Do not stop or get out of the car. Drive to the nearest public place." There you'll be safe and can take your next action, which is to call the police. If you think you're being stalked while on foot, don't wait to be sure. Use your cell phone to call the police immediately. No phone around? "If you're in danger, try to attract attention," advises the Citizens for Crime Awareness, a nonprofit crime prevention organization in Winnipeg, Manitoba. "Scream, run, and yell if you are able."

Repel a potential rapist. You've been attacked by a rapist; sexual assault might be imminent. What's your best plan of attack? According to the Hingham, Massachusetts, police department, your best defense is your common sense. Your goal isn't to fight the rapist, but to make an opportunity to escape from him. This can be done passively by claiming to be pregnant, sick, or having a sexually transmitted disease. You can also try to discourage him by saying that a friend or family member is on the way over.

The website www.safetyforwomen.com says that using items on your person, or in your immediate environment, can be your key to surviving violent confrontations. You can use the most mundane things to defend yourself, including glass bottles, hair spray (throw the can at your attacker, or spray him in the eyes), silverware, sand, bricks, even furniture. ◄

Telephone Tricks and Tips
6 Secret Techniques for Stopping Eavesdroppers and Unwanted Calls

Know how to recognize if someone has tapped your phone. Maybe you're involved in a court case, or work for a high-profile company. Truth is, there are some folks who are often the targets of covert eavesdropping, even in their own home. Signs that someone is eavesdropping on your telephone calls include:

- Strange sounds coming from your phone, like static, squealing, or scratching noises; sounds that come from the phone when it's hung up; volume changes or other odd noises.

- Interference on your home or car radio.

- A telephone repairman shows up when nothing is wrong with your service, or no one called him.

- Friends or business associates know things you didn't tell them—like secret meetings, trade secrets, even personal information that they'd have no way of knowing otherwise.

Block the call-waiting service. Call-waiting can be a problem if you have to make a very important phone call and don't want to be interrupted by telemarketers or Aunt Mabel while you're on the line. Before you make your call, dialing *70 will block call-waiting—anyone calling your number will get a busy signal. This trick is only good for a single phone call; you have to repeat *70 whenever you want to use it. This number might vary depending on your region; check your local phone book for specific information.

Know how tricksters can circumvent your caller ID service. It's quite easy for unwanted callers to get around your caller ID system. They can buy a device or service to install on their phone that will block their number on any caller ID system, or dial *67 before dialing your number. Another trick, which can be done from virtually any phone, says one private investigator, is for the sneak to dial the operator and tell her that he's having trouble getting through to your line. Then the operator will dial the number for him, in which case the original caller's number won't be listed. Your best line of defense? Don't pick up the phone when there's anything other than a familiar name on your caller ID.

Reject unknown callers. Your phone keeps ringing, but all of the numbers are coming up as "private" or "unknown," so you don't want to answer—how annoying! There's a way to keep those calls from getting through to your line in the first place. Dialing up a service called "anonymous call rejection" from your phone means that callers who block their numbers will get a recorded message saying that your line doesn't accept unidentified callers. The way to turn on this call rejection is usually dialing *77 from your phone; turning it off is usually *87. Consult your local phone company for specific advice; there might also be a charge for this service.

Cut off those pitchmen. Reduce the number of telemarketer phone calls by signing up for the National Do Not Call Registry. When you do, most of these annoying pitchmen will be forced to bother someone else. (However, some groups—charities and political outfits, for instance—are exempt.) Sign up by calling 888-382-1222 or visit

www.donotcall.gov on the Internet. When a telemarketer does get through to you, tell him to put you on his "do not call" list. In Canada, residents can ask for a registration number when they tell a telemarketer to add them to the "do not call" list, and they can use this number if they need to file a complaint in the future.

Weed out nonurgent phone calls. If you are constantly being interrupted by a ringing telephone, wean some of your contacts off voice communication and onto e-mail communication. After all, you can respond to e-mails on your own schedule rather than the sender's, it's easier to save e-mails than it is to take notes over the phone, and you can easily delete inconsequential e-mails without offending the sender. Tell frequent, nonurgent callers, "I'm late for an appointment—would you please send me an e-mail on that?" Emphasize to colleagues that e-mail is the best way to get your full attention. Also, have a separate set of business cards printed up with nothing but your name, title, company, and e-mail address. ◄I

How to Know Where You're Calling From

EXPERT INSTANT ADVICE

There's an easy way to determine the number of a unmarked phone in an unfamiliar place: Call the ANAC (automatic number announcement circuit) number—when you dial this number from a landline phone, it reads back to you the number from which you called. A couple of numbers include 800-444-4444 and 800-444-3333; you can find local ANACs by googling "ANAC number" plus your area code. This number may come in handy should you find yourself in an unfamiliar place or other danger; it's the number that telephone repairmen call when they're trying to distinguish between two phone wires.

Identity Theft
8 Surefire Ways to Protect Yourself from Prying Thieves

Guard your Social Security number like the crown jewels. Many businesses act like it's their right to demand your Social Security number whenever they feel like it. It's not. In most cases, even when some form or employee tells you it's "required," it usually isn't. Be *very* selective about who you give this number to, because a Social Security number (or a Social Insurance Number in Canada) is the holy grail for identity thieves. Once they've got yours, they can commit crimes in your name and get rich at your expense.

"Companies are always asking for unnecessary information," says Linda Foley, executive director of the Identity Theft Resource Center, a San Diego-based nonprofit organization that helps identity theft victims. "Your vet doesn't need your Social Security number. The airline doesn't need it to find your lost luggage. The self-storage place doesn't need it to rent you space."

If such businesses ask you for it, simply refuse or offer to supply another identifying number instead, such as your driver's license number. When sweepstakes or contest forms ask for your Social Security number, it's usually to get you on a company's marketing lists. Write in the space that you'll provide the number if you win. Work- and tax-related dealings usually do require your Social Security number, as do credit checks. That's legitimate. But even then, hold out until you're convinced it's necessary. For example, when filling out a job application, ask if for security reasons you can withhold your number until you are offered the job.

Leave your cards at home. Healthcare providers like doctors and pharmacies have you convinced that you've got to have original ID cards with you to use their services. Not true. To start with, never carry around your Social Security card. Memorize the number and keep the actual card at home, or in a safe-deposit box. And don't carry around any other identification card that includes your Social Security number. If you lose your purse or wallet, you're better protected against identity theft.

But what about your Medicare card and other health insurance cards? Don't you need to keep them on your person in case of emergency? Yes and no—you don't need to carry originals, and again, you need to protect your Social Security number. So here's what you do: Copy both sides of your insurance card, and cut the copy down to wallet size. Snip the last four digits of your Social Security number off the copy—it's like a PIN code, personally identifying you. Without these last four numbers, an identity thief can't do a thing. On a third piece of paper, write down the name and phone numbers of two or more trusted friends as medical contacts. Keep all three of those card-size pieces of paper in your purse or wallet instead of your Medicare card. Give the four missing digits to those two or more trusted friends, along with any pertinent medical information about you—medications you're allergic to, drugs you're taking, and conditions you have. Now, if you have a medical emergency, even if you're unconscious,

How I Do It An ID-Theft Expert Destroys Personal Information

Identity theft experts such as Frank Abagnale, Jr., the reformed con man upon whom the movie *Catch Me If You Can* was based, strongly recommend shredding bank notices, credit card offers, or any other documents with potentially vulnerable information on them before you throw them away. And they insist that you use a crosscut shredder—the kind that turns paper into confetti—so identity thieves can't fit the pieces together like a jigsaw puzzle. But one elderly lady convinced an Identity Theft Resource Center caseworker that a simpler, cheaper way to render documents useless to identity thieves works just as well.

"What I do is tear up the papers and put them in a large mixing bowl," she said during a question-and-answer session after an identity theft prevention talk. "Then I pour boiling water over them and leave them overnight. In the morning, there's nothing but pulp."

the hospital personnel have a copy of your Medicare card, a contact to confirm your Social Security number, and access to crucial medical information. That could save your life.

In Canada, you have to pay for medical services if you don't have your original card with you, although you will be reimbursed for most of the costs.

Get updated. Software companies may not like you to use "borrowed" or otherwise illicitly installed computer privacy protection programs, but hackers love it when you do. That's because unlicensed spyware and firewall protection isn't eligible for free software updates. There's a reason all those updates are offered: Identity thieves are constantly finding ways around existing software to get into hard drives to steal your passwords and financial data. Using non-updated protective software is like taking last year's flu vaccine. It won't work. For extra protection, put password protection on files that contain sensitive personal information, like your credit card or bank account numbers. Just click the help button on your computer and follow the instructions.

Check for credit trouble without paying. Companies that charge $50 to $120 a year to monitor your credit rating won't go out of their way to tell you, but if you live in the United States, you have free access to your credit reports. By law (as of 2005), each of the three licensed credit bureaus must provide you with one free report each year if you request it. Stagger your requests and you can review your credit standing every four months, which is usually often enough to make sure an identity thief hasn't run up unpaid bills in your name. What's more, you're entitled to a free report right away if you've been denied credit, or if you suspect you've been a victim of identity theft.

To order a free credit report, go to www.annualcreditreport.com—this is the only site, besides the credit bureaus' sites, that is authorized to process credit report requests. (There's no similar site in Canada.) If you prefer, you can contact the individual credit bureaus directly at:

- Equifax, www.equifax.com, 800-685-1111 (or in Canada, www.equifax.ca, 800-465-7166)

- Experian, www.experian.com, 888-397-3742 (or www.creditbureau.ca, 800-646-5876)

- TransUnion, www.transunion.com, 800-916-8800 (or www.transunion.ca, 800-646-5876)

Whether you order your report online or by phone, you will have to give your Social Security number.

If you spot an irregularity on one of your credit reports, ask the credit-reporting company to place a fraud alert on your report right away. This means that any company reviewing your report must check with you personally before issuing credit in your name. Each credit-reporting company is required to notify the other two credit bureaus, but they aren't always prompt about it. Call the other two agencies yourself to make sure the fraud alert is applied to all three reports. You will probably get a recording that will ask for personal information to verify your identity. It is okay, in this case, to give out your Social Security number.

Trash the junk mail. Most of your junk mail problem will disappear when you "opt" yourself out of marketing offers originating with companies you're already doing business with. It's a little tricky, but you can do it. Look for small print in the bills between May and July, when the companies are required to inform you how to stop receiving pitches. Then you have to send in the request, and usually to a different P.O. box than where you send payments. That's simply to make it harder for you. "They don't want you to opt out," says Foley. "They want to keep sending you offers." (To learn more about opting out of pre-approved credit card offers, see page 234.)

Get your identity back ... without paying for it. If you've been a victim of identity theft, you may be on the hook for a lot of lawyer's or restoration service fees to fix the problem. But did you know that there are free services that will help you get your good name back and your true credit record restored? Believe it or not, your best first step is to contact the U.S. Federal Trade Commission (www.consumer .gov/idtheft). This government agency is set up to walk you through the process of recovering your identity with simple, clear instructions; its website includes a link to a useful PDF: "What to Do If Your Personal Information Has Been Compromised." Yes, you'll have some paperwork to fill out, but you'll have to do that even if you pay a restoration service to help you. On the FTC site, you'll learn exactly how to close accounts that may have been tampered with or opened fraudulently in your name, file a police report, and file a complaint with the FTC. If your problem requires ongoing help, the Identity Theft Resource Center (www.idtheft center.org) can assist you.

In Canada, your best bet for reporting identity theft is to call the Canadian Anti-Fraud Centre's PhoneBusters (888-495-8501), your bank, the local police, and the three credit bureaus (opposite page).

Choose a hack-resistant online password. Just as you wouldn't give your ATM code to a stranger, it's just as important to protect your online passwords—otherwise, computer hackers could have access to your medical and financial records, e-mail account, even your credit card information. Here are a few ways to choose passwords that no one will ever guess:

- Birthdays, kids' names, anniversaries—forget it. These are the first

bits of data that thieves and hackers go to when trying to break into your accounts.

- Don't think that spelling your spouse's name (or any other easy password) backward will work either. Hackers have programs that will detect words spelled out backward and forward.

- Don't use one password for all of your accounts. If online thieves happen upon just one, you're in big trouble.

- Your best plan of action: Choose passwords that have both letters and numbers. Pick a password that's not even a real word—just jumble up some letters and numbers. And change your password frequently.

Be wary of clicking on a link in an e-mail. If you receive an e-mail from your bank, broker, or some other business that you regularly deal with, be aware that the e-mail may not have come from the business in question. It may be a trap designed by an identity thief to get you to click on a link. Instead of taking you to the business, that link will take you to a phony website, cleverly designed to look like the real thing. There the thief will try to extract as much information as he can from you, such as your password, your Social Security number, and your mother's maiden name. If you do get an e-mail from a financial institution, never click on a link in the message. Instead, call the branch you normally deal with and speak with a customer representative. Or if you bank online, go directly to the website by typing the name in your browser. ◄

Auto Theft
4 Ways to Deter Potential Car Thieves and Carjackers

Use a steering-wheel locking device. Any car-alarm vendor will want to sell you the latest high-tech device, like hidden "kill switches" that automatically cut off the ignition, engine, and fuel supply so even the most skilled hotwire pro can't start your car, let alone steal it. But think about it: For the gizmo to work, the bad guy has to already be in your car. Do you really want that? Instead of the kill switch, use an easily installable mechanical device that locks to the steering wheel or steering column. Until you unlock it, nobody can turn the steering wheel, which means nobody can drive the car away. But best of all, these clubs, collars, or J-bars are highly visible, so they act as a deterrent. If car thieves spy a good auto theft device, they're likely to look for another car to steal.

Park using this special trick. Here's how to park so that it's harder for thieves to make off with your vehicle. On the street, park between two other cars (practice that parallel parking!) and turn your wheels toward the curb. Thieves are looking for fast getaways, and the last thing they want to do is waste time maneuvering out of a tight spot. Take your ticket with you when you park in a parking garage—and never leave the ticket in plain sight on your dashboard. Auto thieves look for those tickets so they can take your car out of the garage without having to stop and explain to the attendant how they lost your ticket. If your home has a garage, always use it. A car sitting out on a residential street is an inviting target, even if it's locked. Finally, the more light and traffic around, the safer the parking place. Car thieves hate audiences.

Pay attention to prevent carjacking. Carjacking is a violent crime in which the thieves physically overpower you to take your car—and sometimes you with it.

"Carjackers, like street robbers, depend on the element of surprise," explains security guru McGoey. "I interview victims all the time, and they usually say they never saw the guy coming until he appeared at the car door." Your first line of defense against carjacking (and most other street crime) is to be aware of your environment at all times, and hyperaware at key times. This means not chatting on your cell phone as you walk around, not dawdling before getting into or out of your car, not putting on makeup before getting out of the car. If you're like most people, you do things like that all the time.

"People go out of their homes and they're immediately in la-la land, just oblivious to the world around them," McGoey says. "If you just pay attention to your environment, your chances of being victimized are drastically reduced."

Here are a few strategies to remember:

- Be especially careful when you are approaching or leaving your automobile. Don't park in deserted spots, in areas with obstructed vision (because of trees and walls), near a big van with no windows, or near somebody who's just sitting inside a nearby car.

- Once you park, look around again, scan the area, ready to drive away if anybody approaches. Then get out, lock up quickly, and walk away.

- Reverse the strategy coming back to the car. Never turn your back to load groceries, kids, or anything else. Make it a habit to start your car and drive away quickly. Keep your antennae up in unusual situations. Are you bumped in traffic by a car with a young male inside who gets out to "help"? High alert! This is a common carjacking ploy.

Survive a carjacking. If you're confronted by an armed carjacker, don't resist. Give up your keys, and hand over the money if it's demanded. Don't argue, fight, or chase the robber. These people have no qualms about hurting you. However, never agree to be kidnapped if you can avoid it. Wherever they take you will probably be more dangerous than where they are confronting you. If you're still outside the car, drop the car keys and run for help if you can, screaming all the way. If you're forced to drive, you have to assess the situation and the degree of danger. Consider crashing your car intentionally near a busy intersection to attract attention. ◁

SECRET WEAPON

Disaster Kit

Is your family ready if disaster strikes? The American Red Cross recommends that every family prepare a disaster supplies kit that could sustain you for three days in case of an emergency. The following supplies should be kept in an easy-to-carry container, like a duffel bag or a small plastic trash can:

• Flashlight and extra batteries

• Battery-powered radio and batteries (or a hand-crank powered radio)

• Plastic sheeting and duct tape

• Water (a three-day supply of one gallon (3.7 liters) per person, per day)

• Nonperishable food that's compact and lightweight (granola bars, peanut butter, crackers, trail mix, etc.)

• First-aid kit

• Sanitary supplies (toilet paper, soap, personal hygiene items)

• At least one complete change of clothing and footwear per family member

• Blankets or sleeping bags

• Miscellaneous items like medication, baby supplies, and important family documents (keep the latter in a waterproof container)

You'll find a more detailed checklist at www.redcross.org (click the "Get Prepared" link, then go to "Be Prepared At ... Home").

Getting Legal Advice

4 Secrets for Obtaining Help with Legal Problems Without Paying a Fortune

Start with free legal advice. Can you imagine an attorney telling you, "You don't need to pay for my legal help to solve your problem"? No. But a lot of people needing legal help should hear that. For a lot of legal situations, it makes sense to aim your first call at any one of a myriad of free legal services. That applies especially if you're over 60 in the U.S., because most states have senior legal hotlines that let you talk to an attorney over the phone at no charge. The hotline staff will also review documents for you, prepare letters, and get you whatever legal forms you may need. And if they can't do it all, they may refer you to some other free legal service that can. You'll find a list of these senior legal hotlines, complete with phone numbers, at the federal Administration on Aging website. Just go to www.aoa.gov and search for "legal hotlines." If you're not an Internet person, call 202-619-0724. There are no similar hotlines in Canada, but the government website www.seniors.gc.ca has a legal matters section that will take you to many helpful local links.

Younger folks have other options. If the problem is with a company or public utility, contact the company's consumer service (or complaint) department. They usually don't want legal hassles any more than you do, so you might be able to work something out. Government agencies provide some legal services for consumers; start by calling your state or provincial attorney general's office and asking for the consumer protection department. If your problem is with a regulated industry—say a bank, an insurance company, or a health care provider—look in the yellow pages under your state government for the agency in charge, such as the "Insurance Commission." At the very least, the phone call will glean some additional information, and you might even find a solution.

Check out community groups that make it their business to help people in legal trouble. Civil rights organizations, women's groups, immigrant centers, and a lot of other volunteer agencies will help you out in certain situations. If you're going to search the yellow pages for a lawyer anyway, consider trying one of the free advice services first.

Get your legal advice à la carte. The legal profession may have you convinced that seeking its help involves a major full-time commitment. You must "retain" a lawyer, they say, so he or she can "represent" you and "handle" your case. Well, we'll let you in on a secret: You don't have to do anything of the kind. Instead, think of a lawyer as the legal version of an electrician.

"Just because you need to consult with a lawyer from time to time does not mean you need to retain a lawyer," says Birmingham, Alabama, attorney and divorce mediator Lee Borden, who runs divorceinfo.com. "Just pay for the specific service you need."

Take a simple, uncontested divorce, for example. You can probably handle most of it yourself, but you may need a professional to, say, determine the true value of your spouse's retirement accounts, or to review a particularly confusing document. If that's the case, call your lawyer,

How to Size Up a Lawyer

It's not easy to judge the skills of a potential legal advocate. The reason you're there in the first place is that he or she knows so much more than you do about the subject matter. Intuition and good character judgment help, but so does a list of specific questions. There are no correct answers, but productive questions planned in advance will give you much more to go on than trying to wing a conversation. Try these:

- Do I need an attorney?
- What area of law do you have the most experience in?
- Have you handled matters like mine before?
- What have been the results of similar cases you've been involved in?
- What are the possible outcomes of my case?
- What are the alternative approaches for pursuing my case?
- How long will the case take?
- What are the chances of a settlement instead of a verdict?
- How will you keep me informed of progress?
- How much control will I have to give up to you over the decisions in my case?
- Is mediation or arbitration an option?
- Will you be working on my case personally?
- What are your exact rates and how are they determined?
- How often will I be billed?
- How do you charge for expenses?
- Who else in the office will be working on my case?
- Are there things I can do on my own to help things along, or to save me money?
- What's a ballpark figure for total cost?
- Can I meet any paralegals, junior attorneys, or support staff who will be involved in my case?
- If I am dissatisfied with how things are going, can I "fire" you?

ask how much it will cost you to have that (and only that) done, and proceed accordingly.

This pick-and-choose approach—or "unbundling," as it's sometimes called in divorce cases—has two big advantages for you. It saves a ton of money and keeps you in control of your own case. The help is there when you need it, but you're still making the decisions—in a divorce case, for instance, what issues to negotiate and whether you will discuss things with your spouse (something a retained lawyer usually won't let you do). Obviously, you'll need to dive in and retain full-time legal help if you're dealing with a bitter, adversarial divorce or more serious legal problems, such as criminal charges. Otherwise, don't shun legal advice just because you think you'll get deeply obligated to a lawyer's services. Approach it like conveyor-belt sushi—just grab what you need.

Watch out for additional costs. When you do hire a lawyer, be aware that you may face a lot of unexpected charges. Here are some things to keep in mind:

- You can be charged for telephone calls. Time is money, and phone calls take time. So the meter might be running, no matter who initiates the phone call. That's why legal consumer advocates like lawyers.com suggest you make sure any call to your lawyer is really necessary. If you can get the needed information from an administrative assistant, you'll save money.
- They charge for travel time and transportation costs—even if they're just going across the street. So your lawyer's offer to "drop by" your home or office to discuss your case may be a considerate gesture, but it's seldom a cost-free one.
- The hired help costs money too. Every time a paralegal looks something up in the law library or an administrative assistant types up a document, that's time spent on your case. You can be charged for it.
- Billing rates vary according to the rank of the attorney doing the work. Partners in the firm naturally cost the most. That doesn't mean you're wasting money, though. More experienced partners may resolve your case faster.
- Each time you're billed, you are supposed to get an itemized bill. Insist on it. You can learn where you're needlessly and unknowingly running up expenses. Then you can adjust your interaction with your lawyer accordingly to save money on the next bill.

Beware of ambulance chasers. In a lawyer, initiative and a go-get-'em attitude are not necessarily a good thing—these qualities may mask a serious ethical lapse. Let's say you have been in an accident. If a lawyer you've never met approaches you, already knows about your problem, and offers legal services, say no. This is ambulance chasing, even if there's no ambulance and no physical chasing. Does that mean this person is a "bad" lawyer? It doesn't matter. In most areas, such unsolicited contact violates the normal standards of professional conduct. A lawyer who has no qualms about breaking the rules is not somebody you want acting in your name. ◁

Divorce Cases
5 Ways to Keep the Pain to a Minimum When a Breakup Is Inevitable

Have a kinder, gentler split-up.
Judges, lawyers, therapists, and just about everybody else involved in marital issues tend to see divorce as a knock-down, drag-out battle. They're all wrong. "Despite the common cultural assumption that people going through a divorce have to fight about it, most people end their marriages with dignity and quietly move on with their lives," says attorney Lee Borden. "A cooperative, uncontested divorce is not only a good idea, it's the way most people do it."

So once you decide to split up, the first person you should talk to is not your lawyer but your soon-to-be ex-spouse. The conference agenda: Can we do this together? Can we agree now on the big issues and work out the details as we go along? Can we talk about who needs to end up with what, about where the children are going to live, about who's going to pay how much for their support? If so, what might have been World War III turns into a simple signing ceremony.

Warning: Divorce professionals may try to steer you and your spouse away from the peaceful path. "It's not that they're trying to stir up trouble," Borden says. "They spend most of their time with the nastiest adversarial cases, so that's the way they think divorce has to be."

If your spouse is reluctant to try the cooperative approach, trot out the following facts about contested divorces: They take much longer, they are infinitely more expensive, they create more problems than they solve, and they leave the two of you permanent adversaries.

That can make for a lifetime of tension-packed encounters at your children's school performances, graduations, weddings, and grandchildren's birthdays.

"You don't have to like each other a whole lot," Borden says. "Just be smart enough not to get caught up in all that adversarial stuff if you don't have to."

Keep relatives on the sidelines.
Why do relatives who never gave a moment's thought to your marriage suddenly present themselves as indispensable guides as soon as you start down the road to divorce? Because, they tell you, they "have your best inter-

ests at heart." Because they "know how you feel." Because they "know a good lawyer/counselor/detective/psychic" you simply must see. Because, some will say, they've "been there." And because, all will say, they knew all along what a rat that no-good spouse of yours is.

The only thing they don't seem to know is that this is your divorce and yours alone. You and only you must control it. No matter how well intentioned or well informed your family members are, it is almost always best to accept their emotional support but keep them away from the action.

Sure, go ahead and listen—to your wise uncle, to your parents, to your sisters, and cousins and aunts. Listen to your stylist, to your mail carrier, to your child's soccer coach, to the kid who prepares your morning latte. Then make your own decisions. Your family and your friends can be cheerleaders, but they can't play on your divorce team.

Look beyond a 50-50 split. The idea that splitting everything down the middle is the only fair way to divide marital assets is so entrenched that few people question it. After all, isn't marriage a 50-50 proposition? And don't community property jurisdictions, like Texas, California, and all Canadian provinces, call for a 50-50 split of material assets acquired by either spouse during the marriage? Well yes, but most states are not community property states. The judge's task in those states is to treat both spouses fairly, to "do equity" as the law puts it, and not necessarily to split everything in two. And even in community property states, fairness can take precedence over arithmetic if both parties are willing.

Your lesson in all this, if you're getting divorced, is to avoid getting hung up on some perfect 50-50 solution. Look at the big picture: Are you getting what you want and need, in an overall package that strikes you as fair? That's your goal. That's especially true when it comes to individual assets. A judge, for example, may have a reason for awarding the house to your spouse. Perhaps it was your spouse's father who gave it to the two of you in the first place. Unfair? Not if you weren't planning on living in the house anyway, and you get something else you wanted more. Focus on what you want, not what the calculator says you should have.

Don't let lawyers run wild with the case. Divorce lawyers tend to be set in their ways, going about things as they've been trained to do, which is not necessarily the best way for your particular case. As a result, costs skyrocket, squabbles proliferate, and the case drags on.

That's why neutral divorce law experts advise you to keep control of the proceedings and not let the lawyers turn it into a bigger case than it already is. How? Mostly by doing on your own those things you can do more quickly, more efficiently, and light-years more economically than your lawyer.

For example, both sides in a contested divorce need to know who owns what so that the assets can be divided fairly. Your lawyer is well trained to use the legally intricate "discovery" process to extract this information from your spouse's lawyer, who is just as well trained in finding ways not to provide it. The two of them can go round and round for months, racking up billable hours without much information changing hands. Better for you and your spouse to sit down together like adults and get it done in a day or two. All it takes is a realization that both of you gain—financially and emotionally—from sharing this information, which eventually is going to come out anyway.

Of course, if the two of you hate each other so much by now that you're incapable of communicating like adults, this won't work. It also won't work if one spouse—typically the man, even in this day and age—holds the lion's share of the information about family finances. He may just sit there with folded arms, offering you nothing. And finally, your lawyer may warn you against talking to your spouse under any circumstances until the case is concluded. We would never advise disobeying your legal counsel, but we will tell you what experts say off the record: Most divorce attorneys are secretly grateful when their clients work anything out on their own.

Be wary of potential financial traps. No matter how friendly your divorce is, when it comes to financial matters and divvying up property, it pays to question not only the motives of the other party but also your own. Here are three traps you should avoid falling into:

- *Your spouse has no intention of paying that debt.* No wonder your spouse generously offered to assume the $35,000 joint loan debt in exchange for your letting him have the paid-for Range Rover. He already knew he was going to file for bankruptcy or simply default on the debt. And what can you do about it? File an enforcement petition, perhaps, but that's not going to get you the vehicle back, or pay the debt. Lesson: Never exchange a solid asset for a debt payment unless you're sure that the debt is going to get paid. You're better off taking on your share of the debt while claiming your share of the assets.

- *There's a looming tax burden.* Future taxes are a big-money item that even divorce judges and lawyers often overlook and your spouse might "forget" to mention. So one spouse who thinks he or she did pretty well ends up getting a nasty surprise months or years after the divorce when a humongous tax bill falls right on his or her lap. Make sure you or your lawyer or your accountant considers the tax implications of any asset you're claiming or conceding. You don't want to get hit down the road with something like a capital-gains tax on the sale of property that you didn't even get to keep.

- *Your spouse is not moved by your generosity.* But she or he is more than happy to take advantage of it. This is one of the more heartbreaking mistakes divorced people make. One spouse, still carrying a torch, believes that by being nice and giving up more than necessary, the other spouse will be wooed back to give the marriage another go. It almost never works. You end up just as divorced, but worse off financially than you should be, and more bitter than you would have been. Being civil and cooperative is laudable. Letting yourself get taken advantage of isn't. ◁

Child Custody
3 Unexpected Suggestions for a Clearheaded Custody Arrangement That Benefits the Child

Don't listen to what your kids say they want. Yes, you read that right. It may seem counterintuitive to play down the children's expressed desires at a time when you're fighting for their best interests, but it's the big picture that matters. Many a child-custody arrangement turns unnecessarily complicated because one or both of the separating parents goes out of their way to accommodate little Brittany's Friday-night sleepovers or Jimmy Joe's absolutely nonnegotiable need to take his tae kwon do lessons from the same Mr. Mathers that he started with. But a year from now, Brittany may completely lose interest in those sleepovers, and Mr. Mathers may take a position with an accounting firm on the other side of the continent. Your kids are going to change, their schedules are going to change, and your own situations are going to change. That's true for parents and children in any family situation.

So don't spend time, money, and emotional energy bickering over scheduling details. Focus on the broad outlines of a custody arrangement that works for both parents and places the children where it's best for them to be. Your concern should be with nurturing the best family relationships possible under the new circumstances, not with which parent lives closest to the coolest video game store in town.

Think twice about keeping the house. Your lawyer will promise to fight tooth and nail for you to keep the family house, a prime spoil of the divorce wars. But the same lawyer who will lead you into battle also knows something else—down the road that dear, memory-filled house may be more of a burden than an asset.

So consider at the outset what your situation might be like. Here's a typical one: You're going to be a single mother. You won the house in your settlement, but your income is going to be less than what it was when the two of you brought home money. Still, the house payments, maintenance costs, and property taxes won't go down. You may, in short, be putting yourself into a situation where you're "house poor." Yes, the kids get to live in the house they've always known. But will their—and your—quality of life suffer as you scramble to pay for it?

Living below the standards of your own neighborhood is a tough position for a single parent to be in. And it's tough on the kids too. They know what's going on. They know their friends and neighbors have better toys, better clothes, and better cars. They know that each time they're invited on a ski trip, they probably can't go. They're aware that the family attends big barbecues at the neighbors' houses but such events are never held at their own house.

If it's realistic to keep the house, go for it. But if it's not, bite the bullet, take more cash instead, and start your new life in a financially comfortable situation. Your children will adjust, and they'll feel a lot better about it once you and they take that nice vacation you wouldn't have been able to afford otherwise.

Forget the win-at-all-costs approach. What you think is best for your child may not be worth fighting for.

SECRET WEAPON

Cell Phone

If you're like most parents, you probably cringe at the idea of your youngster carrying around a cell phone. But if you're sharing custody of that child with an ex, a cell phone can be a good tool for harmony and happiness. Here's why: Kids are usually fine with an arrangement that sends them back and forth between Mom's house and Dad's (as long as the parents are fine with it as well). But once they reach the tween-age years, starting about 10 or 11, their peer relationships suddenly become *very* important. Now the constant home-switching can become upsetting to them for the simple reason that their friends get confused about where they are. (If that sounds to you like a minor problem, it's because you're not 11.) A cell phone is the perfect solution. Your child will appreciate the easy contact with his friends, instead of starting to resent the unorthodox living arrangements with his parents.

What's more, the priority in custody negotiations should often be what's best for the parents, not the children. Yes, that's a shocking thing to say, which is why experienced family law professionals are reluctant to warn you. But consider: A sane parent will realize at some point that spending $50,000 in legal fees to come out of the divorce in possession of a $30,000 retirement plan makes no sense. He or she will give up that particular fight, and wisely so. But if the issue has to do with child custody—say, whether the seven-year-old will split time with his parents 50-50 on a weekly changeover or a monthly changeover—parents will spend their last dollar and sacrifice any remaining vestige of goodwill with the other spouse to get what they want.

"It's not unusual for a parent who can-not afford it to spend $100,000 arguing over a child custody issue," says divorce mediator Lee Borden. "In their mind, cost is no object in protecting their child from this ex who grows increas-ingly evil as the fight progresses. They lose contact with reality."

That's self-defeating. For one thing, that $100,000 can put your child through college. Also, the fight itself becomes the focus, rather than the child's welfare. You may be spending more energy on "winning" than on being a good parent. And perhaps most important, the fight is poisoning what's left of your relation-ship with your spouse. That relationship still matters. The two of you are going to be parents together as long as both of you live. That hasn't changed.

If you want what's best for your child, seek peace. That matters more than the actual custody arrangement. "Children don't seem to mind even a seemingly inconvenient arrangement as long as Mom and Dad aren't fighting," Borden says. "If Mom and Dad are fighting, I'm not sure any arrangement is going to be good for them." ◁

Wills and Living Wills
5 Things to Keep in Mind When You Prepare These Two End-of-Life Documents

Don't fear going to probate court. Television dramas and certain elements of the legal profession have given pro-bate—the court proceeding where a dead person's will is carried out—a repu-tation as an expensive, uncomfortable nightmare. That's a bad rap, says Michael Palermo, an estate planning lawyer in Lexington, Kentucky. "Probate is not that big a deal in most places," he says. "In some states, the process is so expedited you may not need a lawyer or even have to go to probate court."

So if it falls on you to handle things after a relative dies, consider going down to the county courthouse with-out paying for a lawyer and filling out some papers yourself to get the proce-dure started. The papers will have a name like "Petition for Probate of Will." Follow instructions, ask what you need to do next, and see if you think you can handle it. Many times you can, Palermo says.

You probably *will* need a lawyer if:

- The deceased lived in the "difficult" probate states of California or Florida.
- There's fighting going on among interested survivors.
- There's any kind of unusual complication.

Even then, Palermo advises, hire your lawyer by the hour. "Don't agree to pay a fixed percentage," he says. "That could cost you thousands of dollars for the handling of what are really some very simple tasks."

Read a will carefully before signing it. Yes, that may be the most ignored piece of advice ever given. After all, aren't we paying lawyers so we don't have to read 75 paragraphs of mumbo jumbo? But here's the reason it's especially important to go through your will before signing it: Although it's not the image law firms like to project, wills are put together from form documents. In other words, your last will and testament is essentially a re-tweaked version of somebody else's last will and testament. With all of that cutting and pasting going on, incorrect information can and does sneak into (or fall out of) the final printout. One lawyer tells of a will that was almost signed even though it had the wrong name throughout. So look it over and don't be shy about chirping up if you see a problem.

Explore what a will won't cover. It's convenient to think that a good will takes care of everything, but it doesn't. Though many a will-maker or heir isn't aware of it, a will only arranges for the transfer of assets that aren't already spoken for in some other way. In fact, a common estate-planning blunder is assuming that the will "trumps" previous arrangements. You can avoid a lot of spats and misunderstandings if you make an inventory of all the "out of probate" money or property you have—that is, assets that automatically go to somebody upon your death regardless of what the will says.

Example: You named Son #2 the beneficiary of your retirement plan when you first opened it, oh, so many years ago. That money still goes to Son #2 even if your will says Son #3 "gets everything." Or if you own your house together with your wife, the terms of your "joint tenancy" agreement probably stipulate that she retains full ownership of the house upon your death, even if you froze her out of the will. Along the same lines, your life insurance beneficiary gets the life insurance money no matter what. And most of the time, the fact that you divorced that beneficiary decades ago doesn't change things. Of course, you can always change beneficiaries and restructure your house ownership or joint checking accounts.

A good time to think of these things is when you're having your will drawn up. The point here, though, is that the will itself doesn't take care of "out of probate" assets. So it's a good idea to put together a document listing these assets,

---

SECRET WEAPON

Checklist

All those leather-bound case-law volumes and mahogany file cabinets lend a law office mystique, but chances are a simple checklist will get the job done when you go in for a will. Wills are usually fairly simple documents, and most are pretty much the same, so lawyers know that by asking a series of standard questions and filling in some blanks, they can draft one up quickly.

"When we go through the checklist, only about 1 in 10 clients needs nonstandard attention and only 1 in 100 needs real heavy estate planning," says one attorney. "For 9 out of 10 people, it's very common to check off a few boxes, give the results to a computer operator, and the will's ready in a day or two." Some offices will actually finish your will while you wait.

noting who gets what when you die, and keeping it with your will. You could be saving all your heirs from confusion, and some of them from disappointment.

Give broad guidelines in a living will. The common advice to "be as specific as possible" when putting together any legal document isn't necessarily the best way to go with a living will. If you try to leave detailed, maddeningly precise instructions on what to do in every possible medical situation when you're unconscious or otherwise incapacitated, you're going to leave some things out. Even with the very specific situations you address, it's impossible to be sure that the actual circumstances will turn out to be exactly what you had in mind. Doctors and family members will still have no idea what to do—as if you had no living will at all.

So instead of a precise list, consider the *Pirates of the Caribbean* approach—guidelines instead of rules. Communicate a broad set of thoughts and convictions about the kind of care you want in extreme circumstances, and under what general conditions (if any) you should be taken off life support. Designate a substitute decision maker—often referred to in legal terms as a "trustee" or, in much of Canada, an "attorney"—to carry out your desires if you're unable to do so. For example, if you leave instructions that in case of debilitating Alzheimer's disease, you want to be set up at the St. Mary's extended-care facility in Room 12B with roast beef for dinner on Tuesday nights, that would seem to outline a clear course of action. But what if putting you in that particular place turns out to be the third-best choice of facilities for your condition? More important, what if your finances by then strain under the expense? Better to instruct a decision maker to, say, "arrange for the most appropriate care without creating a significant drain on the family finances." (Your lawyer, of course, will help find the best language to express your thoughts.)

In other words, leave your decision maker with some discretion. That will make it more likely—not less—that your true wishes will be carried out.

Your spouse may not be the best living-will decision maker. No matter what anybody might assume, your spouse (or another very

How I Do It An Attorney Designates His Life-or-Death Decision Makers

Ontario lawyer Brian Babcock has arranged many a living will over the years, including his own. How did he choose his "attorney," or person who will make medical decisions for him if he's unconscious in an emergency or on life support? "I wouldn't trust my wife as a sole decision maker, because she's way too emotional," he says. "We were able to work things out so that I designated her along with a very close friend who is of a more sturdy, unemotional stock. So if she cannot or will not make the decision, I know he'll be practical about it." In fact, Babcock says, it's usually best to designate two decision makers, though one usually serves as an alternate rather than the co-equal in Babcock's case.

Another option: A committee of three, deciding things with a majority vote. This could work well for parents who have three children, for instance. "Deciding on a two-out-of-three basis sometimes makes good sense because there's less likely to be conflict that way," Babcock says. "And there's less likely to be regret."

emotionally close relative) is not necessarily the best person to carry out the instructions in your living will. Let's say you're a woman who's considering designating your husband as your decision maker because, after all, "he loves me the most." But the very fact that he loves you the most may make the decision making more difficult for him. The inevitably heightened emotions in a medical emergency or a pull-the-plug situation can obviously interfere with the one thing needed most at such a time—clear thinking. That's not to say that your spouse is ineligible to be your decision maker. Many spouses fill the role just fine. But there's nothing automatic about it. Choose the most qualified, responsible, loyal, and clear-headed person, whether you're married to this person or not.

And guess what? Your spouse may not even want the job. "Some view it as a burden they'd rather not have placed on them," says Brian Babcock of the large Canadian law firm Weiler, Maloney, Nelson in Thunder Bay, Ontario. "They know they're going to be too emotionally distraught to think rationally if the time comes, so they'd just as soon you selected another family member or a close friend." But under no circumstances should you try to spare your spouse's feelings by keeping secret your selection of another person to carry out the directive in your living will. The decision maker should consult with your spouse, after all. Also, not discussing your decision with your spouse can lay the groundwork for chaos at the worst possible time.

"We've had cases in which the spouse thinks they have the power and are giving instructions on the spot at the hospital, and then the true designated decision maker shows up with the directive," attorney Babcock says. "That causes a great deal of confusion with the medical staff." ◄

Love and Marriage

4 Easy Ways to Make Romance and Attachment Last

Shop for the right spouse. Did you know that there's actually a formula that predicts whether a marriage will succeed? Beatty Cohan, a psychotherapist in Sarasota, Florida, and coauthor of *For Better, for Worse, Forever: Discover the Path to Lasting Love*, offers these predictors for a successful marriage:

- *Look to the parents.* Check out your beloved's family background, particularly the parents' relationship, to get a good idea of the behavior he's been exposed to. What we learned as kids we often play out as adults.

- *Turn investigator.* Are there signs of alcoholism or other forms of addiction in the family? Be careful—there's often a genetic link. Also watch for a family history of depression or excessive anxiety.

- *Listen carefully.* Identify how your potential partner communicates. Also pay attention to how he or she handles sticky situations and painful emotions.

- *Is there compromise?* If you're forever giving in, then you've got a problem. Compromise is one of the key elements of a healthy relationship.

- *Is there true intimacy?* We're not talking sex here, but the kind of intimacy that comes when he can clean up the vomit when you have the flu; when she invites your mother for Christmas even though she can't stand the woman; when he has a hot bath and glass of wine waiting for you after what he knows was a difficult day.

Don't just tell her you love her—show her. Karen Sherman, Ph.D., author of *Marriage Magic! Find It, Keep It, Make It Last*, offers these hints on little ways you can show your mate how much you love him or her:

- Surprise your partner with her favorite dessert.
- While he's showering, draw a heart or a sexy note in the steamed-up glass.
- Give him a foot or back massage—without him having to ask for it.
- Leave a sexy voice mail, saying, "I'm thinking about you" in a low voice.
- Tuck a sexy note into his briefcase or text it to her cell phone.

Light the Sabbath candles together. Not Jewish? No problem. A study conducted by researchers at Syracuse University finds that couples who participate in and value religious rituals, particularly holiday rituals, seem to have stronger marriages.

Take some "alone time" away from the kids. One of the toughest times in a marriage is when you have young children. Finding alone time (okay, time for whoopee) takes creativity. So how about these creative tips culled from young parents we know?

- *Keep 'em occupied.* If the kids are old enough to play alone in the fenced backyard, throw 99 pennies out there and tell them whoever finds 100 pennies first wins a prize.
- *Invest in hardware.* That would be a lock. For your bedroom door.
- *Set the alarm.* Wake up at 3 a.m., make love, go back to sleep.
- *Hire a babysitter.* Only this babysitter takes the kids *out* of the house while you and your partner steal some much-needed alone time.
- *Take advantage of naptime.* Who says you have to do the laundry while your two-year-old naps? ◁

WHAT YOUR MARRIAGE COUNSELOR DOESN'T WANT YOU TO KNOW ABOUT Compatibility

If you knew these things, you wouldn't need a marriage counselor, would you? This insider info comes from psychologist Karen Sherman and from psychotherapist Wendy Allen, Ph.D., author of *How to Survive the Crisis of an Affair*.

- ☐ Sixty-nine percent of all arguments between you and your partner will never be resolved. So don't try so hard.
- ☐ A couple that doesn't fight is in trouble.

- ☐ Having a "good enough" marriage is the most couples can expect and is actually quite an accomplishment.
- ☐ Letting go is sometimes better than discussing everything to death.
- ☐ Respect, not sex or money, is the most important factor in a happy marriage.
- ☐ There are marital breaches worse than an affair.

- ☐ A therapist cannot teach, train, or guide you to "be happy." That is not a reasonable outcome to expect from therapy.

In short, there's no way you're going to be compatible all the time.

Kids and Teens
12 Keys to Raising Healthy, Responsible Children

Get the TV out of the bedroom. Studies find that kids who have televisions in their bedrooms are more likely to be overweight. But here are other crucial reasons for ditching the tube: When a TV is in a child's bedroom, you have no control over what he's watching, nor do you have any opportunities for family bonding time—when everyone piles onto the couch to watch a favorite show.

Get them used to doing chores from a young age. We know one parent who still makes her high school daughter's lunch every day. Don't find yourself in this situation! By the time your two-year-old begins talking, he's old enough to start helping around the house. Here are some age-appropriate

chores to give your kids to teach them responsibility, and how a household is run:

- *Two to four years old.* Ask them to put toys away, help to set the table, and put dirty laundry in the laundry basket.

- *Five to seven years old.* They should begin emptying the dishwasher (at least putting the silverware away), setting and clearing the table, emptying trash baskets, and doing light yard work with your guidance (like pulling weeds).

- *Eight to ten years old.* Kids should be changing sheets, dusting, vacuuming, putting away laundry, and bringing groceries into the house.

- *Eleven and up.* They're ready for almost any tasks that you can throw at them. This might include cleaning bathrooms, mopping floors, washing and folding laundry, putting away groceries, and simple meal preparation.

Teach them how checking accounts work. If you really want to teach your teen about money, then stop handing over the credit card and the "allowance." Instead, put your kid on a budget, open a checking account for him or her, and let your teen *really* learn to manage money. Tell your kid that all clothing, movies, entertainment, fast food, and cell phone bills come out of his or her checking account (which you fund). If your son or daughter has a job, then cut

How I Do It A Parenting Expert Gets a Child to Behave at a Restaurant

You *can* eat out in a sit-down restaurant with children. Just follow these tips from Stacy DeBroff:

☐ Pick the right restaurant. Chain restaurants are great because they're used to serving families and they're trained to turn over tables fast, meaning you'll get your order in and get fed in a hurry.

☐ Get a booth. It provides the all-important buffer zone between your family and the rest of the restaurant.

☐ Reward kids for good behavior. To get your kids to behave during the meal, tell them you'll take them out for ice cream afterward. Don't offer dessert *at* the restaurant—it just adds to the sitting time.

☐ Bring a "restaurant kit." This would be a bag filled with crayons and paper, small puzzles, Legos (depending on age of child), even a Game Boy or other handheld electronic game (hey, whatever works!).

---

back the amount you're funding by the amount they're making. Just make sure you also set up a savings account for your teen and insist that at least one-third of any savings or money from you be socked away.

Don't interfere with sibling scuffles. Stay out of fights between siblings unless bloodshed is imminent, recommends Stacy M. DeBroff, author of *The Mom Book,* a compilation of tips for moms from moms. She notes that fighting actually teaches siblings valuable skills such as assertion, managing anger, and compromise. If ignoring a fight doesn't work, send them to separate rooms until they cool off.

Limit choices. An inexperienced parent will ask a four-year-old, "What do you want to wear today?" Uh-oh. Offering such an open-ended choice just ensures you'll wind up with a little girl wearing black tights, a pink tutu,

and a sequined top that reads "I'm Hot." Instead, pull out two outfits and ask which she wants to wear. The same goes with food. "Hamburger or spaghetti?" replaces "What would you like for dinner?"

Talk about sex. Get over your embarrassment and let your teen know that he can talk to you about sex without fear of lectures or retribution. The reality is that 85 percent of North American teens have had sex by the age of 19. Open discussions at least ensure that the sex they're having is safe, and may even convince your teen to hold off a while longer.

Monitor your teen's driving speed. If your teenager has a lead-footed tendency, step in and address it. A University of Florida study found that teenagers who break the speed limit are more likely to gamble, use drugs, and drink alcohol than those who don't.

Think of speeding as an early warning sign of worse to come.

Get your teen in the spirit to worship. Encourage your son or daughter to get involved in some sort of religious or spiritual organization. Why? Researchers who tracked 1,182 adolescents from 7th through 10th grade found those who thought religion was important were much less likely to smoke, drink, and use marijuana.

SECRET WEAPON

Dinner

Forget all that psychological baloney about what makes for a healthy child—a box of Hamburger Helper can be your best tool. Studies find that simply sharing a meal as a family helps groom kids who do better at school, have better relationships with their friends, and are less likely to do drugs or become depressed.

Moms, get closer. If you think you're not necessary now that your kid is driving, think again. A large government study finds that the closer Mom is to her teenager, the less likely teens are to start having sex. Some ideas: Set a weekly date for breakfast, lunch, or dinner. Have a mother-kid weekend away a couple of times a year. Start an activity that you can do with your teen, such as tennis, jogging, or even performing together in the local theater. Begin a marathon gin rummy game that goes on until one of you hits 100,000 points (or goes to college). And in the midst of all of this, say the researchers who conducted the study, slip in a few comments about the importance of education—it also helps.

Ban tattoos. So you gave in to the double ear piercing, but when it comes to tattoos for your adolescent, just say no. When researchers studied more than 6,000 junior and high school students, they found those with tattoos and body piercings were more likely to smoke cigarettes or marijuana, go on drinking binges, have premarital sex, get into serious fights, join gangs, skip school, and get poor grades. If your kid is asking for a tattoo, take it as a canary-in-the-mine kind of warning and sit down for a heart-to-heart.

Set your expectations high. Just because you drank and smoked pot in high school, don't think it's reasonable for your kid to follow suit. If you vocalize the expectation that *your* child will *not* drink or do drugs when in high school—and make that expectation known to your teen—you reduce the risk that your child will engage in such behavior.

Visualize the future with your kids. It's never too early to begin talking to your child about his or her future. By age 10, kids are old enough to start looking ahead and figure out the value of an education (for instance, "I go to school so I can go to college so I can get a good job so I can afford that vacation in Aruba"). Why bother? Because studies find that teens who can visualize themselves with a future are less likely to do those things that destroy a future, such as engaging in sex, drinking, drugs, and crime. ◂

7 TIPS ON RAISING
financially savvy
Kids

We've all heard horror stories about kids who go off to college with shiny new credit cards and run up mountains of debt over the first several months. That won't happen to your kids, thanks to these tips from Syble Solomon, the creator of Money Habitudes, a deck of cards used by educators and counselors to identify financial issues in relationships:

1 **Show them money going in, not just out.** If your kids only see you withdrawing those $20 bills from the ATM, they're going to think machines hand out money. Make sure they also see you depositing funds.

2 **Teach them to set goals and save for them.** Label a jar with a set amount of money to be used for something specific. Start small—say, $5 to buy some ice cream and sprinkles. Collect $5 worth of change in the jar and count it out before buying the treat. Keep this money separate when you go to the store, so your child can buy the ice cream himself with the cash.

3 **Differentiate between wanting and needing.** You *need* shoes, but you *want* the trendiest brand. You *need* food, but you *want* to eat out. Apply this rule to anything you buy and to any of their requests for "stuff."

4 **Make choices, not sacrifices.** Instead of saying, "We can't afford that," "That's too expensive," or just saying no, substitute a comment that expresses an intentional choice. Examples: "I want to stay home and visit state parks this year so we can save for a special vacation next year." "I choose to bring my coffee [or water, or soda] with me and not buy it at the convenience store so I can save that money for more important things." Instead of feeling that "no" means sacrifice, scarcity, or embarrassment, children learn that life is about making choices.

5 **Show them you're planning for the future.** In addition to using a change jar to save for special treats, let your kids hear you talk about saving for a new roof, paying off the car, putting money aside to celebrate a birthday, saving for their education, and paying bills on time.

6 **Give to others.** Along with that jar for ice cream, label another jar for charity. Make sure your children put a fixed percentage of their earnings and allowance in it. And make sure they see you giving to others, whether it's tithing to the church, writing a check to a nonprofit, or volunteering for a charitable cause.

7 **Turn off the shopping channel.** Keep TV time to a minimum to avoid the "buy me" ads that dominate. Also point out the marketing tricks that advertisers use, and make sure your kids understand how they try to sell.

Parents and Siblings
5 Secrets to Getting Along Well with Your Relatives

Involve your dad in your life. As we get older, most of our dads tend to blend more and more into the wallpaper. Instead of leaving him to molt into the easy chair while you and your mom chatter like 13-year-olds, find ways to involve him, says Tina B. Tessina, Ph.D., a licensed California psychotherapist and author of *It Ends with You: Grow Up and Out of Dysfunction*. For instance, ask him to flex his handyman muscles by fixing that loose shelf, or ask if he'll give you an opinion on that weird noise in your car.

Digitize, then share the memories. Forget photo albums. Today's memories have gone high-tech, with DVDs and home movies produced on your home computer. So get out your camcorder and start filming, particularly those older relatives who may not be with you much longer. When they do pass on, make copies and send one to each family member.

Make the trust a living one. Probate lawyers won't like that we shared this tip from Kraig Kast, CEO of Atherton Trust in Redwood Shores, California: You need to set up a living trust *now*. Having a living trust ensures that when you die, your financial wishes are immediately carried out without the cost or delay

---

WHAT YOUR PSYCHOTHERAPIST DOESN'T WANT YOU TO KNOW ABOUT Family Stress

You can deal with stressful family situations without seeing a shrink. How do you show grace under pressure? California psychotherapist Tina B. Tessina offers these insider's techniques:

☐ **Put it in perspective.** Will what they're saying or doing be important in an hour or two? A day from now? Most won't.

☐ **Rise above it.** Next time you are totally fed up with your mother, remind yourself of all of the tough times she has experienced.

☐ **Cut yourself a break.** If your mother upsets you by bringing up that failed first marriage again, don't beat yourself up for getting tense about it. Your reaction is normal. It's what you do about it that counts.

☐ **Take a time-out.** If you can't send your uncle Richie to time-out when he's had one vodka martini too many, at least you can send yourself there. Take a walk or go shopping.

☐ **Keep your mouth shut.** One of the most powerful tools you have is silence. Use it!

☐ **Pretend they don't belong to you.** If your in-laws are obnoxious, pretend they're your friend's parents. You wouldn't snap and say something you'd regret to your friend's parents, would you?

associated with probating a will or intestate (no will) estate.

Practice saying no to relatives.
Always find yourself saying yes when your sister asks for money? Then practice ten ways to say no in front of the mirror before you see her. Here's a couple to get you started: "No, I can't. All my money is tied up in retirement accounts and I can't take it out without paying a penalty"; "No, sorry, but I'm going back to school to get my master's and I need every cent"; "I'd really like to, but our water heater just burst and we have to recarpet the basement."

Learn your family's health history.
We know, we know, you don't want to hear another single word about your dad's chest pains, your mom's high cholesterol numbers, or your brother's arthritic knee. But there are good reasons to listen to them besides being a good offspring or sibling and lending a sympathetic ear. As a matter of fact, it's not a bad idea to pursue information on the health of all your extended family members even further by asking about chronic conditions that affected your grandparents, aunts and uncles, and even nieces, nephews, and cousins. Compiling a family medical history will give you and your kin insight into the various diseases and conditions that are common in your family. It can be helpful to doctors in diagnosing a medical condition, determining what medical tests to run and preventive measures to take, and calculating the risk you, your children, and other relatives have of certain diseases. Among the major diseases that the Mayo Clinic recommends that you ask about are heart disease, stroke, cancer, depression, diabetes, Alzheimer's, obesity, blindness, and deafness. Find out the age

the conditions were diagnosed and if they were treated successfully. Allergies, asthma, migraines, and frequent colds are other conditions that families may share as well as problems with infertility, miscarriages, birth defects, and learning disabilities. ◄

Dos and Don'ts on Fitting In with His (or Her) Family

So you just got married and you've got a whole second family. Here's how to survive the transition and thrive long-term, courtesy of psychotherapist Tina B. Tessina:

DO	understand how your spouse relates to his or her parents.
DON'T	assume that family relationship will resemble the one in your family.
DO	take the time to get to know your in-laws—if you're separated by distance, write or e-mail each other.
DON'T	take offense easily—you may just not understand the family dynamic.
DO	check with your partner about family customs. Will his mother expect a hostess gift? A thank-you note? What do they like to eat? What's their sense of humor like? Can you talk about politics or religion in front of them?
DON'T	criticize your partner's family. Rather, ask for explanations of things you don't understand.
DO	be polite and friendly—use your most charming ways around your in-laws.
DON'T	assume they understand how you feel—they may not have a clue. Along those lines, don't take their comments and reactions personally. You may not understand them as they were meant.
DO	think about what will work best for you and your partner before you try to please your partner's family.
DON'T	ignore your partner while you're with your family. You can talk to your sister, but make sure you check in with each other frequently.
DON'T	hesitate to ask your spouse how it went when it's over. A "debriefing" can help both of you.
DO	consider doing something that's time-limited and easier. If you go to dinner in a restaurant, everyone might be a bit better behaved.

Family Pets

7 Hints for Keeping Your Four-Legged Family Members Happy and Healthy

Vacation with your pets. This tip isn't going to make the local kennel happy, but Spot and Fifi don't have to be boarded while you go on vacation. Plan ahead and find one of the many pet-friendly hotels that have sprung up, suggests Dr. Kim Langholz, a community practice veterinarian at Iowa State University in Ames. Just think through the details, she says. And plan early, since it could take six to eight months to get all your paperwork in order before traveling to some locations abroad. Other things to consider:

- What, if any, health papers do you need for your pet, including vaccinations? Take your pet in for an annual checkup and ask the veterinarian which shots need to be updated.

- If you're traveling by plane, where will the airline put your pet? Can you carry him in the passenger

cabin, in a carrier, or must he travel in cargo? If it's the latter, make sure the cargo area is pressurized; while typical on larger planes, it's not always available on smaller commuter flights.

- Make sure the contact information on your pet's ID tags is current, including your cell phone number.

- If you haven't already, have a microchip implanted in your dog or cat. If she runs off while you're away and someone finds her, the microchip contains information that will get her back into your arms.

- Check the legal requirements at your destination. Some municipalities won't allow pit bulls or ferrets, for instance.

Pack for your pooches and kitties. If you're taking Fido to your mother's for Christmas, make sure you take all the necessary accoutrements, says Langholz, including:

- A health certificate, along with information about vaccines, medications, and your vet's telephone number. In fact, why not just ask your vet for a copy of the past two years of your pet's medical records?

- Enough medication for the entire trip. Make sure this is in your carry-on bag.

- Your pet's regular food, unless you're sure you can find it at your destination. Switching food abruptly could give your pet diarrhea—not exactly the best way to endear yourself to Aunt Mabel.

How I Do It   A Vet's Guide to Brushing a Cat's Teeth

Given a study that found cats with oral disease are five times more likely to test positive for feline leukemia and feline immunodeficiency virus (FIV), tooth brushing is no joke. Here's how James Richards, D.V.M., head of Cornell University's Feline Health Center, recommends you do it.

☐ Ideally, start with a kitten or very young cat. The "old dogs/new tricks" adage is just as true of kitties.

☐ Help your cat feel comfortable with having her mouth touched by gently placing your finger in her mouth or on her teeth when she's on your lap or while you're petting her.

☐ Try putting your cat's favorite foods (such as water from a can of tuna) on the toothbrush and letting her get used to it before attempting to brush.

☐ Always offer a special treat after tooth brushing, one that isn't available at any other time.

- Pet favorites, including toys, bedding, and kitty litter. Some people even take along tap water from home!

- A first-aid kit for your pet, available in most pet stores.

Distract them for nail clipping with peanut butter. Nobody enjoys clipping a pet's toenails, but it's a must if you want to save your floors, clothes, and furniture. Kayce O'Brien, a project manager at Johnson & Wales University in Denver, found a way that works for Finnegan, her two-year-old Lab-retriever mix. She smears natural peanut butter on the lower part of her refrigerator (stay away from chunky), and as Finnegan licks away at the luscious treat, she quickly lifts his paws and clips away. This also works, she says, for ear cleaning and fur brushing.

Show your cat who's boss. To do that, you need to do some serious training to make sure your cat doesn't destroy your house. Amy Osete, vice president of marketing for pet products manufacturer Bamboo, suggests the following:

- Get a scratching post covered with sisal rope, corrugated cardboard, or carpet turned wrong side out (if you have the same stuff on both the scratching post and the floor, your cat may think scratching on the floor carpet is okay).

- Spread a paste of cayenne pepper mixed with water or dried orange or lemon peel with water on electrical cords to keep kitty from chewing them.

- Temporarily cover counters and furniture with double-sided tape so that kitty learns not to jump up or curl up on them.

Let someone else handle the mess. Tired of arguing over whose turn it is to scoop up the backyard poop? Just hire it out. Today even the smallest town has at least one poop-scooper for hire.

Give your cat a sense of the outdoors. Even though Buttercup is an indoor cat, she can still get a taste of the outdoor life. What about giving her free rein on the screened porch? Or you could purchase a large dog crate and pad it with soft pillows for sunny afternoons in the backyard. And, of course, you can always put her on a leash. If you want to try walking your cat (and yes, many people do), Belinda Mager, spokesperson for the Humane Society of the United States, recommends the following:

- Use a harness, not a collar.
- Begin the training in the house, when she's hungry. Why the hunger? You'll be using treats as an incentive.
- Start by putting her on the leash for one minute, then increase the time during each training session.
- Once she's comfortable on the leash in the house, it's time to venture outside.
- Stay in the yard and don't go far. This also reduces the risk that you'll run into dogs and other animals.

You can have a pet if you are allergic. Don't instantly blame your pet for all your bouts of sneezing and watery eyes. Sure, you may have a reaction when you are around the cat, but many if not most allergy sufferers are sensitive to more than one allergen. If you react to animal dander, chances are good that you are also sensitive to other common allergens such as dust, cigarette smoke, and pollen or any combination of them. And the effects of these allergens are cumulative. So before you go bundling the family pet off to a shelter, try lowering the overall allergen level in your house. Basically this means controlling dust by cleaning thoroughly and frequently, keeping out pollen by closing windows and running the air conditioning during peak seasons, and by banning smoking inside the house. Consult with your doctor about allergy shots, antihistamines, and other treatments that may reduce your reaction to dander and other allergens.

To specifically reduce allergy symptoms from a pet—provided they are "simply miserable but not life-threatening"—here are some suggestions from the Humane Society of the United States that may let you keep that furry creature that has won your heart:

- Make your bedroom an allergy-free retreat that the animal is never allowed to go into. Install a high-efficiency HEPA air cleaner. Put impermeable covers on mattresses and pillows to keep them from picking up dander brought in on clothes.
- Use HEPA air cleaners throughout the house and cut back on dander-collecting fabric furnishings such as curtains and carpets.
- Vacuum frequently using a HEPA-filter machine or a microfilter bag. Launder slipcovers, pillow covers, and pet bedding regularly.
- Bathe your pet weekly. It's more effective than any dander-control spray. Even cats can be trained to tolerate bathing.
- Some but by no means all allergy sufferers are less irritated by animals with constantly growing hair, such as poodles and bichon frises, so you might want to consider one for your next pet. ◁

OWNING A PET
turtle
or Tortoise

Okay, maybe it's not everyone's choice for the ideal pet. However, turtles don't bark, scratch, or pee on your Persian rug. Here's what you need to know about owning one, says Susan M. Tellem, a representative for American Tortoise Rescue:

Water Turtles (Red-Eared Sliders or Cooters)

What to buy   Choose a healthy turtle at least four inches in length. Any smaller and the person selling it to you is breaking the law.

What to look for   Clear eyes and energy. A runny nose or swollen eyes means you're getting a sick turtle, one likely to carry salmonella.

Where they live   In a pond. Tanks are cruel for these creatures used to traveling from pond to pond in the wild. They need a safe area, protected from predators like raccoons and dogs. Electric fencing is a good option, or a screened cover over the pond.

What to feed them   They're carnivores, so live food like feeder fish as well as prepared turtle food is the way to go.

Where they go   These turtles hibernate underwater all winter and need protection from predators during this time.

Tortoises and Land Turtles

Where to buy them   Not at the pet store—these typically come from the wild. There are lots of rescue chapters around the country that can help you find the right tortoise.

What kind to buy   One that meshes with your household. Smaller ones include Russians or box turtles. Both hibernate and like cooler weather. Larger ones include desert, leopard, or sulcata tortoises. They're vegetarians. If you get a desert tortoise, and live in the U.S., many states require a permit, because they're endangered. For that reason, they're not allowed on the East Coast. Also know that sulcatas can grow to 200 pounds, so you'll need at least a fenced half-acre.

What to feed them   Box turtles are carnivores. Snails and worms work, along with some greenery. The larger tortoises are vegetarian.

Dating and Relationships
5 Ways to Better Your Luck in Love

Online, leave some things to the imagination. If you are dating on the Internet, don't put anything on your site that you wouldn't want up in a PowerPoint presentation given to your coworkers. That's because, office etiquette experts say, that is essentially what you are doing when you post information on a dating site. Your boss doesn't need to know that midnight skinny-dipping is your favorite pastime. Plus, work aside, dating experts say that the people who have the most success with online dating are the ones who use some discretion.

Embrace chivalry on a first date. No matter who asked whom out on that first date, etiquette experts say a man should *always* foot the bill (for same-sex couples, the asker buys). Here's a trick: If you are a woman on a first date and the guy doesn't reach for the check, take a trip to the powder room. If he doesn't pay while you're gone, offer to split the check. If he allows that, find yourself another knight.

Tread carefully with office romance. Twenty percent of us meet our mates at work, says Robin Bond, a workplace etiquette expert and employment attorney in Wayne, Pennsylvania. Because there's nothing other than *American Idol* to talk about at the water cooler, the news about your office romance will spread like wildfire, and the relationship could be quickly construed as inappropriate. To handle an office romance professionally, keep the following rules in mind:

- Most important: *Do not* speak to anyone in Human Resources about the romance. "Despite what the company might tell you about HR being your friend, they are not—do not trust anyone in HR," says Bond.

- Make sure you like the coworker enough to take a risk. If it is just a fling and the person has no potential as the love of your life, end it.

- Assess how much you like the person by hanging out with him or her at group lunches or happy hours.

- Be certain the person likes you back. People are quick to cry sexual harassment these days, so be sure your advances are wanted, Bond says.

Set the mood with food. If you are preparing a romantic meal for the one you love (or really like), certain foods can make the evening more pleasurable for both of you … without your date suspecting a thing.

- *A game animal.* According to historical theory, if you eat a wild animal, you take on some of its wildness. Given that your beloved is not a vegetarian, of course, make something like a wild game hen or roasted duck.

- *Oysters.* Used in ancient times in lieu of Viagra, oysters contain zinc, which is stored in the prostate and is thought to prolong sexual pleasure in men. Enough said.

- *Wine.* This one is a no-brainer when it comes to romance. But keep Shakespeare's words of moderation in mind: "Liquor provoketh the desire but taketh away the performance."

- *Chocolate.* This popular food contains a chemical called phenylethylamine, a compound that the body naturally produces when a person is in love. Your date may instantly feel more amorous toward you after a bite (or a bar).

In love with your friend's ex? Be careful. Most etiquette experts agree that a friend's former boyfriend, husband, girlfriend, or wife is totally off-limits. If you truly feel this ex is your soul mate, there are a few things you can try that may still salvage your friendship. For one, out of respect for the failed relationship and both parties who were in it, wait an appropriate amount of time before you dive in (the rule of thumb for relationship mourning is three months for every year the couple was together up to a maximum of a year or so). Second, if you ask your friend—asking is imperative—and he or she gives you the go-ahead, you are closer to the green light. If your friend was the one who did the breaking up, you are even closer. If your friend is now happily recoupled, you are as good as home free. ◁

SECRET WEAPON

A Bright Tie

At social gatherings where you are likely to meet potential dating partners, wear some distinctive article of clothing or jewelry. It not only makes you stand out from the crowd, but also offers anyone interested in you an excuse to start a conversation. For a man it might be a bright red or unusually patterned tie, while a woman might try distinctive earrings, a necklace, or an embroidered vest or belt.

Parties and Entertaining
7 Ways to Be the Perfect Host (and Guest)

Dress your event up by serving mixed drinks. Most people think that wine is cheaper than liquor. The truth is, serving mixed drinks instead of wine will actually *save* you money on your booze tab. "A bottle of wine yields only five glasses, which will serve only three to five guests at best," says Denise Vivaldo, author of *Do It for Less! Parties*. At an average cost of $15 a bottle, a fairly decent wine adds up if you're having a lot of people over.

Here are a few less expensive (and perhaps more festive) options: For easy, frothy daiquiris, mix a liter of rum with frozen limeade; for a new twist on the classic Cape Codder, combine sparkling cranberry juice with a liter of vodka. (Use one part liquor to three parts juice for both cocktails.) You will get about 30 cocktails out of a liter of liquor, which costs roughly the same as a bottle of wine.

If you don't want to spend the night with a cocktail shaker in your hand, opt for a champagne punch so that guests can serve themselves. A punch made of inexpensive sparkling wine, fruit juice, and soda is cheap, easy, and a real crowd pleaser. Here's how you do it: In a punch bowl, combine a bottle of sparkling wine or champagne with a 12-ounce (355-ml) can of frozen juice and two 12-ounce (355-ml) cans of a light-colored soda such as ginger ale or Sprite. Stir and serve!

Not a drinker? Fake it. Here's the scenario: You don't drink, but you're at a party and you're being pressured to booze it up. Why not ask the bartender for a virgin drink that looks alcoholic?

You can order a soda and ask the bartender to put some fruit and a stirrer in it. If someone asks, just say it's a gin and tonic if you are drinking Sprite, or get a Coke and say that it has rum or whiskey in it. If you are at a barbecue and people are drinking beer out of bottles or cans, dump the beer out in the bathroom and fill it with water. Not comfortable with the drinking façade? It's perfectly acceptable to be firm about refusing liquor.

Rent the dishes yourself. If you're hosting a catered party, ask the catering company to itemize all charges. When you get the figure you'll be charged for such accessories as dishware, silverware, and tablecloths, use it to do some comparison shopping. Chances are, the caterer is renting these accoutrements himself and is just marking up the rental fees. Call several party suppliers in the phone book to see if you can beat the figure your caterer is charging you. The caterer may stamp his feet, but you're in charge.

Keep your pipes clean. Nothing will kill the mood of a great party faster than a backed-up toilet. It's one of those aspects of party planning that no one really talks about, but it should not be overlooked. If you're hosting a sizeable event at your home, prepare for a potential septic challenge by having all toilets that partygoers will use professionally snaked right before the event. It's better to spend $40 ahead of time than risk the embarrassment and expense of an emergency call to the plumber in the middle of your party.

How I Do It An Etiquette Expert Hosts a Fun, Sophisticated Evening

An inventive host will go the extra mile to inject some fun into a party to help people mingle and have a fabulous time, says Liz Scofield, an etiquette instructor at Lehigh University.

"One year, my husband and I gave people secret tasks they had to accomplish throughout the evening," she confesses. "For instance, one person had the task of finding out how old I was. Another guest had the task of making someone tell a dirty joke. And to accomplish their tasks, guests couldn't flat-out ask someone her age or to tell a dirty joke—they had to somehow convince the other person that it was the perfect time for a dirty joke or for an age revelation.

"It was on a sophisticated yet lighthearted level, and it was absolutely wonderful. People were on their toes and on the alert for the tasks. We had prizes at the end of the night for people who completed their tasks—it was a magnificent success. I think communication games like this can really make people interact and have a great time at a party."

Play musical plates. Worried that your party guests will clean out your buffet? Use smaller, 9-inch (23-cm) plates instead of the standard 12-inch (30-cm) size. By shrinking the size of the plates, you will trick your guests into thinking that they're putting more food away than they are. On the flip side, if your dinner is winding down and you don't want leftovers, switch over to larger, 12- or 14-inch (30- or 36-cm) plates and hope that your guests pile them high!

Celebrate diversity at your party. Here's a tip that will not only make you look like a hero for celebrating everyone's cultural background, it will save you from having to make all the food yourself: "To make everyone feel included, request that each person bring a menu item that is representative of his or her religion or cultural background," says Liz Ngonzi, president of Amazing Taste, an event-planning firm in South Orange, New Jersey. For an added bonus, ask them to send you the recipe in advance so you can create a multicultural holiday cookbook for your guests.

Make just one outstanding dish. When you are trying to be the perfect host or hostess, there is a natural tendency to overdo it, to try too hard. And when it comes to a formal sit-down dinner or even a buffet, you want every course or dish to be extra special and perfect. In the process, you can not only bust your budget but also drive yourself into a frenzy. Well, the solution is simple: Make one dish the star of the meal and spend your extra effort and money on that one course. As a matter of fact, if the other parts of the meal are straightforward and simple—but made with fresh, tasty ingredients—they will set off the prize dish rather than compete with it, letting it shine like a diva with a fine but unobtrusive supporting cast. And you'll garner more compliments. ◂

Tying the Knot
7 Special Tips from Seasoned Wedding Coordinators

Hire a wedding coordinator to save you time and money. Most brides think that hiring a wedding coordinator will break their budget. It's a little-known fact that wedding coordinators can actually *save* you money after you get all the discounts and perks they have arranged with partner vendors, says Sharon Naylor, who has written 30 wedding books including *1000 Best Secrets for Your Perfect Wedding*. But use caution when selecting a planner: Anyone can call herself a "wedding planner." Look for someone who is certified by organizations such as the American Academy of Wedding Professionals or the Association of Bridal Consultants (www.bridalassn.com) who have consultants throughout North America.

Read the fine print on your contract. Caterers bank on the fact that most clients won't read their contracts carefully. Read yours, and then read it

SECRET WEAPON

Credit Card

Even if you have a million dollars in the bank, experts will tell you to pay for everything related to your wedding and reception with a credit card. This will protect you should anything go wrong with your vendors. If the first-rate photographer you booked gets hit by a bus the day before the wedding and you put the deposit on a credit card, your money will be refunded. If you had paid with cash, your money would have gone down with the photographer. Your credit card is like a free wedding insurance policy in your wallet, so use it.

again, because they often charge you for things that you don't know you're being charged for: They might have a minimum number of guests they'll serve (i.e., you will be charged for 100 people even if only 75 show up), a per-slice cake-cutting fee, or overtime for waitstaff who stay late (whether you ask them to or not). These fees are often not added until the final invoice, so make sure you get a breakdown of all extra costs before the big day.

Skip the custom-printed invitations. Here's a secret: Most people couldn't care less about other couples' wedding invitations. Your guests will probably never even notice the scalloped edges and silver ink that cost you an extra $2 per print. Therefore, they probably also won't know if you've made your invitations yourselves. Instead of ordering them custom made, use invitation software such as www.mountaincow.com's Printing Press—your whole set of invites will only cost about $40. Although they are the enemy of wedding invitation designers, invitation software packages offer modern fonts and graphics, and they are easy to use.

Book a budding musical talent. If you have always dreamed of having a live string quartet at your wedding but can't afford their fees, hire music students. Your guests don't have to know that the musicians are still perfecting their talents. A local performing arts school, university, or music school will be able to recommend some students; you may also find performers' contact information on bulletin boards at music stores. To avoid disaster, hold a brief audition for your musicians before you hire them, or ask for permission to observe them at another gig.

Focus your flowers. This nugget comes straight from a former florist: "The cost of flowers is minimal—it's the labor it takes to arrange them that costs so much," says Deb McCoy, president of the American Academy of Wedding Professionals. "To save money on flowers, put your money into your bridal party flowers and go with nonfloral table centerpieces at your reception." The flowers in the bride's bouquet and on your mom, dad, bridesmaids, and other relatives are the flowers that will forever be in your photos, so that's where you want to invest. Rather than having floral centerpieces, McCoy suggests something you can make yourself: "Put beautiful, tall candles on the tables and surround them with glass pebbles, or float votive candles in water." You will save a ton of money.

Cut to the cake. Plan to cut your cake and toss your bouquet early in the night. Your wedding guests will never know you've done this to let your photographer and videographer leave early, and it will cut down on the per-hour costs. Plus, after the professional photographers leave, your guests will be more likely to start snapping pictures with the inexpensive, throwaway cameras on their tables (if you provide them).

Don't hire a hat-switching photographer. No matter how fabulous your friend is at shooting photos for CNN, and no matter how hard he tries to convince you that he can transfer that skill to your wedding for decent price, *do not* hire him to save a few bucks on your wedding photos. "Shooting news photography and wedding photography are two totally different skills," McCoy says. "A wedding is a scripted event, and if you go with someone who isn't a seasoned wedding photographer, I guarantee he or she will miss 50 percent of the high points." Think about it this way: Would you rather have 20 beautiful photos of the happiest day of your life or 200 blurry ones?

"Photography is the one thing you can't put a price on—I call it the bite-the-bullet component of a wedding," McCoy says. "Most of the complaints I get from people are about the photography, and the reason I get these complaints is that they shopped quantity instead of quality." Talented wedding photographers are hard to come by, so you are probably going to have to spend a little more than you planned to get a good one. ◁

Caterer Confidential
6 Classy Ways to Serve a Crowd for Less

Check out your caterer at an event. You've found a catering service that you like, and you are ready to go with it, but there are still some lingering doubts in the back of your mind. After all, this is a very special occasion; otherwise you wouldn't be hiring a caterer. You can and should always ask for references, but you can't be sure that you aren't just getting friends of the caterer, who are not going to bad-mouth him. So how do you make sure this particular caterer can do the job you want? Ask the caterer to arrange for you to visit another function he is handling so that you can observe firsthand how he and his staff perform. Be sure to dress properly for the occasion, as if you were an invited guest, and don't overstay your welcome. You can pretty much gauge how well the caterer is doing in a half-hour or so.

Take a seat and save. "Most people are under the impression that buffets are cheaper than sit-down dinners, but that is absolutely not the case," says McCoy. Although some catering companies tell their clients otherwise, the buffet actually requires more food and labor. When you have a sit-down dinner, she says, chefs are exacting in their quantities. They say, "Okay, there are six ounces of meat, five ounces of potatoes, and four ounces of peas on each plate." This helps keep food costs under control. When they put buffets together, they have to plan for guests returning again and again, so they have to make a lot more food. Plus, buffets require constant maintenance—servers have to be there to replenish the food, and keep the area tidy. And you also need people to wait tables to serve drinks and such, which requires hiring nearly double the staff.

The cheapest way to go? Have a sit-down dinner—packaged. "Every hotel, club, and catering facility offers packages where you can get a sit-down dinner including everything from your appetizer to your salad to your champagne toast. Of course, they vary in price depending on the items you choose, but it is your best value," McCoy says.

Serve surf and turf. Even though it may sound more expensive to serve each guest a combination plate, chefs say combo platters can cost up to 40 percent less than dinners at which guests have a choice of seafood, chicken, or beef. The savings come from the planning that goes along with combination platters—the chef knows exactly how much food to buy. No need to get extras in case guests change their minds on site. So go ahead, serve surf and turf—you'll save money, but your guests will think you just won the lottery.

Order up extra bartenders. Caterers will tell you that one or two bartenders will be enough to staff your wedding reception, but unless you want 200 people standing in line for drinks all night, it won't be. Most catering companies will assign one bartender to every 75 guests, but wedding planners in the know say that you should specify in your contract that you want one bartender for every 50 guests during the cocktail hour (when guests will do most of their imbibing), with one bartender for every 75 guests during the dinner hour. It will cost a little extra, but it will prevent your reception from looking like a cafeteria line.

Buy booze by the head, not by the drink. Even if most of your wedding guests are nondrinkers, don't let the caterer talk you into paying by the drink. The secret about teetotalers is that many actually do imbibe when the liquor is free, and what's free for them costs you about $7.50 per cocktail.

"I was pulled into this trap when I planned my stepdaughter's wedding a few years ago," says McCoy. "Because most of the people in my family don't drink much, the catering director persuaded me to pay for the liquor by the glass. It ended up that the liquor bill was more than the food bill." It is almost always cheaper to buy liquor by the head. Caterers "may charge you $20 per head for a four-hour event where guests can drink as much as they want," McCoy says. "With a per-head liquor contract, there will be no surprises when it comes to paying the bill."

Spring for top-shelf stuff. People will remember whether they had Grey Goose or Banker's Club vodka at your celebration, so you may want to spend a little extra for the brand-name booze. Here's the thing: The price discrepancy between shelf and *top*-shelf liquor is only a few dollars per head, but it can make a significant difference in how classy your event is, and how happy your guests are. For 200 people, the cost will only be a few hundred dollars extra. ◁

WHAT YOUR CATERER DOESN'T WANT YOU TO KNOW ABOUT Food Amounts

Your catering director will try to talk you into courses that you just don't need in your meal, warns wedding specialist Deb McCoy. Both an appetizer before your meal, and an extra dessert before the wedding cake, are unnecessary. Skipping them could save you thousands of dollars.

With regard to the appetizer, if you serve hors d'oeuvres during your cocktail hour, no one will be chomping at the bit for an extra course before the entrée. In fact, they will probably be bursting with the mini quiches and cocktail shrimp they just chowed with their vodka tonics. When everyone is seated, jump right to the salad.

Your caterer will also try to tell you that wedding cake is just there for show, and that no one will eat it. Not true. It *is* true that your guests may not eat their cake because they just ate a bowl of cherries jubilee that cost you an extra $5 to $6 per head. Instead of spending the extra money on the extra dessert, spend half of it—$2 or $3 per head—on upgrading the wedding cake. Splurge on a cannoli cream cake, or one with raspberry filling. The last taste your guests will have in their mouths will be a delicious one.

Dinner Parties
5 Secret Ingredients for a Great Evening

Bring a nonedible hostess gift.
The key to choosing the perfect hostess gift: Choose something that will please the hostess without disrupting the flow of the party, says etiquette instructor Liz Scofield. Don't bring flowers—she'll have to leave her guests and go searching for a vase. Don't bring a dessert—she probably already has every crumb of the meal planned out, and she'll feel obligated to serve what you brought in addition to what she already had planned. Instead, present her with something fresh and delightful, such as homemade chocolate, gourmet teas, cocktail napkins, or candles. Better yet, send something ahead of time that will add to the festivities, such as a floral arrangement.

If you are on the receiving end of a disruptive hostess gift, tell the gift giver, "This is great—I will save it for the next special occasion when it can be appreciated on its own."

Pinch pennies with pasta. Pasta will stretch a dinner like no other food—both in terms of cost and quantity, says catering expert Vivaldo. One cooked pound of pasta mixed with grilled vegetables and chicken will serve six to eight guests for just $5 or $10. Compare that to $50 and up for a leg of lamb or other higher-end meat dishes. To hide the fact that you have chosen pasta to cut costs, give your dinner party an Italian theme. Serve Italian wine and bread, throw some red-and-white-checked tablecloths on your tables, and make a tiramisu (or other Italian dessert) to top it off.

Dine with both ying and yang. You may think a dozen guests with similar interests equals one successful dinner party. Not so—the secret to a rollicking evening is usually a quirky collection of opposites. If you want a dynamic, delightful dinner, mix it up a bit. Invite both your conservative neighbor and your bohemian brother-in-law, for starters, and see what happens.

Don't get stuck with the blowhard. If you find yourself stuck at a party with the most boring blowhard you've ever met, excuse yourself to get a drink refill and offer to get him something as well. If he says no to the drink, you are off the hook and can depart with grace. If he says yes, it's still okay if you get the drink, hand it over, and then walk away. Another way to escape? Introduce chatty Charlie to a passing friend and remark on the interest or hobby they might have in common. Then leave.

Master the art of the empty invitation. Learn when to give an empty invitation and learn when an invitation is empty, Scofield says. Few people would admit to giving one, but there are some invitations that are offered purely out of social grace, not out of a genuine desire to see someone again. These "empty invitations" are particularly prevalent at the close of a social event such as a dinner party. "For instance, if you just met someone at a dinner party and they offer to let you stay at their home the next time you come into town, that's an empty invitation," she says. "If you tried to take the person up on it, they would likely tell you their house was full that weekend."

Similar to the empty invitation is the empty parting comment, such as "Let's have lunch" or "I'll call you." These comments really mean, "I like you as a person, but I probably won't call." To avoid confusion, if you are the one giving the empty invitation or parting comment, substitute it with a more general phrase, such as "It was good to see you." ◁

Psst ... Table Manners Still Matter!

If you think people don't care about etiquette at the table as much as they used to, think again. One soup slurp or tooth pick is all it takes to turn some people off. So to stay on your toes, here is a quick—and necessary—table manners refresher course from Louise Fox of the Etiquette Ladies, Canada's Etiquette Experts:

☐ If you are the recipient of a toast, keep your glass at arm's length—never drink from it. Instead, simply nod your head and graciously say, "Thank you."

☐ Never take your cocktail to the dinner table.

☐ Allow your food to cool on its own—never blow on anything.

☐ If you wear lipstick, keep it off your plate and napkin by blotting it as soon as you apply it.

☐ Your napkin is there for you to dab your mouth *only*. Do not use it to wipe off lipstick or (God forbid) blow your nose.

☐ Keep your elbows off the table at all times.

☐ Don't put your purse, keys, sunglasses, or eyeglasses on the table.

☐ Take food out of your mouth the way it went in. If a piece of steak fat went into your mouth with a fork, spit it out onto the fork.

☐ Remove an olive pit with your thumb and index finger.

☐ Taste everything on your plate before you add salt or pepper.

☐ Leave your plate where it is when you are finished with your meal—don't push it away from you.

You'll find even more good-behavior tips at www.etiquette ladies.com.

Class Reunions

5 Time- and Money-Saving Tips for Your Stroll Down Memory Lane

Reunite by sunlight. The caterer may try to talk you into a dinner reunion, but a daytime meal will save a bundle on your reunion (or just about any big event). Daytime meals—breakfast, brunch, and lunch—cost a lot less than evening meals because these foods typically cost less, people expect smaller portions, and you can get away with serving less alcohol. At a daytime outdoor reunion, you can organize games like horseshoes and volleyball that will break the ice and encourage people to interact. Daytime events such as picnics or barbecues are also more casual; for example, you can get away with plastic plates rather than fancy, rented china.

Trick former classmates into pitching in. Sure, it may have seemed like a great idea to run for class president when you were 17, but 10 or 20 years later, you're stuck planning your high school reunion—a *big* responsibility. To figure out how much of this work you're able to delegate to others, survey the group and see if anyone is in the event-planning business. Ask these event planners if they can arrange for a discounted (or free) venue, photographer, or caterer, says Ngonzi. In exchange for your much appreciated discounts, offer to advertise the businesses prominently at the reunion.

Ask attendees for their two cents. Whether you are planning a high school reunion, coworker reunion, or family reunion, one of the best things you can do is to ask attendees for suggestions. Even if you never use their ideas, people love to think that they had a role in creating a fabulous event. Try emailing attendees a survey a few weeks (or months) before the event to ask what their thoughts are on games, activities, and themes. Then you can use the innovative ideas and ignore the lame ones.

How to Make a Memorable Entrance

EXPERT INSTANT ADVICE

Psychologists say most people form impressions of others within the first four minutes of meeting them, and 80 percent of those first impressions are based on nonverbal behavior. Making a dignified entrance at an event might just be more important than the conversations you have later.

When you make your entrance, the best way to draw attention to yourself in a tasteful way is being attractive, charming, witty, and memorable, says Scofield, the etiquette teacher. To turn heads and leave good impressions, pay attention to:

- **Your walk.** As you enter, walk with confidence, but not arrogance. Keep your head up, your shoulders back and down, and smile. No swaggering!

- **Your clothes.** Your clothes should be stunning without being over the top—fashionable without revealing too much skin.

- **Your placement.** When you first pass through the door, pause, step to the right, and survey the crowd. People watch the front door, so you'll be in plain view.

- **Your sociability.** Do not make a beeline for safety nets such as the bar, food, or people you already know. Instead, move from group to group and introduce yourself. If you are confident and friendly, people will naturally be attracted to you.

Spark a prom déjà vu. For a great high school reunion favor, create a replica of the champagne flute you got at your junior prom. It's a little-known fact that giving out these flutes can also save your event organizers some money! If you request that guests drink all alcoholic beverages out of the flutes, you will cut down on alcohol consumption (those flutes don't hold much in the way of beer or cocktails). Also, if your high school reunion is being held in a public place, the flutes will deter reunion crashers on the prowl for free drinks.

Find an affordable reunion space. Looking for a place to hold your class reunion? Renting a hall, a dining room at a restaurant, or a conference room at a hotel can be an expensive proposition. And if you are the chief organizer, you not only have to make an upfront down payment on the space but also have to nudge your former classmates into paying their fair share. And to be quite frank, many of your classmates are probably deadbeats—they think they've done their part just by showing up. But finding affordable space is really not that difficult.

- First off, chances are at least one of your former classmates has gone into the restaurant, bar, or hotel business and would be more than willing to offer a special deal, especially if he or she is the owner or manager.
- If that doesn't pan out, talk to the administrators at the school itself to see if there is any way to make an arrangement to use the school gym, cafeteria, or even the schoolyard if you're thinking of a warm-weather gathering. Colleges, eager to endear themselves to future donors among their alumni, are more likely to offer

a venue; just call the alumni affairs office at your college.

- For outdoor get-togethers, check the parks department for available space; some even have pavilions you can rent for a moderate fee.
- If you end up having to go to a commercial source, make bars, not restaurants, your first choice. Bars often have large back rooms that they will rent out inexpensively. ◁

Plan a Big Event from Your Laptop

Party and event planners don't tell people about event-planning software packages. That's because many of them use such software themselves and fear that if the secret gets out, they'll lose business. Instead of hiring a party planner or wedding coordinator, you can spend the $75 to $200 for software and do it yourself. Here are just a few good packages:

- ☐ **Mountain Cow's Printing Press.** Printing Press is an invitation software package that helps you design and print perfect invitations or "save the date" cards. Features modern fonts and graphics. Available at www.mountaincow.com.

- ☐ **My Wedding Companion CD.** The longest-selling wedding planning software on the market, My Wedding Companion organizes every aspect of your wedding, from the registry and seating chart to your honeymoon. Available from Amazon.com or Amazon.ca.

- ☐ **B'nai Mitzvah.** This bar and bat mitzvah planning software can also be used for planning other types of parties and events. Can be purchased at www.castlecomputer.com.

- ☐ **Reunion Planner Software.** Helps you organize a reunion celebration; keeps tabs on your budget, contact information, name tags, and seat assignments. Available at www.reunionplanner.com.

- ☐ **The Ultimate Wine and Cheese Pairing Guide.** Never be confused about wine again. This software has lists of the most popular white, red, and dessert wines, as well as classic food pairing matches for each. Available from Amazon.com or Amazon.ca.

Dining Out
6 Tricks for Having a Memorable Meal When You Eat Out at a Restaurant

Fine-tune restaurant recommendations. Hotel concierges are all too happy to recommend a restaurant to a stranger in town. What many don't want you to know is that they get referral fees in exchange for steering customers to certain eateries. That doesn't mean the place they pitch won't be good, because they do want you to be happy. But it does mean it may not be the best choice for what you had in mind. So ask some specific questions about the food, prices, and atmosphere. Kids welcome or romantic? Quiet or lots of music? Local style or haute cuisine?

Get a second opinion about restaurants. Your concierge isn't the only source of restaurant tips when you're out of town. The hotel teems with savvy locals. But remember about different strokes for different folks. If you're looking for upscale dining, hotel waiters may be plugged into the scene. But asking most other hotel staffers could backfire; they probably can't afford to frequent such places and don't want to be reminded of it. Hotel bar customers are a better bet. Even if they're from out of town themselves, they often have experiences to share. But if it's 100 percent local food and atmosphere you're after, the staff is a gold mine of advice. "Where do the locals eat?" is a question that can lead to unexpected pleasures.

Watch out for terms indicating fat. The folks who write restaurant menus are trying their darndest to sound enticing while dancing around the fact that many of their offerings are dripping with hidden fat—much of it the artery-clogging kind. You probably already know that words such as *creamy, breaded, buttery, crisp, pan-fried, cheese sauce,* and *stuffed* are indicators of fat—often saturated or trans fat. Other words to look out for are not as obvious: *Thermidor, Newburg, Parmesan,* and *scalloped.* But it's the foreign words that can really fool. For example, the innocent-sounding *au gratin* added to oysters or whitefish turns a lean, heart-healthy food into a plate of saturated fat.

Also from the French we get *au lait, à la mode, au fromage,* and *sautéed*—meaning, respectively, "with milk," "with ice cream," "with cheese" and "pan-fried in fat." On an Italian menu, beware of *Alfredo, carbonara, saltimbocca, parmigiana, lasagna,* and *manicotti,* which indicate heavy amounts of cream and cheese. (On the positive side, *griglia* indicates a heart-healthy grilled approach.)

In a Mexican restaurant, watch out for *chimichanga* (a fried burrito), *chalupas* (small deep-fried tortillas), *milanesa* (breaded and fried), and *con queso* (with cheese). *Relleno* means stuffed, which is always risky. For example, a chile relleno is actually a breaded chile pepper deep-fried in oil or lard and stuffed with cheese. Not what cardiologists recommend.

Rule of thumb: If you can't translate a menu word into a specific English word yourself, ask your waiter what it means, exactly. Better to appear unworldly than walk away less healthy.

Forge an alliance with your waiter. A discreet, professional waiter would never mention it, but the truth is that most of the foul-ups at a restaurant are not the waiter's fault. He or she is only the most visible link in a chain that includes chefs, sous-chefs, line cooks, prep staff, bussers, cleanup crew, hosts, managers, and owners. It's not the waiter who overcooked your veal, or forgot to hold the onions, or sat you at the table by the restrooms. But most customers will jump all over the waiter when things go wrong.

That's a mistake. The waiter is on your side. Nobody has more at stake in your satisfaction. So let your waiter know early on that you consider him or her your ally, not those others. Don't say, "Waiter, you brought me the wrong dressing." Say, "They put the wrong dressing on this, didn't they?" Even if the first statement is truer than the second, your server will appreciate your sympathetic approach and take better care of you.

Make dinner conversation interesting. If conversation makes the meal, avoid making a common mistake when you're dining with another person, or several others. Somewhere along the line it became common wisdom that the key to being a good dinner partner is to keep the conversation focused on the person you're with, and then "be a good listener." So now, who knows how many restaurant meals consist of one diner having to answer 75 questions before she or he has buttered the first roll. "Yes, you do have to listen," says Susan RoAne, a California business networking consultant and author of *What Do I Say Next?* and *How to Work a Room.* "But if all you do is ask questions, I'm going to clam up and my attitude becomes, 'What's it to ya?' "

Instead of grilling the person across the table from you, bring something to the party yourself. Good conversation strikes a balance between giving and

How I Do It   A Restaurant Manager's Tip on a Great Seat

Karen Beban, the manager of a northern California seaside restaurant and a frequent restaurant customer, has a favorite way to enjoy great service while having a wonderful time when she dines out. "Eat at the bar," she says. "I recently read a complaint from a woman who felt she was getting the single-woman treatment when the host suggested she eat at the bar. Wrong. Eating at the bar is more fun, whether you're single or a couple."

By way of example, Beban relates a recent dining experience: "A friend and I tried a fairly new restaurant in Sausalito with a good reputation. We sat at the bar, of course. Carol immediately learned the bartender's name, and we asked him about the new chef. Connection made. We ordered martinis before lunch, asking him to suggest an appetizer. Rapport established. We let him suggest the glass of wine with our entrée—pinot grigio for her, zinfandel for me."

At the bar, there's a more open camaraderie with the diners and drinkers around you, not to mention having your "waiter" standing right there the whole time. "Besides having a great time, we got extra scallops and our wineglasses refilled at no charge," says Beban. "When we go back, we'll make it a point to remember the bartender's name and ask him about the vacation he told us he was about to take. And he'll remember the large tip we left, and how much fun we were."

Beban offers a few cautions for maximum bar dining pleasure. Don't sit at the bar with a large party. A bartender counts on turnover for tips, and that can't happen if diners take up all the seats. Don't sit at the bar if all you're having is herbal tea and salad. And if you're out with the kids, stick to the main restaurant floor. Bars are for adults.

receiving. "Naturally you want to show you're interested in your dinner partner," RoAne says. "But you want to be interesting too."

Don't nitpick; relax and enjoy.
Anyone who works the floor of a restaurant knows something you don't, but should: It's not the food that determines whether a customer has a good time, and it's not the service. The biggest factor is the attitude of the customer himself. Sure, a high-priced entrée that disappoints, or a Simon Cowell wannabe as a waiter, can ruin your evening. But more often than not, waiters say in private, disgruntled customers walk into the restaurant poised for battle and ready to have a bad time. They usually find it.

So here's a tip for your dining pleasure: Relax and have a good time. Don't make a big deal out of small things. If there's a piece of cork floating in your wine, you can raise a stink, alienate the serving staff, and poison the atmosphere for the rest of the evening. Or you can just take the piece of cork out. The wine's still fine. Leave the nitpicking to the professional restaurant reviewers. They get paid for finding problems. You, on the other hand, are paying. So decide to have a good time. No restaurant's perfect, and it doesn't have to be for you to enjoy it. ◁

Wine Secrets
4 Things to Consider When You Order Wine with Your Meal

Order wine by the bottle.
Restaurants love it when you order your wine by the glass. That's because they make more money per bottle that way, and you usually end up paying more per sip. How? Do the math. You and your date each order a glass of wine, typically five ounces. So far, so good. You liked it, so you each order another glass. You've now probably paid a few dollars more than what a bottle costs, and if you had bought a bottle, there'd still be another glass left—which you don't have. So unless you're purposefully tasting around—that is, trying different wines, a glass at a time—or you're sure you'll each order only one glass, buy a bottle. It's a better bargain and more fun to boot.

Serve your own wine. Do you really need your waiter controlling the wine bottle all meal long and refilling your glass every time you take a sip? Before you answer, be aware that the motive isn't entirely good service. As often as not, all that fussing and pouring is mostly about pushing the wine at you so you'll drink more and order more. So unless you honestly enjoy the extra attention, take control of your own consumption by telling your waiter after the wine is first served that you'll be pouring for yourself throughout the meal. After all, it's pretty easy to do.

BYOB (bring your own burgundy).
Restaurants in the U.S. aren't crazy about customers toting in a bottle of wine to drink with their meals, and the industry as a whole has fostered the impression that you can't do it. But in fact most restaurants in all price ranges will let you bring your own bottle, but they'll charge a "corkage fee." That fee might be $10 per bottle or it might be $50 or more. Not only does corkage vary from restaurant to restaurant, it sometimes varies from table to table in any one restaurant. At the end of the day, they can charge whatever they want.

So call ahead, let them know what you're bringing with you and ask about the corkage fee. That way you get a fee nailed down in advance, and they usually appreciate the heads-up. If you plan to drink a second bottle, consider buying that one from the house. Sometimes when you do that, the corkage fee on the first one goes down or even gets waived. In several Canadian provinces—like Quebec and Ontario—some restaurants are designated "Bring Your Own Wine" establishments and customers are encouraged to bring their own. Wineglasses are supplied free of charge and no "corkage fees" are applied. However, waiters expect a better tip for these services.

Doggie-bag that merlot, please.
Hesitant about ordering that second bottle of wine because you're not sure the two of you can finish it? Go ahead. In the United States, it's perfectly legal in most states to take the unfinished portion home with you, properly sealed and bagged by the restaurant staff. Problem is, "recorking" is not something restaurants are in the habit of suggesting, and most diners are unaware that such a thing exists. But now you know, so get that wine to go. ◁

HOW TO ORDER
wine
Without Worry

Nearly everyone knows by now that rules about wine were meant to be broken. Some white wines go well with meat and some reds with poultry and seafood dishes. But it's still important to wait until everyone has decided on a main course before selecting wine in order to get one that goes well with everything. Here are some tips on handling the wine-ordering ritual.

☐ If you know which wine you want, order it. If you don't, tell the waiter or wine steward how much you want to spend and have him or her recommend one. Then accept the recommendation gladly, knowing your chances of enjoying the wine are better than if you'd taken a shot in the dark.

☐ Take advantage of the wine list—not just to find a bottle to order but to point to your choice if you can't pronounce the name. The waiter will nod knowingly and say the name perfectly. And then you *still* won't be able to pronounce it, but it doesn't matter. Your only job is to drink it.

☐ If you chose your wine off the list, check the label when the bottle comes to make sure you're getting what you ordered. That includes the year. A 2001 might cost a lot more than the 2003 you asked for, but if you drink it, you can be charged the higher price.

☐ When the waiter pulls out the cork and then puts it down in front of you, stick it in your ear and say, "Sounds good." Are we kidding? Yes. But it's no more ridiculous than the cork-smelling routine that some folks feel obliged to perform. All you need to do is make sure the cork's not moldy or decaying. If it's moist on the bottom, that's good; it means the wine was stored correctly. Otherwise forget about it. It's just a cork.

☐ If you ordered, you'll get a splash in your glass to taste. Relax. It's not a test. If the wine's gone bad, you'll know. First look: You don't want brown or cloudy. Then smell and taste. Remember, you're not judging at a wine tasting. You just want to be sure the wine hasn't oxidized (turned vinegary) and the cork didn't go bad (musty taste). If it's bad, don't be shy about telling the server. Suggest the server taste it to confirm. Trust us, he or she won't take it personally.

☐ Tell the server out loud that the wine's okay. Something like, "Nice wine, thanks for the suggestion" will work fine. He appreciates the verbal confirmation, because it's like a contract that you agree to pay for the bottle.

Having a Drink

5 Tricks for Getting on the Barkeep's Good Side When Out for a Quick One with Colleagues

How to get a free drink. You won't see a sign on the wall announcing it, but a bartender has some (limited) leeway to offer a round on the house. There's no guarantee that you'll get one, but these "buybacks" go to customers who (1) have been ordering multiple rounds, (2) have been tipping well, and (3) aren't acting like jerks. But even if you qualify on all three counts, you have to help the barkeep know it.

First, if the bar's crowded, the bartender's more likely to connect you to what you've been buying if you (and your party, if there is one) order the same drink each round. A bartender may not always remember a face or name, but will always remember making a manhattan and a whiskey sour on the same ticket four times.

Second, unless you're a known regular, tip as you go—in cash, even if you're on a tab, and even if you'll be paying with a credit card. That puts your tipping on record, and servers prefer tips in cash anyway.

Finally, go out of your way to ingratiate yourself with the bartender. Thank him or her for the attention, hand out a compliment on the drink preparation, or (if it's not too busy) strike up a light conversation. Sympathize subtly with the beleaguered bartender, sharing in the eye-rolling over obnoxious customers. The idea is to establish your non-jerk credentials.

How to get another free drink. Always tip your usual amount on the free round. Most bar customers don't, thinking free means completely costless. That drives bartenders crazy. You still come out ahead when you tip your buyback, and you greatly increase your chances of getting another one.

How to get to the front of the line. What do you do when you need to order directly from the bar but it's already crowded with patrons waiting to do the same thing? Try politely asking if they'd mind if you went first. Tell them why you need to go ahead of them, and you'll be surprised at how often they'll step aside, says Susan RoAne.

Maybe your husband spilled his drink back at the table and is very upset about it. Maybe the movie you're going to starts in 20 minutes. Maybe the babysitter has to go home and you barely have time for a nightcap. Maybe you really have to go to the bathroom but your table is waiting for you to bring the drinks first. "If you give a reason for your request, reasonable people will usually accept it," RoAne says. "Most people are actually very nice."

One caveat, though. It helps if the reason you give is actually the truth. Otherwise, you'll have to carry a guilty conscience back to the table along with the drinks.

Be decisive when ordering. Cocktail waitresses and bartenders frequently encounter the type of customer who comes into the bar presumably to have a drink but then acts completely stumped when asked what he or she wants. If that's you, then you should know your server's secret thoughts: This table is going to waste a lot of my time, so I'm staying away from it as much as I can. Since being ignored is exactly what you don't want, make sure you have something to say to your server as soon you sit down. One way to do that is to think about what you'll have well before you reach the place. You can browse through a bartender's guide or poke around the Internet for ideas. If you're still clueless when the moment of truth arrives, order what somebody else in your party is ordering. If that's not an option, tell your server you'll start off with a soda water for now. That "for now" is a signal for your server to come back soon, and buys you time to make a decision.

Think like a bartender. To competent mixologists, the bar area is their personal fiefdom, over which they exercise absolute authority. It is not a democracy, and it is not always fair. Once you realize this mind-set, you'll get better service. "The bartender decides who is served and when," says Karen Beban. "If you feel you've been slighted, don't make an issue out of it if you want to drink at all." Show some patience, don't take things personally, tip, and you'll soon break through the service barrier and will usually be treated well.

The bartender has a lot to consider that is not always obvious to you. For example, pushy twenty-somethings may be passed over at first. That's not because the bartender thinks they're jerks; if that were the case, they'd be served quickly so they'll go away sooner. The bartender is more likely buying time to figure out if they're too drunk to be served. Or a male bartender may serve some lovely lady ahead of you. There's a good reason for that, according to Beban: "He's a man and he can't help it."

The point is that when you sit down at a bar, you've entered into a bartender's unique domain. Take a few minutes to absorb the vibes, reserving judgment until you have a take on where the bartender's coming from—his or her quirks, concerns, and competence. You'll usually avoid a lot of unnecessary anxiety that way. ◁

5 Secrets for Having a Great Time When You Go Out to See a Hit on the Silver Screen

Buy your movie tickets in advance. On a typical Friday night hundreds of people line up for tickets to some huge blockbuster that everybody wants to see at once. Half of them are in the ticket-holders line by mistake, and the other half have no guarantee the darn thing won't be sold out before they reach the ticket seller. But others just walk up to a machine, swipe their credit card, grab the tickets that pop out, and walk right in. That's because they're the ones who knew enough to buy their movie tickets in advance online or over the phone.

Most people don't yet realize that in some cases it makes no more sense to wander ticketless into a movie complex than it does to show up at a visiting performance of the Bolshoi Ballet and hope to get in. You might, but you'll more likely find yourself all dressed up with nowhere to go. Moviegoing has changed, and the planned evening out, complete with advance tickets, is more and more the way to go. The online buyer who takes advantage of that today is way ahead of the clueless masses who will follow tomorrow—and wait in line in the meantime.

The two main sources for online tickets are MovieTickets.com and Fandango.com. They sell tickets at the same price as the theater box office, but charge a fee of $1 or $1.50 per ticket. That's worth it if:

- It's the opening weekend or early in the run of a major release, such as *Superman Returns Yet Again* or *Son of Titanic*. Tickets for these blockbusters (the real ones, not the names we just made up) are often available several weeks in advance.

- It's a Friday or Saturday night in a major and always crowded theater complex.

- You have an evening planned around a major new movie across town and you don't want to risk any surprises.

Register at both online ticket sellers. Both major online movie-ticket sellers—MovieTickets.com and Fandango.com—make purchases easy, displaying info about what's playing where in your area and then taking you through a quick and simple point-and-click process to buy the tickets. But you'll often find that you can't get tickets for the movie you want to see. That's because of a quirk in their operations that they don't tell you about, namely that each has exclusive arrangements with the movie theater chains. So if the movie you want is playing at, say, an AMC theater, you need to purchase it at MovieTickets.com. But if it's showing at a Regal theater, only Fandango.com will offer it.

Once you know this, the way around it is obvious. Just punch up the other service if you strike out at the first one. Of course, neither is going to say, "Please see our competitor for tickets to this movie." So it makes sense to be registered at both sites, registration being a simple matter of giving them basic information such as your name, age, and credit card number.

Sidestep all of those pre-movie ads. Plenty of moviegoers are convinced that the very idea of a theater running soft drink and credit card commercials before a movie portends the decline of civilization as we know it. Alas, the ads probably aren't going away anytime soon. A captive audience of mostly young adults with nothing to do but stare at the screen is too mouthwatering for advertisers, and the exhibitors need cash any way they can get it. But you can cheat the system in three ways.

The first is simply to frequent movie theaters that don't show ads. And yes, there is such an animal. Some upscale theaters proudly announce they don't run commercials—it's part of their package of extras that lets them charge $2 to $6 more per ticket. More economically, seek out smaller or older theaters that never did run ads and still don't. Call ahead to find out.

Another ploy is to time your arrival to a minute or two before the true,

---

announced showtime. If you're just going to be sitting there chomping on popcorn and waiting, why not chomp and wait in the lobby, watching people instead of commercials? This strategy works best in uncrowded theaters; otherwise, you might end up in the front row.

The most rebellious response to commercials is to ignore them. The no-talking rule is sacred in a movie theater, but it doesn't kick in until the lights go down. These days, most of the advertising is packaged into what's euphemistically called "pre-show entertainment," which generally runs with the lights on. So chat away until the lights dim for the trailers. Talk about how much you hate ads in movie theaters.

Snack before or after the show. The food they sell you at the movies is expensive, messy, unhealthy, and only available at the end of a long wait while the kids behind the counter move in slow motion. The theaters constantly try new tricks to keep us spending $14 for junk we'd never buy anywhere else, but they ignore the solution that will work best. Are you ready for a radical new approach to dealing with movie food? Here it is: Just don't eat the stuff. Have a nice meal before or after the show instead.

Most of us eat popcorn and candy at the movies despite the hassles because … well, we've always eaten popcorn and candy at the movies. But it wasn't always thus. "You know, for a long time there was no food, because the movie palaces didn't want their rugs and tapestries and upholstery ruined by gum and chocolate and spilled drinks," says Ross Melnick. "You really didn't have much food in the better theaters until after World War II." So consider boycotting the snack bar as an act of nostalgia for the golden age of cinema.

Try a drive-in theater for a change. Few moviegoers realize that the number of drive-in theaters is actually increasing, and everybody connected to the walk-in movie business would prefer that they never realize it. That's because drive-in picture shows make for a great alternative, offering everything a standard theater offers except matinees. And they do it without a lot of the problems of the megaplexes. To wit:

- *High ticket prices?* Drive-ins generally charge only $5 to $8 dollars per person, and you almost always get a double feature.

- *Parking hassles?* By definition, you don't pay extra for parking at a drive-in. And once you park, you're already in your seat.

- *Expensive snack foods?* Drive-ins are the only movie venues where you can pack in anything you want. Carry in a rack of lamb with mint jelly and a few bottles of pinot noir, if you like. As long as the driver doesn't drink the wine, it's perfectly fine. And if you don't want to bring your own, a drive-in's food selection is usually much more ample than what a walk-in offers.

- *Poor sound?* Those tinny speakers you hang on the window are relics of the past. Instead, you tune into a low-frequency station on your car radio. If your speakers are decent, the sound is wonderful.

- *Talkers?* The only ones you have to worry about are right there in the car with you.

- *Antiseptic atmosphere?* Are you kidding? Parked under the stars enjoying a big-screen movie with your family or friends in the private comfort of your automobile? That's as good as it gets. ◂

WHAT **MOVIE THEATERS** DON'T WANT YOU TO KNOW ABOUT DVDs

All the hype surrounding the release of a blockbuster movie is designed to get you to rush out to your local multiplex as soon as possible. But unless you just have to be the first on your block to see the latest multimillion-dollar production from Hollywood, it pays to be a little patient. The time between a film's release in the theaters and its release on DVD is growing shorter and shorter. It used to be six months, but recently it has dropped to a matter of a few weeks. And indeed, some movie companies are talking about releasing them simultaneously, since the filmmakers now make much more money from DVD sales and rentals than from theaters. If a movie is really good, it will be just as enjoyable to watch at home in a few weeks as in a theater now. This is especially true now that more and more homes have large-screen televisions that show off those spectacular special effects as well as the downsized screens at the multiplex. And if you miss the theater experience, just hook your TV audio to your stereo, make some popcorn, turn down the lights, and settle down. By the way, new blockbuster DVDs are often discounted heavily (to less than the cost of two movie tickets) during the first week of their release at outlets like Best Buy and Circuit City. Go on Tuesday—the day of the week when DVDs are released.

Live Events

5 Ways to Live It Up and Make the Most of Special and Pricey Live Entertainment

How to get tickets when they're "sold out." Never take it literally when it's announced that there are no more tickets left for a major concert, show, or sporting event. "Nothing's ever really sold out," says Kenneth Dotson, chief marketing officer at TicketsNow. " 'Sold out' just means that face-value tickets at the box office are gone. There are always tickets available for any hot event." And he should know. His is one of a growing number of reputable online ticket brokering sites that hook up ticket-seekers with licensed ticket resellers. And most of the time there are tickets to be had right up to the last minute. Just go to the site, see what's still there, and buy the ticket right then and there. The cost? Don't ask. But a lot of sold-out concerts are once-in-a-lifetime events that you might be willing to splurge on. For example, as we've been hearing since 1972, the next Rolling Stones tour will probably be their last one.

Get a good seat by paying more. The cruelest deception foisted on the public is that good seats for big-time concerts or sporting events are available at the box office if you jump on them fast enough. Forget it. The bigger a show is, the less likely it is that any significant number of decent seats are going to be sold through the standard channels. They all go to promoters, advertisers, underwriters, sponsors, and a host of other insiders with enough pull to get first shot at big blocks of tickets. In other words, you didn't miss out on the good seats; they were never there in the first place.

But that doesn't mean you can't get your hands on them. You can, on what's called the "secondary market." While most regular folks assume they're doomed to the nosebleed section, the smart ones are snapping up the choice location tickets that the insiders turned around and unloaded to licensed resellers. Those prime tickets are sitting there at online ticket broker sites, waiting for you to point, click, and buy. You'll pay considerably more than what's printed on the ticket, of course, but that price was an illusion to start with. These days, face value has given way to market value. That has created controversy, but right now it's the way it is. At least you can be assured that what you're paying for good seats is exactly what they're worth on the free market.

So if your team looks like it could make it to the World Series, or Coldplay's coming to town, ignore what the ads say and go directly to a reputable online ticket brokering site like TicketsNow that guarantees you're not being sold fraudulent or stolen tickets. You'll be in a privileged position, because the entertainment and sports industries still maintain the farce that tickets in the 21st century are sold like they were in the 20th. No ad says, "Good seats available on the secondary market." But for major events, that's the only place they're available.

Get loads of free info at ticket sites. Broker websites help their customers pick and choose by displaying all kinds of information and graphics about the concerts, shows, and sporting events they offer tickets for. For example, they'll have seating charts of major venues across the continent, and schedules of upcoming events. The displays are ostensibly for paying customers, but it turns out you don't have to be one to gain access to them. Just Google up online ticket brokers, find a site with good information, and find out all you need to know.

Phone in your order and get special info. Ticket brokers like you to do your shopping online, because there's virtually no labor cost involved. So they don't shout too loud about the call-in service they might also offer that lets you do your purchasing over the phone. This is worth taking advantage of, and it's not just for the Internet-challenged. TicketsNow, for example, has more than 100 "customer care representatives" available who can often give you something that the site alone might not—answers to your personal questions. Which is the shady side of the venue? What are the bathrooms like? Do they sell Coke or Pepsi? And, of course, they can sell you the tickets. The site will probably have an 800 number in plain view, but the "Contact Us" button might give you more direct access to the customer service phone connection.

Plan ahead and sell those unused season tickets. Do you own the right to season tickets that have been in your family for decades? Wouldn't it be a tragedy to have to give them up because of soaring prices? That particular tragedy is happening a lot these days, but you can avoid it thanks to the secondary market. Here's how:

Unless you're a mega-fanatic with no work schedule and a thermonuclear

passion for your home team, you probably won't be attending all 81 baseball home games, or all 41 basketball or hockey home games. In fact, if you're typical, you probably spend stressful hours arranging to give away the ones you can't use. So go ahead and get your season tickets, check the schedule and plan the games you'll be going to. Then check the Internet for a licensed ticket reseller who will buy the rest en masse. True, you can't anticipate those unexpected great mid-season matchups, and you do run the risk of later wishing you had some tickets back.

But consider the payoff: In one stroke, you've kept the season tickets in the family, drastically reduced your total cost, removed the headache of constantly dealing with extra tickets, and still guaranteed yourself entry to most of the games you'll want to see. Not bad when you think about it. And you've done nothing involved with scalping, as long as you sell your ducats at face value to a legitimate licensed reseller, who must follow state or provincial laws. ◁

6 FREE LIVE
performances
You'll Enjoy

There's a good reason live entertainment seems so outrageously expensive these days: It is. But if you can accept the radical notion that there's solid entertainment to be had without megabuck superstars, you can live it up for free. Start with these ideas:

1 Art openings

The best entertainment bargain on the planet. Free admission, free wine, free hors d'oeuvres, free people-watching, and free mingling with the artist, who is obligated to be nice to you. You might even like the paintings or other art.

2 Free concerts in the park

Instead of passing by these things as you usually do, plop yourself down on the grass as close to the musicians as possible, and get into the sounds. Let yourself go. The players are usually pretty good, or the city wouldn't let them be there. If the music's not your bag and you get bored, watch the drummer if there is one. See if you can follow what he or she is doing.

3 Community theater

Human beings will travel thousands of miles and spend hundreds of dollars to see a Broadway play. Why not try walking a few blocks to see amateurs or semi-pros do basically the same thing—but from closer up? Ask about being a volunteer usher. Free admission is your pay.

4 Open-mike night

Small venues have them on off nights, where anybody can get up there and sing or play or do a comedy routine. Don't smirk. A lot of artists started their careers this way—performers that people now pay $500 to see from 45 yards away in a football stadium. And if some poor deluded wannabe is really awful, that, too, can be entertaining.

5 Author readings

You read the book, now hear the writer. Or the other way around. Big-time and semi-big-time writers often make the rounds to local bookstores to read from their work, sign books, and schmooze with readers. Check the bulletin boards at your area's bookstore or those piles of flyers at the checkout counter. Contrary to movie-comedy stereotype, authors are usually not boring.

6 (Very) small-time sports

True lovers of baseball or any other sport can re-create a no-cost version of major-league spectator pleasure by grabbing a free bleacher spot at a muni-league, high school, or even Little League game. Pick a team to root for (or allow one to pick you). Return a few times, and you'll find yourself experiencing the same thrills and emotions that would cost you two days' salary at the pro stadiums. It ain't the New York Yankees, but as Shakespeare should have said, "The game's the thing."

Casino Games

12 Secrets for Enjoying Gaming and Limiting Your Losses Against the Unfriendly Odds

Be a high roller—for a few minutes. When you enter a casino and start playing for the first time, make your initial bets higher than what you would normally use as a minimum bet. The pit boss assumes that this is your usual betting pattern, and will use it to calculate your comp eligibility—that is, what kind of freebies the house might offer. Not surprisingly, the hotel's generosity when it comes to meal and room discounts is a direct function of how much it thinks you're going to bet per hour. You can always settle into your more modest wagering habits as time goes by. The pit bosses rarely have time to check in on you later.

Check the odds on video poker machines. Casinos don't make it obvious which video poker machines pay off better. So every day a good percentage of push-button suckers are feeding extra coins to the house without knowing it. Avoid being one of them by taking a look at the payoff chart that's right there on the machine. Almost all will range from a high payoff of 250-1 for a royal flush down to even money (1-1) for jacks or better. What you want to notice are the two payoffs right in the middle. If a full house pays 9-1 and a flush 6-1, you're in the right place. It's what the pros call a "full pay" machine.

But a lot of them (and all of them in some states or provinces) will pay just 8-1 for a full house and 5-1 for a flush. That means that when you insert a silver dollar and then get lucky enough to punch up a boat—say, three queens and two 8s—the full-pay machine will drop 9 silver dollars

into your tray and the short-pay machine just 8. No big deal? Well, over the long run it's a very big deal, upping the house's advantage by a significant 2.2 percent. Why give away your money?

Cough up the coins now instead of later. It may seem like you're extending your chances of winning—or at least getting to play longer—when you drop in only a single coin with each hand in video poker. That's just what they want you to believe. The truth is, by putting in the full number of coins with each hand, which is usually five, you increase your chances of being ahead in the long run by a full 12 percent.

Here's why: When you play five coins instead of one, you of course get the same proportional payoff each time you win. For example, if you put in one coin and hit a flush, you get five coins back. If you had put in 5 coins, you would have received 25 coins back. It's like having made five flushes at a time.

Obviously, that comes out as a wash because you also lose five times as much when you pull bust hands. Where the advantage comes in is with an extra-high payoff for that fifth coin with the best hand you can get—a royal flush. The payoff for a royal flush—a straight from the 10 to the ace, all of one suit—is 250-1. (If it's less, don't play that machine.) It stays that way with the first four coins you play. That is, you'll get 500 back if you bet two, 750 back if you bet three, and 1,000 back if you bet four. But if you bet five, the payback jumps to 4,000, the equivalent of 800-1, if you're using a full-pay machine, as you should be. And if you play video poker long enough, you will get a royal flush with any luck. By betting five, you can milk that magic moment to the max.

Never take the craps dealer's suggestion. "The bets to stay away from at the craps table are the ones the dealers try to get you to make," says Bill Burton, author of *1,000 Best Casino Gambling Secrets* and the gambling expert at About.com. "When they encourage you to make certain bets, it's not because they care about you." What they care about is steering you toward the "side" or "proposition" bets where the house has the biggest advantage. These are the bets you place in the middle of the table that usually have to do with what will happen on the next roll of the dice rather than whether the shooter will make the point or not. They're sucker bets—easy, fun, and the surest of losers over a short time.

WHAT THE CASINOS DON'T WANT YOU TO KNOW ABOUT Your Odds

- There's a difference between the true odds of your winning any particular bet and the odds the casino actually uses to pay you if you do win. That difference is always in the casino's favor and it's the reason casino owners (always a government agency in Canada) are rich and you're not.

- Because of the house edge, the casino will always win in the long run, no matter how smart you are, how good you think your system is, or how lucky you are. The Las Vegas strip is paved with the losses of innocent fun-seekers who don't know that.

- Some of the games have a much smaller house advantage than others, so your chances of walking away a winner after playing them are higher. This assumes, however, that you play the best strategy and that you're able to walk away while ahead.

- If gamblers only played blackjack, mini-baccarat, pai-gow poker, live poker, the sports book, and bingo, they'd lose a lot less money. Those are games with a house edge of less than 3 percent.

- The casino loves to see you playing games like Caribbean Stud Poker, Let It Ride, Red Dog, single-deck 21, and those undignified spectacles like the Big Wheel or Wheel of Fortune. The house edge on these is astronomical.

- Playing keno is the equivalent of making a charity donation to the casino ownership. Yes, the young keno ladies are friendly and they need the tips. And yes, it's simple and kind of fun to try to divine some numbers while you're at the coffee shop or buffet or bar. Just be aware that the house advantage in keno can run as high as 50 percent. You're better off playing the state or provincial lottery—it's essentially the same game, but at least you're donating your money to the public good instead of business magnates.

The side bets on a craps table suck away cash that would be better placed on the pass line, where you have a decent chance of coming out ahead. On this basic and better bet, you're simply going with the shooter, hoping he or she will roll anything but a 2, 3, or 12 on the first toss of the dice. If it's a 7 or 11, you win. If it's anything else (4, 5, 6, 8, 9, 10) you win if the shooter repeats that number before rolling a 7. It pays even money, and at 1.41 percent, the house advantage is relatively low.

But the friendly men or women who run the table—called dealers even though they don't deal any cards—will hype plays such as the Big 6 or Big 8. These are side bets that wait for you in a corner of the layout like a black widow spider. Put $6 on the Big 8 and if an 8 is rolled before a 7, you win $6. Put the same $6 on 8 over at the "place" area— for all practical purposes the same bet—and you win $7. How unfair is that? So unfair that in Atlantic City, Big 6 and Big 8 are outlawed.

Rule of thumb: Avoid any bet a dealer wants you to make. "That's especially true for craps, where there are about 40 possible bets, a few of them with decent odds and all the rest terrible," Burton says. "But it also applies to games like Let It Ride and Caribbean Stud."

Getting odds better than most at craps. Talk about forbidden knowledge! There's a bet you can make at the craps table that offers the most favorable odds in the entire casino, but it doesn't even appear on the table layout. That's right—no marked area to place the bet in, no mention of it anywhere, and, you can be sure, no information about it forthcoming from the dealers. It's called the "odds bet" and it's the only play available that actually pays in proportion to the risk, with no house advantage at all.

You are eligible to make an odds bet if you have a bet on the pass line, gambling that the shooter will make the "point" by rolling that number again before rolling a 7. If you have $5 on the pass line, you can put up $5 more as an odds bet, or $10 if the casino offers "double odds." You do this by placing the chips a few finger widths directly behind your pass line bet, outside the back line of the pass bet area.

How much you get if you win depends on what the point number is, but it's always better than the even money pass line payoff. If the point number is 6 or 8, the payoff for an odds bet is 6-5. So if you bet $5 on the pass line and added on a $10 "double odds" bet, your payoff is $5 for the pass bet and $12 for the double odds bet. You invested $15 and got that $15 back plus $17 more.

If the point made is a 5 or 9, the payoff is slightly better at 3-2. The odds-bet payoff when the shooter makes a point of 4 or 10 is the highest at 2-1. That's because there are fewer possible rolls of the two dice that can add up to a 4 or 10.

Choose the crowded roulette table. Roulette's not a game you're likely to win at. The house edge is simply too big. But hey, it's so much fun that folks are going to go for some spins anyway. What's the point of hitting a casino if you can't whoop it up and high-five your fellow players around the wheel, with free drinks to boot? So go ahead and play. But play slow.

Why? Because the more time between spins, the longer it will take for you to lose your money. That sounds negative, but the unvarnished truth is that only the house wins at roulette over the long haul. So what you want to do is shorten the haul—not in time spent at the table but in the number of spins that take place in that time, and therefore the amount of your hard-earned money you're risking.

You can't slow the pace on your own, of course, no matter how much you pretend to fumble in your pocket for chips or act distracted. Instead, choose the most crowded roulette table in the room. At a full table, it takes up to three minutes between spins of the wheel. Now, full tables look like something the casino prefers, with more money riding on each spin. But the house actually doesn't care for full tables, precisely because they result in the slower play you the customer are looking for. They're likely to suggest some move to a less crowded table, or open up a new one in hopes of evening things out. But stay put. At the full table, you'll have more fun, lose less money, take just as many free drinks, and maybe—just maybe—get lucky and win.

Seek out the single-zero roulette tables. They're not everywhere, and even where they do exist, the casino wants you on the double-zero table. However, the smart roulette player will stick with the lonely 0.

The reason is simple. A typical roulette table has 38 numbers—1 through 36, plus a zero and a double zero. Your chances of hitting one are 37-1, but the payoff is only 35 to one. A single-zero table also pays 35-1, but your true odds are better at 36-1, because there are only 37 numbers. That slight difference shifts the house edge downward significantly. You'll still lose in the long run, but not as fast.

Watch the odds at blackjack. Cruise the Vegas strip and you'll see a growing number of places shouting the wonderful news that they pay 6-5 for a natural blackjack. That means if you're dealt an ace along with a 10 or face card at the blackjack table, you immediately win $6 for every $5 you put up. Not bad, huh?

Actually, it's terrible. Because throughout modern gaming history, a natural blackjack has paid 3-2 just about everywhere in the United States and Canada, and it still does in most casinos. If math wasn't your best subject, take our word for it that a 3-2 payoff is much better for you than 6-5. So much better, in fact, that the shift to a 6-5 natural blackjack payoff ups the casino's advantage by so much that it turns a fairly customer-friendly game into a bad proposition. So before you sit down at a blackjack table, make sure that natural blackjack pays 3–2. If there's no indication, ask the dealer what the payoff is. If it's 6-5, go somewhere else.

But don't go to the video blackjack machines. They're even more likely to short-change you in their natural blackjack payoffs, sometimes going even lower than 6-4 down to even money. So unless you find machines that pay 3-2, forget about video blackjack.

Consider the difference: If you have a $50 bet up and get dealt an ace and a king, you'll win $75 at an honest 3-2 table, but only $60 at a 6-5 table and a piddling $50 at an even-money machine. The casino counts on hordes of clueless gamblers not knowing or caring about the difference. But from now on you're not one of them.

Don't go by what you see on TV poker tournaments. Seasoned veterans of the casino poker rooms love the televised poker tournament fad more than they'll ever let on to you. That's because they know that television-educated players are usually easy marks. Inspired by the Joe Hachems and Chris Moneymakers they see on ESPN2, they rush to the table full of enthusiasm … and soon leave it with no money. Here's what the table vets know that television-educated players don't: Casino poker isn't like television poker.

So keep two things in mind. Unless you're well off enough to qualify for a *Forbes* magazine listing, you'll probably be playing with a limit that's too low to bluff anybody out the way they do on TV. And unlike TV tournaments, your game won't be edited so that all the hands are fascinating or decisive. Casino games are more like arduous grinds that reward stamina, patience, and most of all, knowledge.

That doesn't mean you shouldn't play. Poker is a fun challenge, and unlike most casino games, a certain percentage of customers have to be winners, since they're playing against other customers instead of the house. Remember, though, that the winners aren't the ones who pull off spectacular stunts, but the ones who have mastered the odds so they know the right move to make in all situations. You can't learn that from TV. You need a book to learn the percentages from, and lots of practice.

SECRET WEAPON

Player's Card

The first thing you do when you walk into a casino is go straight to the players club and ask for a player's card. Do this even if you're planning on staying for three minutes, and even if you don't intend to come back for 15 years. This card is free money. It's your ticket to all kinds of hotel discounts, and even comped rooms and meals. But about half of casino gamblers ignore it, either because they can't be bothered or don't know about it. Once that card's in your possession, take advantage of it:

Flash it. When you approach a table to play, give your card to the dealer or directly to the pit boss. They'll use it to enter your playing time and estimated total bets into the computer.

Insert it. Don't play the slots or any other machine game without inserting your card in the indicated place and making sure a light indicates it's been accepted. You'll get "credit" for your betting.

Ask. If you've been playing more or less steadily for much of the day, ask for a casino host and see if the casino will comp you a meal or offer you a gift shop discount. They won't think you're being presumptuous. If the answer's no, they'll probably indicate how much more you need to play to be eligible. Unless you're a high roller, the casino isn't going to come up to you and say, "Gosh, you've been a good customer—let us buy you dinner." You have to ask.

Take a shot. Before you pay your bill and go home, ask the casino host if you've played enough to get a break on the room rate. If you put in your time at the tables, you just might get it.

Try again. When you make a reservation at a casino hotel that you've played at before, give them your card number and ask them to review your play record. See if you can get your room comped (that is, free) or at least get in at the "casino rate," which is usually a healthy discount.

Understand that player's cards won't jinx you. One of the myths in Atlantic City and Las Vegas is that players who use their casino-issued gaming cards (see Secret Weapon box) to play the slots are at a disadvantage. As you may know, the cards are used to track your play, and then the casinos are able to offer you deals and discounts in order to keep you in the casino, and get you back to the gaming floor. The prevailing theory is that if you're doing too well at the slots, the machine and the card will recognize this, and your three cherries will turn into a bunch of blank spaces. Don't believe it. According to one casino executive, slots are always 100 percent random; if they weren't, these gaming meccas would quickly lose their licenses.

Use your player's card, no matter how little money you're gambling with. Even $100 poured into a slot machine will garner you freebies in the mail, from free meals to free money.

Bump your bet up at just the right moment. It's easy to rack up points for free meals, rooms, or entertainment on your casino card when you're playing the slots. It's much harder when you sit down at any of the gaming tables, like blackjack or poker. As a general rule, expect to have to play $25 hands for about four hours over the course of your trip to start to see the free offers come your way. There's a way to beat that system, according to one casino executive: Bump up your bets when you see the pit boss come around. His job is to track who's betting what. So if you're betting 10 bucks a hand, and you see the pen and pad coming your way, bump your bet. The higher the better. This way, it will appear you're a high roller when, in fact, you're just taking advantage of your good timing.

Negotiate your "comp" points. Casino executives won't ever tell you this, but it's possible to get casino points on your card just by asking. Virtually all casinos run their comp programs the same way: With frequent play, you accumulate "points" on your comp card, and your points are then converted to free perks. Well, mid- to top-level casino employees—basically, everyone in the casino who is not a dealer—have discretionary "banks" of points they can dole out to players. So if you're looking for a free room, it's worth asking the pit boss if he could spare some points for you. And after you get that free room? Lounge around and hit the nickel slots. They won't know what hit them. ◂

Family Outings
3 Savvy Ways to Make a Day with the Kids an Enjoyable Treat for All

Prep for the fest. Plopping your family into the midst of a daylong festival, carnival, or amusement park can be tricky indeed. Opportunities abound for the kids to get cranky and dispirited, all while money is flowing out of your wallet like a river of green. A little advance preparation will make all the difference:

- Get a map of the festival grounds and an event schedule in advance. Plot out strategies for parking, a walking route through the attractions, and top-priority activities. Make a mental note of the bathroom and food stall locations.

- If you're arriving at an amusement park right at opening time, make a beeline for a favorite ride at a part of the park that's farthest from the main entrance. You will be able to start the day by taking your favorite ride several times before any line at all builds up.

- If your chosen venue will allow it, pack along parent-approved snack foods and a bottle of water for each person. Because provisions are typically outrageously overpriced at festivals and amusement parks, this will seriously reduce the cost of the trip and will ensure that the day is not a complete nutritional disaster.

- Have a plan for killing small amounts of time. Take along books or small games to entertain the kids during waiting times—while standing in line, for instance, or to occupy five-year-old Susie while ten-year-old Zack gets to go on the roller coaster.

- Some valuable survival items to pack: hats, sunglasses, sunscreen, camera, a lightweight picnic blanket, disposable wipes, and a change of clothes.

Picky kids? Let them plan. Ever feel like you can do nothing right—in the minds of your kids, anyway? If choice of family activities is a constant sore point among your children, try this tactic: Let your kids plan the family outing once in a while. You can set broad parameters—budget, distance, time frame, and such—and leave the rest to your children to plot out. The planning will be a great life lesson for the kids, and if the outing is not completely to their liking, they will only have themselves to blame.

Take Harry Potter along for the ride. Anytime a family trip requires an hour or more of driving, you're confronted with the age-old quandary: how to entertain the kids. Books and puzzles will only take you so far. Same goes for cow-counting or license plate games. Giving them unlimited Game Boy time doesn't feel responsible. And just letting them scream and shout will give you a migraine. One of the best solutions around: books on tape. An engaging children's story will keep the kids quiet for hours on end. The story becomes a shared family experience—something you can all talk about over lunch. Best of all: Your local library has a mountain of recorded books that you have access to for free—enough variety to appeal to every taste, from Winnie the Pooh to Star Trek to Sherlock Holmes. ◁

Planning Your Trip

5 Things You Should Know About Getting the Best Travel Bargains

Go directly to the airline. There was a time not so long ago when, if you wanted to book a flight, you had two choices: Either book directly with the airline, or book through a travel agent. Then came the Internet, and airline pricing became a much more competitive game. Prices on Internet travel sites offer some pretty great deals, and now the airlines themselves have taken back the game. In many cases, the airlines can meet or beat the rates on the most popular websites. Always check those airline websites or to give them a call on their 800 numbers—you may be surprised.

World traveler? Talk to an agent. If you think all travel agents charge more for airline tickets than the airlines themselves, think again—especially when it comes to around-the-world travel. And while airline consortiums offer these tickets, it's almost always best to go through a third party. "For a myriad of complex reasons, you'll typically find the lowest rates for this type of travel through travel agents," says Edward Hasbrouck, author of *The Practical Nomad: How to Travel Around the World*. He says tickets purchased through airlines could be twice the price offered by travel agents who specialize in these global adventures. Hasbrouck says the main reason for this is the regulation of international airfares.

Talk the hotel manager's prices down. Here's something the big hotel chains will never advertise: You can negotiate with them. There's always someone in the hotel who is authorized to cut a deal, and doing so is easy. Just tell them you'd love to stay there, but their price is high and you'll probably end up staying somewhere else. If there are empty rooms in the hotel, you can bet you'll get a deal. Another surefire way to get a better rate is to ask, "Is there a lower rate I qualify for?" The hotel manager could, on the sly, give you the military rate, or the friends and family rate, or any other "special" rate he has. In the end, hotel managers prefer selling you a heavily discounted room to leaving it empty.

Know your ABCs. Hurricanes not only do major damage, but they also scare the heck out of tourists. So what to do? The best place for a Caribbean vacation are the ABC islands: namely, Aruba, Bonaire, and Curaçao. They all lie outside the path that hurricanes have been following for hundreds of years. So next time you book that summer getaway, be sure to sneak a peek at these less-traveled gems.

Buy now, visit Cinderella's Castle later. You know that a vacation to the Magic Kingdom is in your future, but you just haven't decided precisely when yet. A never-expiring pass might be just the ticket for you. A seven-day park-hopper pass costs about $250 (at the time of this writing) and expires after two weeks. But for an extra $75 or so, you can get a pass that doesn't expire. This is a good idea because it allows you to get some of your travel arrangements out of the way now; you can work on the scheduling later. Also, Disney ticket prices go up every single year. If you know you'll be heading down there eventually, you could spend now and save big later. ◁

Cabdrivers

Mark Zwick, one of the partners of PhillyTrips.com, takes at least four big trips a year to destinations all over the United States and Canada. You would think he'd go broke buying guidebooks, but he doesn't.

"I always depend on the taxi drivers," Zwick says. "They always know the places to go, the things to see."

As an added bonus, many taxi drivers work in tandem (and on the sly) with restaurants, bars, and nightclubs. Many times a taxi driver will have special coupons for his favorite places, and he'll be more than happy to let you have them. Why? Because he gets a kickback from the establishments.

So let those taxi drivers take you to some places where they get a little something extra, because most of the time you'll be getting something extra as well in the form of discounted meals or drinks.

Using the Web
6 Ways to "Net" a Great Trip by Making the Most of Travel Websites

Search solo even for a group. Airline search engines mess with your head a little when it comes to booking your family's travel. Consider: If you're booking a flight for you, your spouse, and your cousin Larry, you're going to type "3" when the site asks you how many tickets you want to buy. The truth is, sometimes you'll get a cheaper rate by booking seats individually, because single seats can easily go unsold (especially middle seats in the back of the plane). Airlines jump at the chance to get rid of them. See what happens when you book seats individually.

Discount airlines are not on big travel sites. The main travel websites like Expedia, Orbitz, and Travelocity

don't carry JetBlue or Southwest Airlines tickets in the U.S., or Zoom in Canada. Why? Those low-cost airlines never release their inventory to the online travel superstores. Quite frequently, their fares are less expensive than those of other carriers. No matter how many comprehensive travel sites you may visit, make sure you check their prices against those offered by JetBlue and Southwest or Zoom before you buy.

Trash your cookies. You're shopping for a flight on the Web and the flight prices seem to keep going up, not down. Why is that? Many Internet sites install "cookies" on your computer when you visit. A "cookie" is a collection of information that will almost certainly include your user name and the date and time you visited the site. Sometimes travel websites use this information to increase their prices if you repeatedly run the same searches for airlines or hotels. If you price a flight, and go back to the site a few hours later only to find that the price has increased, it's probably a cookie at work.

Before you buy a ticket, erase the cookies from your computer. This is easy—methods vary by browser, but you can usually do it by going to "Tools" at the top of your browser and selecting "Internet Options."

Check out this website for travel pros. So you've checked the airline for price quotes, done the requisite Internet searches at Orbitz, Expedia, Travelocity, and the rest, but still you remain unsatisfied with the selection and price. Out of luck? Not just yet. Check out www.itasoftware .com, a website used by travel agents, travel websites, and the airlines themselves. While you can't book your tickets through this site, it does offer lots of other benefits. You're allowed to choose where you fly from and where you're flying to just like the other sites, but you can also search airports up to 300 miles away from your destinations. In addition, you can see available flights on the days before or after your target dates. It's an awesome tool, too, if you're flying to three or more destinations. Here's an example: New York to Miami to Bangkok, Thailand, and back to New York. Within a minute, we found more than a dozen airline combos, ranging from $1,982 to $8,722.

Once you find the flights you need, booking is a snap. You simply click the "details" icon, which then gives you the flight numbers, booking codes, and fare codes for each flight on your itinerary. At this point, you simply call a travel agent—or call the airlines directly—with the information.

Find Disney savings online. The easiest way to save money on your trip to Disney World is to trim the price of those full-price park passes. Before you plan your trip, it's worth visiting a few Disney-centric discount websites, like www.themouseforless.com and www.mousesavers.com. These and other sites list discount coupons and codes for the Disney theme parks, hotels, cruises, and anything else Mickey-centric. They're at your fingertips with a few clicks of the, uh, mouse.

Sit where you want. Don't let those sneaky airlines put you in the middle seat of a three-seat row. You want to know where the *good* more-legroom, exit-row seats are? SeatGuru.com lists virtually all planes and their seating charts. What's more, with input from fellow travelers, the site tells you where *not* to sit—in other words, which ones have little legroom and are close to the bathroom. The site is an invaluable tool for anyone looking to fly. ◁

Bid—and Win!—with Priceline.com

If your departure city is within the U.S., Priceline.com is a great way to save some dough. Some folks may be intimidated by the "name your own price" gimmick. Here's how you can get the best deal from the site:

☐ As soon as you know what your travel plans are, go straight to www.biddingfortravel.com. This site has a very active online forum at which frequent travelers post their winning bids, and the hotels and neighborhoods with which they've had success. This is a mandatory visit before you bid on anything!

☐ When booking airline tickets, remember that Priceline can place you on any flight (3 a.m. *does* count!) during the 24-hour period of your departure date. For this reason alone, it's best to skip Priceline when booking short trips; you can easily lose two days in travel time.

☐ Booking hotels on Priceline is probably the site's most popular feature. To do so, you bid for a hotel and pick the section of the city and the star level you want. One caveat: If you don't get a hotel at the price you bid on, you can't bid again using the same parameters for 72 hours—you can only bid if you change your search criteria (neighborhood, star level, or price).

☐ A good rule of thumb for hotels: Check other online travel agents, find out how much that kind of hotel costs, subtract 20 percent, and use that figure as your bid on Priceline. You're virtually guaranteed a room.

☐ Car rentals are also a fantastic deal on Priceline. It's a rare day when a $20 bid won't get you an economy rental anywhere.

Airline Confidential
10 Special Ways to Score First-Class Savings, Seats, and More

Redeem your miles wa-a-a-y in advance. "Frequent-flier miles" is a misnomer. When the airlines make them almost impossible to use, they're more like infrequent-flier miles. Well, here's something the airlines won't be advertising anytime soon: They release their booking schedules a whopping 330 days in advance, according to Anne Banas, the editor in chief of www.smartertravel.com. So what does this mean? If you want to use your frequent-flier miles during a peak travel time—say, Christmas—you should start dialing up those airlines on Valentine's Day.

Mix and match airports. It's sometimes cheaper to take a return flight to a different airport than the one you flew out of. Try this little trick: Say, for example, you want to fly from Newark, New Jersey, to Los Angeles. Just for kicks, search for a return flight to a different airport in the region, such as JFK in New York. You'd be surprised to find that it's cheaper to fly back to a different airport than the one you took off from. (Of course, this plan doesn't work if you've parked your car at Newark.)

Get a first-class ticket on the cheap. Airlines don't exactly promote this fact, but it's possible to book a business-class or first-class ticket for the same price as a regular (not discount) coach seat. They're called Q-up, Y-up, or Z-up fares, and they all amount to first-class upgrades of coach fares, according to Laura Powell, a longtime travel journalist and expert. The fares were created by airlines to help business travelers, many of whom work for companies that don't allow them to buy first-class tickets. The website www.farecompare.com helps you search for these fare deals.

Change your ticket penalty-free. Airline employees would probably get in trouble if they ever admitted it, but know this: The fees you're charged when you have to change your airline ticket are negotiable. It happens to everyone— you have your travel arrangements all set, but something comes up, and you either have to add or subtract dates to your trip. So you call the airline, and you're hit with penalty fees, often well over $100 per ticket. Well, don't take it lying down, as the fees can be sliced, diced, and, if you're lucky, waived altogether.

Here's how you do it: When changing the ticket, simply ask the agent if it's possible the fees can be waived. The agent's first response will usually be "No." Ask to speak to the supervisor, and once you do, make your story a good one: Tell them your kid's got a dance recital that you just can't miss. Ask, be nice, and you might just get those tacked-on fees waived. It doesn't cost them anything to do this for you. But what's the airlines' motivation for doing this for you? In some cases, they make even more money if you're changing your ticket from a crowded flight to a less-crowded flight—they can sell that popular seat to someone else at a premium.

Don't settle for the first "bump" offer. You're on an oversold flight, and the gate agents are starting to tempt passengers with $100 in flight coupons if you'll agree to be "bumped" from your seat and take a later flight. Never accept the agents' first offer. What they're not telling you is that they have the discretion to give you even more money. Waiting patiently will be rewarded well during peak travel times, such as spring break or the Christmas holidays: Other travelers will be less likely to want to get bumped when Grandma (or a warm beach) is waiting for them. Make sure you get what's coming to you.

Bump yourself preemptively. If you want to reap the rewards of being bumped from your flight but the gate agents haven't made the offer yet, here's a way to make sure you get to the front

of the line. If you sense the flight is overbooked, go to the agent and offer to be bumped before any announcement is made. How can you tell if a flight is overbooked? One frequent traveler recommends that you observe the gate agents' body language. If they look harried, if there are weather problems at your destination or at the airport from which you're departing, or if there seem to be a lot of people milling about, it's a good time to start the bumping process.

Ask for a free lunch. Who says you can't get a free meal nowadays? Airlines don't advertise this, but if you've been bumped from a flight, you can usually get a meal out of the carrier. As you're being bumped, ask the gate agent if she'll give you some food vouchers so that you can eat while you wait. Most of the time, the gate agents will give you and your party up to $25 in vouchers. These vouchers will be honored at any restaurant n the airport. Not a bad deal for a few hours' wait.

Upgrade your flight experience.
It's every traveler's dream: You buy a discounted coach ticket, ask at the gate if you can be upgraded, and before you know it, you're in a big, comfy seat with a flute of champagne in your hand. Stop dreaming—it's not going to happen that way. But if you're willing to spend a little extra money, it's worth asking the agent to "split the difference" on the price of the first-class ticket. If first class isn't booked, which usually happens on less-traveled routes on off-peak travel days, the agent has some discretion when it comes to moving people into first class. Some airlines also let you use your frequent-flier miles to "purchase" an upgrade.

Get your problem solved *after* **takeoff.** Airlines want you to have a pleasant flight—not because they care about you, but because they don't want you ruining the flight for everyone else. They don't want any part of bad word of mouth. So how does this help you? Once you're on the plane, and once the plane is in the air, it becomes a thousand percent easier to get what you want. Bad seat? Noisy neighbor? The person known as the chief purser can handle all these annoyances. The pilot may be the one flying the plane, but the chief purser is the person running all the other aspects of the flight. Get the

WHAT **AIRLINES** DON'T WANT YOU TO KNOW ABOUT Frequent-Flier Miles

Have you ever tried to cash in your frequent-flier miles? It's nearly impossible sometimes. Here are some secrets that your mileage program may not tell you:

☐ Not all flights allow you to use miles for reward travel. Don't even bother trying to redeem miles during high season to top destinations. Some airlines are now being more up-front about these blackout dates, and are listing them on their websites.

☐ It's easier to use your miles for upgrades on tickets you've already purchased than on free tickets.

☐ If you have frequent-flier miles on an airline that is either in bankruptcy or headed that way, use those miles quickly. Even if the carrier goes out of business before your flight, it may still honor the tickets you "bought" with your miles.

☐ Call the airline directly if there's a specific flight for which you want to redeem miles—even if the airline has already said you can't use your miles on that flight. If the day of the flight draws nearer and the plane isn't near capacity, the airline may let you cash your miles in.

chief purser's attention—it's his or her job to make sure you're happy.

Let's say you had a horrible experience at the gate. Let the chief purser know. He may offer you a free drink, or food from the first-class menu. He might even offer you an upgrade into first class. "It's important to speak with reason and not look like an air rage customer," one former chief purser said. The longer the flight, the better chance you have of getting moved into first class or business class. (Having an angry customer on board for a two-hour flight is annoying, but having an angry customer for a 14-hour overseas flight is a nightmare for the chief purser.) Ask nicely, explain your situation, and don't be surprised if you end up with more legroom and a filet mignon.

Spill something and get a better seat.
Have you ever been stuck with a bad airline seat? Maybe it's next to the bathroom, or next to a screaming baby, or next to a particularly chatty seatmate. How can you escape? "Accidentally" spill something onto your seat. As long as there's another open seat somewhere on the plane, you will be moved. If you don't want to do this, complain about something—anything—that is wrong with your seat. Maybe the headphone jack is loose, or the tray table is shaky. Complain nicely and the flight staff will do their best to accommodate you. ◂

Cruise Control
4 Steps to an Inexpensive, Hassle-Free Sail on a Cruise Liner

Stick to one cruise line. All cruise lines have loyalty programs, and the more you vacation with one company, the better the perks will get—they could be anything from $100 cruise vouchers to private cocktail parties or free bottles of wine. In addition, once you prove that you're a loyal customer, many of the big lines will allow you to skip from brand to brand within the same company and still retain your standing in their frequent-cruiser program. For instance, Royal Caribbean and Celebrity are part of the same corporate structure; once you're a return customer at one, ask if you can use your loyalty points on the other line. Chances are, you can.

Get a group together. Want a free cruise? It's easy. On virtually all major cruise ships, if you can get eight other cabins booked, the ninth one is free. And that one, of course, would be yours. Keep in mind that you don't necessarily need to know the other people in your

---

Learn the Advantages of Touring by Train

EXPERT **INSTANT** ADVICE

While traveling by train in North America is not the most popular choice, it's the way to go when traveling abroad, especially in Europe. If you really want to become an expert at this type of travel, you must go to www.seat61.com. It's the most comprehensive site out there when it comes to trains the world over. Don't board without first checking it out.

Wrinkle Spray

Hotels are more than willing to charge guests an arm and a leg for the dry-cleaning service to revive suitcase-squashed clothing. A relatively new product called wrinkle-release spray is an inexpensive solution to hotel laundering. You just hang up your clothing, spray it, smooth out the wrinkles with your hands, and let it air-dry. Several brands are available, including Wrinkle Free, Austin House, and Downy. Look for them in the laundry products section. Or you can try making your own by mixing 1 tablespoon of fabric softener and 1/4 cup of unscented rubbing alcohol with 1 cup of distilled water. Put it in a travel spray bottle and gently mist the garment about a hand's length away.

group. Hang an ad in your church, at the local gym, or anywhere people congregate. Maybe you'll get lucky and get a group together. At worst, maybe you'll make a friend or two.

Haggle with your travel agent. Most people book their cruises either through websites or travel agents. Here's a significant fact that may change the way you book your next cruise: The cruise lines are getting more and more inflexible with their pricing. In the past, cruise lines would quote their prices to travel agents, and the agents would be able to work within a set of parameters. For example, a cruise line would tell a travel agent that a particular cruise should cost between $2,000 and $2,500. Travel agents would be able to negotiate prices with their clients. Now, cruise lines tell agents exactly how much a cruise costs.

Any rebate your travel agent is offering you is coming straight out of her commission. "Cruises don't rebate on their product anymore," says Sheila Gawel, the owner of GalaxSea Cruises and Travel in Toms River, New Jersey. "They believe they have a good product, and they choose a price and stick with it."

What does this mean for the cruise consumer? Well, no matter where you go to book your cruise, the price of the cruise will remain constant—it's the commission fees that will change. So while you can't easily negotiate prices with the cruise lines or websites, you can certainly negotiate prices with your travel agent. Commissions on cruises are normally 10 to 20 percent of the price of the cruise; when you speak to your agent, tell him you want a deal, or you'll go home and book the cruise on your computer.

If there's a problem, just tell someone. Cruise ships have the best customer service you'll find anywhere in the travel industry, according to one veteran of the business. The reasoning is simple: There is plenty of competition for your cruise dollar, and bad word of mouth can sink a ship. So if you ever find anything not to your liking while on board, be sure to speak up. You will be taken care of. Don't like the people at your table? Speak up. Is your cabin too close to the disco? Dance on over to someone in charge. Any problems you encounter are worth discussing with cruise personnel. ◁

Business Travel
4 Tricks for Taking Drudgery and Mishaps Out of Work-Related Trips

Get a practical lightweight carrier. Yes, a leather briefcase looks dapper and professional. However, it's not the most practical piece of luggage when you have to walk several city blocks or a mile of airport corridors. The conventional briefcase is heavy, it's not designed to accommodate the items a modern businessperson needs to carry, and the weight imbalance it creates on your body will wreck your shoulders over time. Instead, buy a bag that is designed to hold your laptop (including an envelope of padding), has pockets for your cell phone and chargers, and can accommodate a change of clothes and a file folder or two. Make sure it's lightweight and—most important—has two backpack-style shoulder straps as well as a handle.

Carry on your laptop. On the upcoming flight, you think you won't need your laptop computer. So why not just wrap some cushy clothing around it and stick it into your checked luggage? That's a bad move, say seasoned business travelers. You not only increase the chances that it might go astray for a few days, but baggage-handling systems have perfected laptop-smashing to a fine art. It may add weight and bulk to your carry-on, but that inconvenience is nothing compared to the hassle of replacing your computer.

Change for a long flight. Aren't you tired of getting off an airplane after several hours and realizing that your suit and dress shirt or blouse look like you've slept in them—because you *did* sleep in them? The solution is to pack a pair of long, lightweight workout pants and a T-shirt in your carry-on luggage. When you get on the plane, change into these informal clothes and put your dress clothes on a hanger. Near the end of the flight, change back again—your clothes will look crisp and clean.

Tame those receipts. Visit an office supply store and buy a small organizer "wallet" about the size of a legal envelope—one with several dividers inside. Make this a staple in your luggage for organizing business receipts. During the day, just stuff all receipts for business-related expenses into the same place—a jacket pocket, for instance. Every night at your hotel, put the day's receipts into the compartments within the organizer, sorted by the categories required by your employer. At the end of your trip, filling out the expense sheet will be a breeze. ◁

SECRET WEAPON
Ethernet Cable

Just about any hotel today will tell you it offers wireless Internet access, and many say they also have Ethernet cables in every room if you prefer a direct hookup. The sad truth is that the quality and reliability of wireless connections vary widely from one hotel to another, and Ethernet cables disappear from hotel rooms as quickly as those little shampoo bottles. In self-defense, drop by a computer or electronics store and buy your own Ethernet cable. Never again will you get caught in your pajamas at night, unable to access your e-mail.

Resorts and Hotels
4 Savvy Ways to Make Your Visit Less Costly and More Enjoyable

Watch those "resort fees." You shopped around for your vacation hotel—maybe even used a bidding website such as Priceline.com. But when you get to the registration counter, you find out that you will be charged an extra $10 to $15 per day as a "resort fee," supposedly to cover such amenities as the swimming pool and fitness club. This is nothing but a ruse to make a hotel's rates appear lower at the time you are scouting for a room, say industry insiders. The hotel knows that by the time you arrive, fatigued from travel and dragging your luggage and kids along, there's no way you're going to refuse your hotel room because of an add-on fee. So at the time of booking, scan the fine print of your agreement and ask the hotel about any fees that are not included in the quote. If you're surprised by such fees at the registration counter, call your credit card company after checking in and ask it to get the fee waived.

Skip resort-area crowds. If you have decided to vacation in a highly touted resort area, here's a rule of thumb from travel insiders: Schedule your vacation for less popular times of the year. For instance, in central Florida—theme park center of the universe—skip the conventional summer season, as well as the holidays and spring break. Mark your calendar for sometime between the end of August and the middle of December, or from January to the middle of February. You will find the traffic, crowds, and line waits markedly reduced—and you'll save a bundle with the off-season rates as well.

Don't get soaked ordering drinks. You might not want to sound like a penny-pinching weenie every time you place an order during your travels, but never assume that prices will be within some range that you have fixed in your mind. At a resort-town restaurant your repeat business might not be important to the management. One tourist reports that a waiter offered the "helpful" suggestion that his group buy margaritas by the pitcher. Later they were flabbergasted to be billed $35 per pitcher—and they had consumed two! Even if the waiter suggests water, make it clear that you're looking for a glass of tap water (free) as opposed to a bottle of water.

Get your government briefing. Your resort may have that safe-and-secure look that you are accustomed to back home, but that could be an illusion. Before you jump on an airliner to that idyllic foreign vacation spot, if you're American, check the U.S. State Department's travel website, www.travel.state.gov. Click on the "Consular Information Sheet" for your destination, print it out, and take it with you. If you are Canadian, go to the Department of Foreign Affairs, Consular Affairs, Information and Assistance for Canadians Abroad (www.voyage.gc.ca). Both sites provide a wealth of information about your destination. Pay particular attention to the security, safety, and crime passages, and heed the warnings you find there—carrying a minimum of cash, for instance, not taking rides with strangers, locking all hotel doors, and using the hotel safe for valuables and documents. ◁

Money on the Road

3 Strategies for Getting the Best Transaction Deals When You Go Abroad

Play your bank cards right. If you have been faithfully ordering traveler's checks every time you hit the road, give up the habit. These days, ATMs are far easier to use. But having a bank card already in your wallet does not mean you are ready to fly overseas. A tiny bit of homework will make the handling of money during your trip go much more smoothly:

- The most economical way to manage money in a foreign country will probably be withdrawing currency from local ATMs as needed with a bank card. But be sure to ask your bank in advance what fees are charged for international transactions. There could be a flat fee, as much as a few dollars per transaction, and it may also charge a percentage point or two for converting the currency. To lower the impact of a significant flat fee, make larger, less frequent withdrawals during your trip.

- Ask your bank of it has a no-fee arrangement for ATM withdrawals from certain banks at your destination. If so, gravitate toward those automatic tellers during your travels.

- Keypads on North American ATMs have letters as well as numbers, which some people use to help them remember their PIN. The ATMs in many other countries have numbers only, so be sure you know your PIN in numeral form before leaving.

- Tell your bank roughly when and where you will be traveling. (Your credit card company, too, for that matter.) You don't want a security-conscious banker freezing your account because a computer tags some unusual transactions.

- Ask your bank if there's a limit on the number of ATM withdrawals you can make during any one day. You don't want to get stuck with an empty wallet because you have "been to the well" too many times.

- Take a backup bank card with you, and keep it in a separate place. You won't get stranded if your original card gets demagnetized. Of course, if you are a couple and each has a bank card, you have an automatic backup.

Trim those transaction fees. Some popular credit card companies tack on as much as three percent in foreign transaction fees. Before you depart on an overseas trip, shop around for a card that offers low fees or even no fees on purchases you make in foreign countries. Make sure it's a card that's commonly accepted in the country you intend to visit.

Don't pay in dollars. Oh, those friendly overseas merchants! Many stores in destinations that are popular with North Americans obligingly post two different prices on products—a price in the local currency and a price in U.S. dollars. Here's the catch: The price posted in U.S. dollars is typically a few percentage points more expensive for you than the going exchange rate. So decline to have your merchandise rung up in dollars. Either pay cash in the local currency, or charge it on your credit card—which, if you followed our advice above, will automatically do the conversion at a much more friendly rate. ◄

Early Schooling

5 Strategies for Helping Your Child Develop the Skills to Succeed in School and After

Start good habits early. We hear all the time from parents of high schoolers that they still have to get on their teenagers to do their homework. Sheesh. What are these parents going to do—go to college with their kids? First grade is the time to start setting the habits that will stay with your child through graduate school. From the moment said child walks in the door after school, have a routine in place that rarely, if ever, varies. A cuddle, a conversation about school, a small snack, and then homework. Only after homework is complete can video games, soccer practice, and other activities occur.

Create the right work space. You wouldn't do your work at the kitchen table, so why should your kids? Set them up with a dedicated space to do their homework and studying, says former New Jersey teacher of the year Tom Kraeutler, who now hosts the nationally syndicated radio show *The Money Pit*. You don't have to spend big bucks at those teacher specialty stores, he says. You can pick up a desk and chairs secondhand, and the rest of the accoutrements at big-box discount stores and home improvement stores. Your shopping list should include track lighting with halogen bulbs or overhead can lights to complement the ambient lighting found in most homes, a storage center, and a dry erase board and bulletin board to enhance visual learning. Choose a dedicated spot that is a different space from where your kids play video games or watch TV, so they learn to associate that space with learning, not entertainment. Also make sure there's adequate airflow and proper temperature to keep the space comfortable.

Keep a file of accomplishments. Beginning in middle school, make a file and label it with your child's name, suggests Annette Riffle, general manager of Kaplan Premier Private Tutoring programs. Start saving all your child's good work (projects, essays, artwork) in this portfolio, and also use it to keep track of all extracurricular activities, awards, volunteer activities, and accomplishments. Also maintain a list of teachers and other adults in your child's life you can call on for recommendations.

Help your kid conquer tests. As a parent of a school-age child, you'd like nothing more than to go into that classroom on Fridays and take your fourth-grader's spelling test for her. Or your eighth-grader's algebra quiz. Get over it! Your job is to raise independent children capable of standing on their own—and taking tests on their own. That doesn't mean, however, that you can't help with tests:

- Make a test calendar. Every Monday, list all of the tests for the following week. Then with your child's help, develop a study schedule—including all reading assignments—so he's not freaking out the night before.

- Speaking of freaking out—don't do it in front of your kid. The cooler you stay about impending tests, the cooler she'll stay. Focus on the fact that it isn't the grade that's important, it's knowing she did her very best.

- Send your child to bed an hour early the night before the test. Sleep is one of the best tools available to

Evaluating a School—Beyond Test Scores

You've just been transferred halfway across the country, and before you can even think of looking for a house, you have to find the best school district. Forget about test scores, says Eileen Gale Kugler, author of *Debunking the Middle-Class Myth: Why Diverse Schools Are Good for All Kids.* Instead, focus on:

- **The school's overall tone.** For instance, do the educational leaders publicly and privately champion the value of diversity? Do students work on a wide range of topics visible throughout the school? Do students coexist in tension or have they become one community celebrating their diversity?

- **The staff's expectations of students.** What do the principal and teachers expect from the kids? Does the curriculum provide challenge for all students? Are there targeted initiatives aimed at reducing barriers to achievement and decreasing the achievement gap? Are students of color well represented in enrichment activities and rigorous classes?

- **The teachers' active participation.** Do teachers collaborate across grades and across the curriculum? Are they given the opportunity to take part in relevant professional development opportunities? Are they part of collaborative decision-making bodies at the school level and district-wide?

- **The school's resources.** Are there enough books and school supplies? Do teachers have to pay for their own supplies? Are parents and community members motivated to donate time and materials, and are these used in a coherent way that meets the goals of the school?

- **The school's relation to the community.** Is the school a focal point of the neighborhood? Do parents and community members feel welcomed as collaborative partners in the school's success? Does the school use innovative outreach strategies to partner with parents of diverse backgrounds? Does the school have vibrant partnerships with community and business organizations?

consolidate learning and hard-wire it into memory.

- Fix a good breakfast the morning of the test. That doesn't mean a sugary cereal that will leave your child groggy and light-headed just as the teacher hands out the work sheets. Fix something like whole-grain toast with cheese and a piece of fruit. The fiber in the fruit and bread, along with the protein and fat in the cheese, slows stomach emptying and helps maintain steady blood sugar levels.

- When your child brings the test home, go over the test with him so you can both see what he did right and wrong. Then focus on those areas when it's time for the next test.

Be alert to subtle warning signs. Sometimes you really can't be sure how well your kid is doing at school, especially at a new school or the beginning of a new year before you have had any parent-teacher meetings or received a report card. And you know if you ask your child how things are going, you'll get the standard reply: "All right." But there can be subtle signs that trouble is brewing, and the earlier you are clued in on the potential trouble, the sooner you can try to do something about it. Keep an ear out for how your child describes teachers and courses. A statement that he "hates" a certain teacher or that the teacher is going too fast or gives homework that's too hard may indicate your child is having trouble with the subject and may need a little extra help from you. But be leery of contacting the teacher directly without your child's okay; he may resent your interference, especially if he is in middle school or above. And your whole effort could backfire, because he'll hate the teacher and the subject even more. ◄

Getting Into College
9 Ways to Get an Inside Track on the College Admissions Process

Start gathering recommendations in middle school. Every time your child connects with a mentor or teacher, ask for a letter of recommendation at the end of the school year. That eighth-grade drama coach will write a much more passionate letter just after the play closes than four years later, when your kid is applying to drama school. Your portfolio of recommendations will come in handy for both the admissions and the scholarship processes.

Start looking early. Your sophomore year of high school isn't too soon to begin exploring colleges, says Deborah Spinney, executive director for student development at the University of Indianapolis in Indiana. So get out from behind the video game controls and start attending college fairs, requesting literature from places of interest, and doing some online investigating. Don't feel pressure to make decisions, she says. Just gather as much information as possible to begin getting a sense of your preferences.

Create a timetable with deadlines. Many high school seniors move slower than the federal government when it comes to completing the plethora of forms involved in college applications. Instead, Kaplan Test Prep and Admissions consultant Joan M. Pagano recommends creating a timeline in your child's junior year that includes deadlines for everything from applying to take the SAT (twice) or other admissions tests to submitting a list of supplies needed for freshman year. Link rewards (or punishments) to each deadline. For instance, if your kid meets every deadline through December of senior year, he gets a laptop computer for college. If the "assignment" is due Friday and the kid is late, he loses the use of the car for the weekend. Not only will the tasks get done, but you'll be teaching your child the valuable time management and responsibility skills he needs in college.

Do a few extracurricular activities well. If you're a high school student interested in lining up a good résumé for your college applications, limit your extracurricular activities. That's right—limit them. The majority of college admissions officials say a long list of extracurricular activities is of little or moderate interest to them. They would rather see you specialize in two or three outside activities, do them well, and exhibit leadership and commitment. So focus yourself and go deep. You'll also wind up with more energy for your studies.

Work toward your future. If you already know what you want to do after college, get a head start in high school. For instance, planning to become an architect? Make sure the college admissions staff knows you spent your summer working construction, learning how to build a house from inside out.

Do community volunteer work. Top of your class, president of the student council association, and founder of the French club isn't enough. Today's admissions officers want to see a good measure of community service on your résumé. So volunteer at a soup kitchen, become an aide at a nursing home, offer to become a Big Brother or Big

Sister. Not only does it demonstrate that you're an active and responsible citizen, but volunteering exposes you to different peoples, cultures, and organizations in your community.

Don't get sticker shock over high fees. Sure, college in most parts of the U.S. is going to cost some bucks. But those enormous price tags that schools like to wave around on their websites and in brochures—$30,000 a year, $40,000 a year, etc. etc.—are about as realistic as the pricing in a used-car lot. "Students almost never pay that sticker price," says Spinney. Financial aid and other arrangements will make whatever college you choose to attend much more affordable than you think.

Go beyond the campus tour. Visiting colleges is fun, but if all you see of the campus is what the goody-goody in the suit and tie wants to show you, then you're not getting a real sense of what life is like there. Arrange to sit in on a couple of classes in your area of interest, schedule an interview with a professor, go have lunch in the student cafeteria and get kids to tell you what life's really like there. Most admissions offices will even arrange for you to spend a night in the dorms.

Factor in a possible change in interests. You might be 100 percent positive that you're going to be a pre-med major in college, but people change, and nowhere will you change more than during the first year or two at college. So don't choose a college based on your probable major, says Spinney. Instead, make sure the school has strong programs in three or four areas that appeal to you. ◄

LEARNING THE ART OF *SAT* Preparation

Given that the class of 2006 posted the sharpest drop in SAT scores in 31 years, it's clear that there's trouble in test-taking paradise. Joe Jewell—a Rhodes scholar who scored a perfect 1600 on his SATs, was a contributing editor for the book *Up Your Score: The Underground Guide to the SAT*, and is cofounder of prepme.com—offers this advice for SAT takers.

Be comfortable with your calculator

SAT day is not the day to first try out that fancy graphing calculator. Plus, there's nothing on the test that requires anything more than a simple four-function calculator, so stick with the one you use every day in school.

Keep a vocabulary journal

Create a running list of words during your sophomore and junior year. Put three new words on it a day and memorize those words. That's 1,000 new words in a year! Make sure you reinforce the old vocabulary with a monthly review, and try using these new words in conversations with your parents and teachers and in school essays. The more you use the words, the more likely you are to remember them on test day.

Don't practice in the ideal test-taking environment

How will you react on test day if the kid behind you keeps kicking your chair? If the room is too hot? If you didn't get enough sleep the night before? Simulate distractions when you're taking practice tests so you can focus no matter what's happening around you. Try taking practice SATs in a coffee shop or anywhere else with ambient noise. Do this enough and nothing will distract you come test day.

Guess for success

Most questions have one or two answers that are obviously wrong. Eliminate those and then guess from the remaining choices. Don't leave any questions blank, particularly if you can rule out even one answer.

Don't be creative on the essay

Graders score hundreds of essays and scan your essay looking for the same elements: a basic four- or five-paragraph essay with a thesis, topic sentences, specific details and evidence, and a conclusion that restates your thesis. Make sure everything in your essay ties back to the thesis and supports it with evidence.

Paying for College

11 Tricks for Getting Financial Aid When You Head Off to the Halls of Ivy

Grab up local scholarship dollars. When you hear about a national-level $40,000 scholarship, sure, your eyes are going to light up. But you'll shock all the other students and parents when you stack up the mountain of cash from this secret—gleaned from the most successful scholarship hunters: Students can quickly accumulate a six-figure educational nest egg by approaching all of the clubs, community organizations, and businesses right in their vicinity. It's much easier to snatch up $1,500 here and $2,000 there from nearby organizations where there's less competition and a local student is more likely to be a standout.

Search beyond the Web. Every prospective college student on the planet knows to scour the Internet for scholarship dollars. Which means that there will be enormous competition for any scholarships you find there. By all means go after that money. However, while the masses are fighting it out, you'll be scooping up tuition money more quickly if you mine sources that aren't so well publicized. Ask for the financial reference books at your local public library. These are big, fat books full of scholarship opportunities offered by groups that couldn't care less about publicizing themselves on the Internet.

Move fast to apply early. You know the old saying—"The early bird ... " Well, it's especially true when it comes to financial aid, says college planning specialist Alisa LeSueur. For instance, you can submit the Free Application for Federal Student Aid (FAFSA) required for government and private funding as early as January 1 of your child's senior year in high school.

Be wary of school-aid consultants. Paying a financial aid consultant may be a waste of money better spent on college expenses, says Francine Jackson, director of financial aid at Harrisburg University of Science and Technology in Pennsylvania. "There are a lot of scams out there that prey upon families seeking financial support to pay for college," she says. Instead, she recommends that students build relationships with the financial aid professionals at the university to which they've been accepted to ensure

Getting Scholarships for Your Kid

Here's advice for landing free money for your child's college education, provided by Alisa LeSueur, a certified college planning specialist based in San Antonio, Texas.

- College scholarships are available for children as young as six! Meaning, it's never too soon to start.

- Use the Internet for free resources. A good one: weeklyscholarshipalert.org. But limit the personal information you provide. Some sites sell this information for mailing lists.

- Read the small print. Parents often miss eligibility information on scholarship applications, meaning they miss out on the money.

- Meet the deadline! 'Nuff said.

- If there's an essay or art project required, ask to see what past winners submitted. This tells you what the judges are looking for.

- Look in the local paper for scholarship announcements. Then get the application so you can apply for your kid next year.

- Don't give up! There are thousands of scholarships, and you can't win them all.

they're receiving the funding they're entitled to. Be especially cautious about agencies and consultants that guarantee any specific level of scholarships and those that charge fees. A more legitimate arrangement is a consultant whose fee is a percentage of the aid he helps your child obtain.

Don't overreport your financial status. You know how lawyers tell their clients to just answer yes or no when they're on the witness stand? Well, that's what we're telling you when it comes to completing financial aid forms. If they

don't ask about your mother's antique jewelry, don't tell them! Just identify and report the value of the assets you're required to.

Submit an addendum. While you shouldn't reveal assets you don't have to, you *should* reveal hardships *not* requested on financial aid forms, says LeSueur. For instance, if you just got hit with $100,000 in medical expenses for your wife's breast cancer treatment, say so. Ditto if you're funding four college educations at the same time—including one medical school stint. Just make sure you have the documentation to back it up.

Refile every year. You may think your situation hasn't changed, but even a small increase in debt or reduction in assets can make a big difference. So resubmit your financial aid forms every year. And check the date on the financial aid form to make sure you're using the right one; they change every year.

Keep claiming your kid on your taxes. If you stopped claiming your child as a dependent on your income tax form in the hope you'll get more financial aid, you've just left hundreds of dollars sitting on the table. "Many parents are under the incorrect impression that their income and assets will not be considered in the financial aid calculations if they stop claiming their student on their tax return," says LeSueur, but that's simply not true. The only way children are considered independent in terms of financial aid eligibility is if they're married, have a dependent child of their own, are 24 or older, are in or have been in the armed services, are orphans or wards of the court, or are graduate students.

Early decision can mean less aid.
If you need help paying for college, stay away from the "early decision" admissions process. This is the system in which a university will admit a student months before the rest of the crowd is considered. Yes, this gives the student a better shot at the university he or she most wants to attend. However, you're also making that admissions officer's eyes sparkle: By committing to that one college, you're tipping your hand. Early admission students typically get lower amounts of financial assistance because there's no need for the college to woo them.

Never go "off-season" in your sport. If you're a student hoping to get an athletic scholarship, don't wait until your sport's season to play. Get involved throughout the year—in sporting camps and intramural leagues. Whether you coach younger athletes or participate in a traveling league, the year-round training will show your dedication to the sport and pay off with improved skills too.

Land an inside job at college.
If you're working your way through college, you might as well have a job that dumps bucketloads of cash in your lap rather than a trifling hourly wage. Colleges that offer their students work-study programs get low-cost student labor to help with office work or running the front desk at dorms. What the insiders aren't telling you is this: If you have any choice in the matter, snap up that job in the financial aid office. You'll get a great overview of how the entire tuition-funding system works and you'll get early notice of any scholarship opportunities. You'll have a definite edge over anyone else. ◁|

WHAT KAPLAN DOESN'T WANT YOU TO KNOW ABOUT SAT Prep

The SAT—formerly called the Scholastic Aptitude Test—is an often scary fact of life for students applying to colleges in the United States. Scoring well on it can give you an extra edge when it comes to getting into the school of your choice. Tutors and test-prep courses want you to pay as much as $900 for six weeks of practice sessions. But you can prepare for the SAT free of charge: Just go to www.collegeboard.com, the College Board's official website, and you can take a free, full-length practice test, and receive a free skills report and a detailed explanation of all the test questions. If you want more practice, the College Board also offers a four-month self-study course online for $70, much less than Kaplan or Princeton Review.

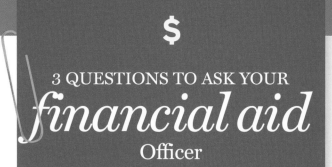

3 QUESTIONS TO ASK YOUR
financial aid
Officer

Sure, it was nice of your financial aid office to recommend a student loan company, but what's in it for them? To make sure you're getting the best deal, ask the financial aid officer the following questions, says Raza Khan, president and CEO of the student loan company MyRichUncle (myrichuncle.com).

1 Which loan company offers the lowest rate?

When the financial aid official recommends a certain lender, it doesn't necessarily mean that that lender is offering the lowest rate.

2 Are you making any money from this loan?

Just as Realtors get a cut when they refer you to a mortgage company, so, too, do some financial aid offices when they refer you to a specific lender. It can come several ways:

- Revenue sharing. The office gets a percentage of any profits made from the loan.

- School-as-lender. The school gets a percentage of the profit made when federal Stafford or PLUS loans are sold to lenders.

- Override pools. The financial aid office gets a portion of the profit from your loan to use to pay for other students' tuition. Why should you be paying for other students? Get a lower rate instead.

- Old-fashioned kickbacks. These are just what they sound like: cash or gifts given to school officials for referring the lender to you. Khan says she saw some financial aid administrators receiving digital music players, DVD players, gift certificates, and designer briefcases at the 2006 National Association of Student Financial Aid Administrators conference. Just as fancy dinners and Caribbean cruises were often used by the pharmaceutical industry to influence doctors to prescribe certain drugs, these gifts can influence which lenders make it onto a college's preferred lender list.

3 How did you choose this list of lenders?

Why *these* lenders and not others? And are you prohibited from going outside this list to find your own lender? If the financial aid office won't give you copies of any "agreements" between the school and lenders, then something fishy is going on.

Succeeding on Campus
6 Easy Ways to Get Ahead at College Both Academically and Socially

Go with debit, not credit. More than half of all college students have at least one credit card billed to them, according to the American Council on Education, and about 40 percent carry a balance from month to month. Since you're likely graduating with student loans to repay, why would you also want to be saddled with credit card debt at 18 percent or higher interest? Here's an easy way to avoid it. You need to establish credit in your own name, so go ahead and get a card. Then use it once for a purchase, pay off the bill immediately, and cut up the credit card. At the same time, get a debit card that looks like (but doesn't act like) a credit card. In other words, you can't spend more than you have in your checking account. Just make sure you track your debit expenses, or you'll find yourself paying some hefty fines in overcharges to the bank.

Check out student housing in person. Before you request the residence hall with 12 rooms over the suite-like dorms, take a tour. Talk to students currently living there about the pros and cons of the living arrangement and the type of students who tend to choose that particular living arrangement. (Jocks? Brains? Frat boys?) Will you absolutely die of embarrassment if you don't have a private bathroom? Do you want to be stuck in the dorm for meals too? Is a single-gender dorm important to you? Do you want the new dorm with the air conditioning or the old dorm with the fireplace? The more carefully you think through these issues the happier you'll be, says Harlan Cohen, author of *The*

Naked Roommate: And 107 Other Issues You Might Run Into in College.

Talk to your roommate *before* September. Most middle-class kids today have never shared a room—until they hit college. So the idea of living with someone else's mess, smells, and personality in a room the size of your closet back home can be, well, quite disconcerting. Never fear! Here's advice for future roommates from Matthew Paul Turner, author of *Everything You Need to Know Before College:*

- Try to meet in person if possible. If that's not possible before school starts, set up a phone call, *not* an instant messaging conversation. Talking is important here, because you're going to be discussing some important issues.

- Have a conversation about cleanliness. If you dust every afternoon and your roomie only changes his underwear every week, there will be problems. Find out now so you can switch before school starts.

- Only share the big stuff. Initially, you might think you should go halfsies on everything in the room—from comforters to pillows and bookshelves. Don't bother. You may never see this person after the first year—or even the first month. Instead, just split the cost of the big items, such as the TV, the refrigerator, and the microwave, and keep the receipts. If you split up, it's easy enough for one of you to buy the other out.

- Decide up-front about sleepovers. If you're fundamentally opposed to premarital sex and your potential roommate has a very involved boyfriend who will be visiting every weekend—and staying in your room—now is the time to either set parameters or switch roommates.

Get to school early on check-in day.
If you want the best closet, the best bed, the desk near the window, and the dresser near your side of the room, get there first, recommends college-life author Harlan Cohen. Your best bet? Stay in a hotel near campus the night before, so you're first in line when check-in starts.

Try the A student's playbook.
Those competitive students running around with perfect 4.0 grade point averages have a handful of test-taking secrets that they would just as soon keep to themselves. You already know to do the reading and the homework, review the class materials regularly, and to get plenty of sleep the night before the exam. But here are some techniques that separate the A students from the other kind:

- If you're going to skip the occasional class, that's your business. But always attend the class that's just before a test as well as review sessions (if they're at another time). This is when you'll get the best hints about the content of the test. Always ask the instructor to get as specific as possible about the material that will be covered.

- Always find out whether answering incorrectly is any worse than not answering at all. If they're the same, you might as well guess when you have to.

- Eat a light meal or snack before the test so you'll have energy and be able to keep your eyes open. Avoid heavy food.

- Take a watch to help you pace yourself. As soon as you receive your test, scan through it quickly and plot out how much time you will devote to each section.

- Give first priority to the easy questions and those that will earn you the most points.

- Don't let any question bog you down. Skip it for the moment and see if anything else in the test provides helpful information.

- After the test, listen carefully as the instructor reviews the answers. This will give you valuable insight about what the instructor will want on the next test.

SECRET WEAPON

Open Door

Okay, so you're getting along great with your roommate. What about the rest of the dorm? If you want to make friends you'll have for life, leave your dorm door open, says author Harlan Cohen. Other students will be more willing to stop by if there's no barrier that suggests "Don't bother me."

Parents, learn to let go. There's a new phrase circulating among college administrators: "helicopter parents," those who swoop in whenever their kid needs a helping hand. Well, it's time to turn off the engines, Mom and Dad. Instead, follow this advice from Rodger Summers, vice president for student affairs at Binghamton University in Binghamton, New York:

- Don't call the president of the college or university!

- Acknowledge your own feelings about your child leaving and address them, either on your own or with a trained therapist.

- Be familiar with the university resources available and where your child can get help, as well as where you can find answers.

- Keep all contact information and resource material in your night table drawer or in a central location.

- Support and demand degrees of independence from your student. Remember: At age 18, your student is an adult.

- Develop expectations for communication and talk about them before your child leaves home.

- Have a life of your own and recognize that others depend on you besides your college freshman.

- Be supportive but not "hyper" when it comes to your child's college life.

- Celebrate your accomplishments and let go! ◁

5 Most Common Freshman Mistakes

You've heard of that weight-gain hazard called the Freshman 15? This is the Freshman 5—the five most common mistakes freshmen make, courtesy of Deborah Spinney, executive director for student development at the University of Indianapolis in Indiana.

☐ **Assuming college is an extension of high school.** Many students aren't prepared for the quantity and complexity of college work and rely on their high school study habits to get by. A good rule of thumb: Spend the same amount of time studying for a course each day as you spend in that class. If you need help with study skills, seek help from your university's academic support office right away. Don't wait until you're mired in midterms.

☐ **Trying to save money by not buying books.** Do you have any idea how much reading is required in college? If you think you're going to check out the book from the library and save a few bucks, think again. You'll quickly fall behind on your reading assignments and your grades will suffer. Instead, search out bargains online and from students who already took the class.

☐ **Being overly ambitious.** A heavy course load in high school may have been manageable, but it could overwhelm you in college. Set yourself up for success by taking no more than 12 to 14 hours of classes your first semester so you have time to acclimate.

☐ **Ignoring e-mails.** Yeah, yeah, you think e-mail is for ancient people like teachers and parents. Well, here's a news flash: Professors and school administrators use it too. They're not going to instant message or text message you about assignments, grades, tuition deadlines, and the weekend parking ban. So check your e-mail regularly!

☐ **Over- or under-socializing.** If your calendar holds more party dates than class dates, you're overdoing it. Conversely, if your idea of a hot Saturday night is when the air conditioning breaks in the library, you're underdoing your social life. You can't have the ultimate college experience if you never get out of your room. So find activities you enjoy beyond schoolwork—just keep it all in perspective.

Acknowledgments

The author wishes to gratefully acknowledge the help and information supplied by the following sources:

Jim Abbott, handyman franchise owner, Aurora, Ontario

Katie Albright, Sierra Club environmentalist, Ottawa, Ontario

Jennifer Appel, landscape designer-landscape architect, Houston, Texas

Brian Babcock, attorney, Thunder Bay, Ontario

Linda Bacon, Ph.D., nutrition expert, Davis, California

K. George Beck, professor of weed science, Colorado State University, Fort Collins, Colorado

Cheryl Bell, M.S., R.D., L.D.N., healthy living advisor, Chicago, Illinois

Stephen J. Berne, chair restorer and wicker expert, Vancouver, British Columbia

Robin Bond, workplace etiquette expert and employment attorney, Wayne, Pennsylvania

Walt Borchers, vice president, MovieTickets.com, Santa Monica, California

Lee Borden, divorce lawyer and mediator, Birmingham, Alabama

Kathy Brownfield, bathroom fixture industry expert, Richmond, Virginia

Susan Burke, R.D., nutrition expert, Fort Lauderdale, Florida

Bill Burton, casino gambling authority and author, New Britain, Connecticut

Gene Bush, owner, Munchkin Nursery, Depauw, Indiana

Rita Carey, gardener-gardening advisor, Kapat Garden Center, Squamish, British Columbia

Michelle Cederberg, fitness trainer, Calgary, Alberta

Harlan Cohen, college expert and author, Hackensack, New Jersey

Dan Collins, public relations professional, Baltimore, Maryland

Charles Cox, freelance handyman, Beaver Falls, Pennsylvania

William Davis, M.D., medical director, Milwaukee Heart Scan

Stacy DeBroff, mothering expert, Chestnut Hill, Massachusetts

Nancy and Glenn Deines, gardeners for over 50 years, Platteville, Colorado

Jason Denton, author of *Simple Italian Sandwiches* and owner of a panini restaurant, New York City

Laure Dixon, innovative amateur cook and certified wine connoisseur, Nashua, New Hampshire

Kenneth Dotson, chief marketing officer, TicketsNow, Crystal Lake, Illinois

Alison Doyle, former human resources director, Saratoga Springs, New York

Howard Dvorkin, president and founder, Consolidated Credit Counseling Services, Fort Lauderdale, Florida

Steve and Annette Economides, a.k.a. "America's cheapest family," Phoenix, Arizona

Linda Eremita, TreePeople Forestry Educator, Beverly Hills, California

David Felton, executive chef at Pluckemin Inn, Bedminster, New Jersey

Jodi Fitzpatrick, kitchen and bath designer, Fresno, California

Linda Foley, executive director of Identity Theft Resource Center, Washington, D.C.

Louise Fox, etiquette coach, the Etiquette Ladies, Manitoba

Eugene Fram, marketing professor, Rochester, New York

Michael Fugate, furniture sales veteran, Auxvasse, Missouri

Sheila Gawel, owner, GalaxSea Cruises, Toms River, New Jersey

Kevin Gianni, fitness expert, New Haven, Connecticut

James Gibbs, hardware store manager, Richmond, Virginia

Phil Goodin, head of Cherry Creek High School (Colorado) Plant Lover's Club, Englewood, Colorado

Mary Hardy, M.D., director of integrative medicine, Ted Mann Family Resource Center at the University of California, Los Angeles

Edward Hasbrouck, travel writer, San Francisco, California

Mikki Hopcroft, furniture salesperson, Richmond, Virginia

Jan Horsfall, owner of Gelazzi, Denver, Colorado

Douglas Husbands, certified clinical nutritionist, San Carlos, California

Francine Jackson, financial aid director, Harrisburg, Pennsylvania

Daniel Jalkut, software developer, Somerville, Massachusetts

Jennifer James, nurse and long-time gardener, Lafayette, Colorado.

Ingrid Johnson, professor of textiles, Fashion Institute of Technology, New York City

Val Jones, owner, Orchard Park Travel, Kelowna, British Columbia

Charles Joseph, labor lawyer, New York City

Susan Joyce, computer security expert, Marlborough, Massachusetts

Marina Kamen, fitness expert, New York City

Larina Kase, Psy.D., M.B.A., psychologist and author, Philadelphia, Pennsylvania

Kraig Kast, financial expert, Redwood Shores, California

Francine DiFilippo Kent, president, Celebrate a Hero!, Sarasota, Florida

Stanley Kershman, author and debt expert, Ottawa, Ontario

Raza Khan, student loan expert, New York City

Shelley Kincaid, yard-sale maven, Denver, Colorado

Peggy Koontz, remodeling professional, Fresno, California

Brian Korte, computer consultant, Richmond, Virginia

Tom Kraeutler, education supply expert, Lincolnshire, Illinois

Eileen Gale Kugler, education expert, Springfield, Virginia

Dale Kurow, career and executive coach, New York City

Michael Laimo, longtime staffer for Mercury Beach-Maid, a New York City sportswear wholesaler, and also a horror novelist

Katherine Lawrence, professional declutterer, Richmond, Virginia

Alisa LeSueur, certified college planning specialist, San Antonio, Texas

Hugh Lobban, drapery cleaning expert, Lorton, Virginia

Enga Lokey, gardener and part-time landscaping professional, Natimuk, Australia (also part-time resident of Salida, Colorado)

Tom Long, stay-at-home dad, Elkins Park, Pennsylvania

Wanda Martens, appliance repair expert, Mound, Minnesota

Kristina Matisic, bargain hunter, Vancouver, British Columbia

Greg McArthur, Ph.D. in plant ecology, biology professor, part-time garden center employee, Denver, Colorado

Susan McCausland, landscape installation and garden maintenance expert, Beyond Gardens Inc., Boulder, Colorado

Deb McCoy, president, American Academy of Wedding Professionals, Palm Beach, Florida

Jonni McCoy, frugality expert, Colorado Springs, Colorado

Chris McGoey, security consultant, Los Angeles, California

Paul McKinzey, appliance expert, Richmond, Virginia

Ross Melnick, cofounder, Cinema Treasures, West Hollywood, California

Isadore B. Mirsky, C.P.A., Wayne, New Jersey

Donna Montaldo, bargain expert, New Orleans, Louisiana

Susan Louisa Montauk, M.D., professor of clinical family medicine, Cincinnati, Ohio

Birgit Mueller, Emmy Award-winning costume designer for television, based in Los Angeles, California

Brian Muntz, veteran computer consultant, Ajax, Ontario

Sharon Naylor, author, *1,000 Best Kept Secrets for Your Perfect Wedding*, Madison, New Jersey

Stephanie Nelson, frugality expert, Atlanta, Georgia

Marion Nestle, professor of nutrition, New York City

Brent Newbold, CFO, Holy Cow cleaning products company, based in Rocklin, California.

Susan Newman, Ph.D., social psychologist and author, Rutgers, New Jersey

Liz Ngonzi, president of Amazing Taste, an event-planning firm in South Orange, New Jersey

Jeff Novick, director of nutrition, the Pritikin Longevity Center and Spa, Aventura, Florida

Anne Obarski, customer-service expert, St. Charles, Missouri

Robert O'Shea, real estate attorney, Petaluma, California

Joan M. Pagano, Kaplan Test Prep and Admissions consultant, New York City

Michael Palermo, estate planning lawyer, certified financial planner, Lexington, Kentucky

Ryan Peif, landscape design and installation professional, Greeley, Colorado

Gary Peterson, auction expert, Hudson, Quebec

Bruce Powell, Pappy's Motorhome Rentals, Salt Lake City, Utah

Wanda Prychitko, executive secretary, Citizens for Crime Awareness, Winnipeg, Manitoba

Wendy Reed, EPA energy expert, Washington, D.C.

Rick E. Ricer, M.D., family medicine specialist, Cincinnati, Ohio

Annette Riffle, tutor, New York City

Susan RoAne, career counselor and networking authority, Greenbrae, California

Clark Robins, architect and home remodeler, Richmond, Virginia

Nancy Rosebrock, furniture conservator, Asheville, North Carolina

Ron Rupert, chef at Seasons 52, Orlando, Florida

Harvey M. Sachs, Ph.D., energy efficiency expert, Washington, D.C.

Prentice St. Clair, Detail in Progress auto detailers, San Diego, California

Noah Scalin, founder of a community-supported agriculture organization, Richmond, Virginia

Karen Schaffer, career coach, Halifax, Nova Scotia

Lou Schlachter, Ph.D., R.N., teacher of herbal and folk medicine, the College of William & Mary, Williamsburg, Virginia

Liz Scofield, etiquette teacher and director, Zoellner Arts Center, Lehigh University, Bethlehem, Pennsylvania

Brette McWhorter Sember, parenting expert, Clarence, New York

Sheri Sheets, heating and plumbing contractor, Stuarts Draft, Virginia

Karen Sherman, Ph.D., psychologist, Long Island, New York

Kevin Reid Shirley, real estate stager, Washington, D.C.

Frank Silva, manager, Schwartz's Hebrew Delicatessen, Montreal, Quebec

Viviana Simon, Ph.D., director of scientific programs, Society for Women's Health Research, Washington, D.C.

Beth Smerek, assistant manager and bedding plant specialist, Sturtz & Copeland, Boulder, Colorado

Connie Smith, manager, Sturtz & Copeland garden center, Boulder, Colorado

Syble Solomon, financial expert, Rockville, Maryland

Susan Sommers, author and fashion coach, based in New York City

Deborah Spinney, student development executive, Indianapolis, Indiana

Jyl Steinback, senior editor, *Looking Good NOW!* magazine, Scottsdale, Arizona

Bobette Stott, clothing designer, Los Angeles, California

Jeffrey Strain, frugality expert, Cupertino, California

Rodger Summers, vice president for student affairs, Binghamton University, New York

Tina B. Tessina, Ph.D., psychologist and author, Long Beach, California

Mathew Paul Turner, college expert and author, Nashville, Tennessee

Denise Vivaldo, author, *Do It for Less! Parties,* Los Angeles, California

Anna Wallner, bargain hunter, Vancouver, British Columbia

Louise J. Wannier, CEO, Internet clothing retailer myShape, Inc.

Brian Wansink, director, Food and Brand Lab, Cornell University, Ithaca, New York

Lindsay Wombold, health educator, Indianapolis, Indiana

Alan Zell, a.k.a. "The ambassador of selling," Portland, Oregon

Mark Zwick, owner, Phillytrips.com, Philadelphia, Pennsylvania

Also Available from Reader's Digest

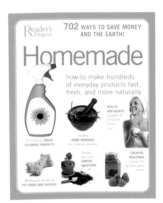

Homemade

Discover 702 all-natural replacement recipes for your favorite name-brand products and save 95 percent off retail prices. Plus reduce the amount of environment-damaging waste-spray bottles, jars, and cans-and use ingredients that are safer for drains, sewage, and septic systems.

ISBN: 978-0-7621-0904-3 • $15.95

Free Money, Free Stuff

Welcome to the great big world of bargains! Here is a practical collection of more than 1,000 legitimate free giveaways and super bargains-money-saving offers available for the assertive shopper and savvy computer user, and all carefully researched and fact-checked for validity and accuracy.

ISBN: 978-0-7621-0903-6 • $15.95

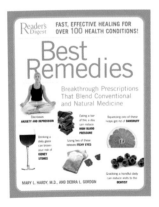

Best Remedies

Combine the strength of conventional medicine with the wisdom of natural healing and get powerful solutions to improve your health and achieve total relief from 103 of the most troubling medical conditions-from the flu to migraine relief, from ulcers to cancer-with more options than you'll actually use.

ISBN: 978-0-7621-0899-2 • $15.95

Reader's Digest Books are distributed by Penguin Group (USA) Inc. and can be purchased through retail and online bookstores nationally.

FOR MORE INFORMATION OR TO ORDER BOOKS, CALL 1-800-788-6262.